2016

The Year Book of OPHTHALMOLOGY®

Editor-in-Chief

Christopher J. Rapuano, MD

Professor of Ophthalmology, Sidney Kimmel Medical College at Thomas Jefferson University; Director, Cornea Service; Co-Director, Refractive Surgery Department, Attending Surgeon, Wills Eye Hospital, Philadelphia, Pennsylvania

Wills Eye®

ELSEVIER
MOSBY

ELSEVIER
MOSBY

Vice President, Global Medical Reference: Mary E. Gatsch
Acquisitions Editor: Jennifer Flynn-Briggs
Developmental Editor: Colleen Viola
Production Supervisor, Electronic Year Books: Donna M. Skelton
Electronic Article Manager: Mahalakshmi Nithyanand
Illustrations and Permissions Coordinator: Vasu Parthasarathy

2016 EDITION

Composition by TNQ Books and Journals Pvt Ltd, India

Editorial Office:
Elsevier
1600 John F. Kennedy Blvd.
Suite 1800
Philadelphia, PA 19103-2899

International Standard Serial Number: 0084-392X
International Standard Book Number: 978-0-323-44690-7

Editorial Board

Carol L. Shields, MD

Professor, Sidney Kimmel Medical College at Thomas Jefferson University; Co-Director, Oncology Service; Attending Surgeon, Oncology Service, Wills Eye Hospital, Philadelphia, Pennsylvania

Kiran S. Talekar, MD

Assistant Professor of Radiology, Neuroradiology Fellowship Program Director, Sidney Kimmel Medical College at Thomas Jefferson University, Thomas Jefferson University Hospital, Philadelphia, Pennsylvania

Contributors

Preema Mehta Buch, MD

Ophthalmology resident, Department of Ophthalmology, University of Pennsylvania, Scheie Eye Institute, Philadelphia, Pennsylvania

Nicole Fuerst, MD

Ophthalmology resident, Department of Ophthalmology, University of Pennsylvania, Scheie Eye Institute, Philadelphia, Pennsylvania

Rahul Hegde, MD

Neuroradiology Fellow, Sidney Kimmel Medical College at Thomas Jefferson University, Thomas Jefferson University Hospital, Philadelphia, Pennsylvania

Benjamin J. Kim, MD

Assistant Professor, Department of Ophthalmology, University of Pennsylvania, Scheie Eye Institute, Philadelphia, Pennsylvania

Marisa Lau, MD

Ophthalmology resident, Department of Ophthalmology, University of Pennsylvania, Scheie Eye Institute, Philadelphia, Pennsylvania

Daniel Lee, MD

Fellow, Glaucoma Service, Wills Eye Hospital, Clinical Instructor, Sydney Kimmel Medical College at Thomas Jefferson University

Akosua A. Nti, MD

Ophthalmology resident, Department of Ophthalmology, University of Pennsylvania, Scheie Eye Institute, Philadelphia, Pennsylvania

Wasim A. Samara, MD

Fellow, Ocular Oncology Service, Wills Eye Hospital, Philadelphia, Pennsylvania

Keirnan Willett, MD

Ophthalmology resident, Department of Ophthalmology, University of Pennsylvania, Scheie Eye Institute, Philadelphia, Pennsylvania

Table of Contents

Journals Represented

Journals represented in this YEAR BOOK are listed below.

Acta Ophthalmologica
American Journal of Cardiology
American Journal of Ophthalmology
Annals of Neurology
Archives of Pathology & Laboratory Medicine
British Journal of Ophthalmology
Canadian Journal of Ophthalmology
Cornea
Cytopathology
Eye
Eye (London)
International Journal of Pediatric Ortorhinolaryngology
Investigative Ophthalmology & Visual Science
Japanese Journal of Ophthalmology
Journal of American Association for Pediatric Ophthalmology and Strabismus
Journal of Cataract & Refractive Surgery
Journal of Neuro-Ophthalmology
Journal of Pediatric Ophthalmology & Strabismus
Journal of Refractive Surgery
Journal of Sexual Medicine
Journal of the American Medical Association Neurology
Journal of the American Medical Association Ophthalmology
Journal of the Neurological Sciences
Lancet
Molecular Immunology
Neurology
Neurosurgery
New England Journal of Medicine
Ophthalmic Plastic and Reconstructive Surgery
Ophthalmic Surgery, Lasers & Imaging Retina
Ophthalmology
Plastic and Reconstructive Surgery
Radiologia Medica
Retina
Rheumatology (Oxford)
Survey of Ophthalmology
The Ocular Surface
Thyroid

STANDARD ABBREVIATIONS

The following terms are abbreviated in this edition: acquired immunodeficiency syndrome (AIDS), cardiopulmonary resuscitation (CPR), central nervous system (CNS), cerebrospinal fluid (CSF), computed tomography (CT), deoxyribonucleic acid (DNA), diopter (D), electrocardiography (ECG), health maintenance organization (HMO), human immunodeficiency virus (HIV), intensive care unit (ICU), intramuscular (IM), intravenous (IV), magnetic resonance (MR) imaging (MRI), ribonucleic acid (RNA), ultrasound (US), and ultraviolet (UV).

Note

The Year Book of Ophthalmology® is a literature survey service providing abstracts of articles published in the professional literature. Every effort is made to assure the accuracy of the information presented in these pages. Neither the editors nor the publisher of the Year Book of Ophthalmology® can be responsible for errors in the original materials. The editors' comments are their own opinions. Mention of specific products within this publication does not constitute endorsement.

To facilitate the use of the Year Book of Ophthalmology® as a reference tool, all illustrations and tables included in this publication are now identified as they appear in the original article. This change is meant to help the reader recognize that any illustration or table appearing in the Year Book of Ophthalmology® may be only one of many in the original article. For this reason, figure and table numbers will often appear to be out of sequence within the Year Book of Ophthalmology®.

1 Cataract Surgery

Changes in intraocular pressure after cataract surgery: Analysis of the Swedish National Cataract Register Data

Zetterström C, Behndig A, Kugelberg M, et al (Blekinge Hosp, Karolinska, Sweden; Umeå Univ Hosp, Sweden; et al)

J Cataract Refract Surg 41:1725-1729, 2015

Purpose.—To analyze changes in intraocular pressure (IOP) after cataract surgery based on data from the Swedish National Cataract Register (NCR).

Setting.—Ophthalmic surgery units in Sweden.

Design.—Prospective database study.

Methods.—Data for 2012 through 2014 were obtained prospectively from the NCR. The outcome register of the NCR has collected data on IOP before and a mean of 37.7 days ± 29.1 (SD) after cataract surgery since 2012.

Results.—The analyses were based on 20 437 cataract extractions reported during 1 month each year to the outcome registry of the NCR. Cataract surgery was found to reduce IOP by a mean of 1.46 mm Hg, which was statistically significant ($P < .001$). A larger IOP reduction was seen in cases with a higher preoperative IOP ($r = 0.557$, $P < .001$). Older patients and shorter eyes had a greater IOP reduction after surgery ($P < .001$ and $P = .001$, respectively). Women had a greater IOP reduction than men ($P = .04$) When high IOP was given as an indication for surgery, the IOP reduction after cataract surgery was 5.50 mm Hg compared with a reduction of 1.40 mm Hg in patients for whom this indication was not given ($P < .001$). Patients with glaucoma or pseudoexfoliation (PXF) had a more pronounced IOP reduction than patients without these diagnoses ($P < .001$).

Conclusion.—Cataract surgery had an IOP-lowering effect, in particular in older patients, women, short eyes, eyes with high preoperative IOP, and eyes with glaucoma or PXF (Table 4).

▶ Modern small-incision phacoemulsification cataract surgery leads to a decrease in intraocular pressure (IOP). This prospective database study examines outcomes of all cataract surgery in Sweden during the month of March of 3 consecutive years, yielding a total of more than 20 000 cases for analysis. The study is limited to a single snapshot in time for each patient, at about 30 days postop. At that point, average IOP reduction ranged from 1.4 mm Hg in patients without glaucoma or risk factors, to 5.5 mm Hg in patients who had elevated

TABLE 4.—Reduction in IOP After Cataract Surgery in Eyes With Indication of Elevated IOP, Glaucoma, and PXF According to Data From the Swedish NCR (indications) and the Outcome Registry of the NCR (Outcomes)

Characteristic	Patients (n)	IOP Reduction (mm Hg) Mean	95% CI	P Value*
Indication of elevated IOP				<.001
Yes	286	5.50	4.68, 6.33	
No	20 151	1.40	1.35, 1.45	
Glaucoma				<.001
Yes	1842	2.28	2.04, 2.53	
No	18 595	1.38	1.33, 1.43	
PXF				<.001
Yes	1903	2.30	2.09, 2.51	
No	18 534	1.37	1.32, 1.42	
Glaucoma and pseudoexfoliation				<.001
Yes	490	2.53	1.98, 3.07	
No	19 947	1.43	1.38, 1.48	

CI = confidence interval; IOP = intraocular pressure; PXF = pseudoexfoliation.
*Independent-samples *t* test.
Reprinted from Zetterström C, Behndig A, Kugelberg M, et al. Changes in intraocular pressure after cataract surgery: analysis of the Swedish National Cataract Register Data. *J Cataract Refract Surg*. 2015;41:1725-1729, with permission from ASCRS and ESCRS.

IOP as an indication for surgery. The difference was statistically significant for patients with elevated IOP, pseudoexfoliation, or glaucoma (Table 4). This result should help surgeons predict the expected benefit from cataract surgery alone in patients with glaucoma or preglaucoma and improve planning for simultaneous adjunctive procedures such as minimally invasive glaucoma surgery or trabeculectomy.

M. F. Pyfer, MD

Cataract surgery outcomes in corneal refractive surgery eyes: Study from the European Registry of Quality Outcomes for Cataract and Refractive Surgery

Manning S, Barry P, Henry Y, et al (Mater Misericordiae Univ Hosp, Dublin, Ireland; St. Vincent's Hosp Group, Dublin, Ireland; VU Univ Med Ctr, Amsterdam, the Netherlands; et al)
J Cataract Refract Surg 41:2358-2365, 2015

Purpose.—To analyze visual outcomes after cataract surgery in patients with previous corneal refractive surgery.

Setting.—Cataract surgery clinics in 18 European countries and Australia.

Design.—Database study.

Methods.—Cases of cataract extraction with corneal refractive surgery eyes (corneal refractive cases) were identified from all cataract extractions reported to the European Registry of Quality Outcomes for Cataract and

Refractive Surgery database over a 5-year period. Preoperative and postoperative measurements and trends over time were analyzed.

Results.—Of 807,220 cataract extractions, 1229 (0.15%) were corneal refractive cases. There was a significant increase, over time, in the number of corneal refractive cases ($P < .001$). Corneal refractive patients were younger than patients without corneal refractive surgery (nonrefractive patients) (62.9 years versus 74.0 years; $P < .001$) but had similar mean preoperative and postoperative corrected-distance visual acuity (CDVA) (preoperative logMAR 0.44[6/16] for both [$P = .286$]; postoperative logMAR 0.06[6/7] for both [$P = .245$]). Postoperative CDVA was worse than preoperative CDVA in 35 (4%) corneal refractive and 8,999 (1.5%) nonrefractive patients ($P < .001$). In all, 74 (8.5%) of 873 corneal refractive versus 16,566 (2.8%) /584,496 nonrefractive patients, having cataract surgery, had preoperative CDVA of logMAR 0.0[6/6] or better ($P < .001$). Nineteen (54.3%) of 35 corneal refractive case patients who had worse postoperative CDVA had preoperative CDVA of logMAR 0.0(6/6) or better.

Conclusion.—Cataract surgery has been reported with increasing frequency in corneal refractive surgery patients, since 2008. These patients had preoperative CDVA similar to those of patients without previous corneal refractive surgery but were younger and were at higher risk of worse postoperative CDVA, especially if they had preoperative CDVA of logMAR 0.0(6/6) or better.

▶ This is an example of the type of study that is facilitated by using electronic medical records (EMR) with reporting to a central registry. This so-called big data revolution is poised to transform health care. It will affect decision making by physicians, as well as policy setting and reimbursement rates for government programs and private insurers. However, it is critically important to interpret the aggregated statistics carefully with awareness of the limitations of the underlying data set.

This article reports on a small subset of more than 800 000 cataract extractions reported to the European Registry over a 5-year period. Patients with prior refractive surgery amounted to only 0.15% of those having cataract surgery during the time period. This number increased slowly each year. Patients with prior refractive surgery were more likely to have a decline in best corrected distance visual acuity (BCVA) at a single time 2 months after cataract surgery, especially if they had preoperative acuity of 20/20. The reasons for this cannot be determined from this study because no further information is recorded in the database. However, surgeons should carefully counsel their cataract patients who have had prior refractive surgery and consider delaying surgery until the cataract becomes more visually significant to avoid a loss of BCVA.

M. F. Pyfer, MD

Toric Intraocular Lens Versus Monofocal Intraocular Lens Implantation and Photorefractive Keratectomy: A Randomized Controlled Trial

Nagpal R, Sharma N, Vasavada V, et al (All India Inst of Med Sciences, New Delhi, India; Iladevi Cataract and IOL Res Centre, Ahmedabad, India; et al)

Am J Ophthalmol 160:479-486, 2015

Purpose.—To compare the outcomes of phacoemulsification with toric intraocular lens implantation vs phacoemulsification with monofocal intraocular lens implantation followed by photorefractive keratectomy (PRK) for correction of pre-existing astigmatism.

Design.—Randomized controlled trial, 6-month study.

Methods.—Setting: Institutional.

Study Population.—Sixty eyes of 52 patients with age-related senile cataract and regular corneal astigmatism ranging from 1.50 to 3.00 diopters, enrolled and randomly allocated in 2 groups based on computer-generated random number table.

Intervention.—Group 1 patients underwent phacoemulsification with toric intraocular lens (IOL) implantation and Group 2 patients underwent phacoemulsification with monofocal IOL implantation followed by PRK 3 months later.

Main Outcome Measures.—The main outcome measures were uncorrected distance visual acuity (UDVA), corrected distance visual acuity (CDVA), residual cylinder, contrast sensitivity, glare acuity, pain score, and higher-order aberrations.

Results.—At 6 months 53.3% of eyes in the toric IOL and 60% eyes in the monofocal IOL with PRK group attained UDVA of 20/20. Median residual refractive cylinder value was higher in the toric IOL group (toric IOL = −0.5, monofocal IOL with PRK = 0; $P = .02$). Mean root mean square value of total aberrations (5 mm pupil) was higher in monofocal IOL with PRK eyes (toric IOL = 1.02 ± 0.44, monofocal IOL with PRK = 1.28 ± 0.5; $P = .04$). Mean contrast sensitivity values were comparable. Mean toric IOL rotation was 1.3 ± 2.1 degrees. Mean glare acuity was better in toric IOL eyes (toric IOL = 0.46 ± 0.16, monofocal IOL with PRK = 0.73 ± 0.12; $P < .001$). Median postoperative pain scores were higher in monofocal IOL with PRK eyes.

Conclusion.—PRK yields lesser residual cylinder compared to toric IOL. However, it causes greater postoperative pain and corneal aberrations, and poor glare acuity.

▶ This prospective randomized trial provides meaningful information to compare the outcome of toric intraocular lenses (IOLs) versus monofocal IOLs combined with photorefractive keratectomy (PRK) in patients with both cataract and astigmatism. The data are mixed, showing lower residual refractive error and better uncorrected vision for the PRK eyes, but lower total aberrations and better glare acuity in the toric IOL eyes. What would have helped to differentiate the results is to include a subjective measure of vision from the patient's perspective, such as the vision-related quality-of-life metric.

Most studies show patient satisfaction after cataract surgery is most closely related to peak visual acuity and minimal residual refractive error, so this would support the combined IOL plus PRK technique. The obvious disadvantage to this, besides added risk and discomfort with PRK, is the need for a 2-step procedure with an unavoidable delay in between. Light adjustable IOLs, if they perform as expected when finally approved, may make this a moot point.

M. F. Pyfer, MD

A Proposed Minimum Standard Set of Outcome Measures for Cataract Surgery

Mahmud I, Kelley T, Stowell C, et al (International Consortium for Health Outcomes Measurement, Cambridge, MA; et al)
JAMA Ophthalmol 133:1247-1252, 2015

Importance.—Aligning outcome measures for cataract surgery, one of the most frequently performed procedures globally, may facilitate international comparisons that can drive improvements in the outcomes most meaningful to patients.

Objective.—To propose a minimum standard set of outcome measures for cataract surgery that enables global comparisons.

Design, Setting, and Participants.—A working group of international experts in cataract outcomes and registries was convened, along with a patient advocate, to agree on a consensus of outcome measures for cataract surgery. In a modified Delphi process, the group met regularly between November 10, 2012, and November 21, 2013, to discuss which outcomes to include in a standard set. Included factors were based on extant literature, existing registries, and the experience of group members. Similarly, a series of consensus discussions were held to determine a set of risk factors to be gathered for each patient. The final shortlist was compiled into a standard set. Analysis was performed from November 22, 2013, to April 5, 2014.

Main Outcomes and Measures.—Development of a recommended standard set encompassing preoperative metrics including patient risk factors, intraoperative factors including surgical complications, and postoperative cataract surgery outcomes.

Results.—The recommended standard set encompasses all patients treated for cataracts by 1 of 4 surgical approaches (phacoemulsification, sutured manual extracapsular cataract extraction, sutureless manual extracapsular cataract extraction, or intracapsular cataract extraction). The recommended metrics to be recorded preoperatively include demographics, ocular history and comorbidities, preoperative visual acuity, and patient-reported visual function. The recommended outcomes were split into intraoperative and postoperative metrics. Intraoperative outcomes include capsule-related problems, dislocation of lens nucleus fragments into the vitreous, and other complications. Postoperative outcomes include visual acuity, refractive error, patient-reported visual function, and early and late complications of surgery. The suggested follow-up for collection of postoperative outcomes is up to 3 months.

Conclusions and Relevance.—A minimum standard set of outcome measures for cataract surgery is important for meaningful comparison across contexts. The proposed data set is a compromise between all useful data and the practicalities of data collection.

► This is the consensus report from a panel of international experts convened by the International Consortium for Health Outcomes Measurement (ICHOM). They propose a standard set of preoperative, intraoperative, and postoperative measures for cataract surgery outcomes (Table in the original article). Most of the measures are already recorded in standard clinical practice, so for ophthalmologists using electronic medical records (EMRs) and reporting data in the United States through a registry service, few changes would be needed to implement this system. However, the study group calls for recording patient reported visual function in a standard metric before and after surgery. This is not done routinely in US clinical practice and would require extra work to implement. Also, intraoperative events would have to be transcribed into the office-based EMR system because most surgeons currently use either paper records or a different electronic system for surgical event recording in the operating theater.

One notable omission from the proposed measures is the type and position of the intraocular lens implant, and I strongly encourage adding this crucial information on cataract surgery to the minimum standard.

Clearly, with the ongoing transition to quality and outcomes based reimbursement models for physicians in the United States, this type of standardized outcome measurement for surgery is here to stay.

M. F. Pyfer, MD

A Comparative Cohort Study of Visual Outcomes in Femtosecond Laser-Assisted versus Phacoemulsification Cataract Surgery

Ewe SYP, Abell RG, Oakley CL, et al (Tasmanian Eye Inst, Launceston, Tasmania, Australia, et al)

Ophthalmology 123:178-182, 2016

Purpose.—To evaluate visual outcomes after femtosecond laser-assisted cataract surgery (LCS) with phacoemulsification cataract surgery (PCS).

Design.—Prospective, multicenter, comparative case series.

Participants.—Consecutive patients undergoing femtosecond LCS or PCS with intraocular lens insertion.

Methods.—A total of 1876 eyes of 1238 patients (422 male and 772 female) who underwent cataract surgery between January 2012 and June 2014 were included in the study: 1017 eyes from center A and 859 eyes from center B. Cases underwent clinico-socioeconomic selection. Patients with absolute LCS contraindications were assigned to PCS; otherwise, all patients were offered LCS and elected on the basis of their

TABLE 2.—Visual Outcomes Between Laser Cataract Surgery and Phacoemulsification Cataract Surgery Groups

Postoperative Visual Acuity	LCS (n = 988) % or Mean (SD)	PCS (n = 888) % or Mean (SD)	*P* Value
Mean UCVA (logMAR) (1 mo)	0.23 (0.21) VA 20/34	0.23 (0.29) VA 20/34	NS
Change in logMAR (UCVA)	−0.11 (0.33) 5.5 letters gain	−0.19 (0.47) 9.5 letters gain	<0.001
≥20/40	82.0% (809/986)	82.6% (728/881)	NS
≥20/30	63.2% (623/986)	67.3% (593/881)	NS
≥20/25	33.6% (331/986)	35.2% (310/881)	NS
≥20/20	19.9% (196/986)	29.6 (261/881)	<0.001
Mean BCVA (logMAR)	0.09 (0.13) VA 20/24.5	0.12 (0.22) VA 20/26.4	0.001
Change in logMAR (BCVA)	−0.25 (0.27) 12.5 letters gain	−0.29 (0.43) 13.5 letters gain	0.018
≥20/40	96.6% (891/922)	93.9% (784/835)	0.009
≥20/30	89.7% (827/922)	84.2% (703/835)	0.001
≥20/25	68.0% (627/922)	58.8% (491/835)	<0.001
≥20/20	53.3% (491/922)	53.1% (443/835)	NS

BCVA = best-corrected visual acuity; LCS = laser-assisted cataract surgery; logMAR = logarithm of the minimum angle of resolution; NS = nonsignificant; PCS = phacoemulsification cataract surgery; SD = standard deviation; UCVA = uncorrected visual acuity; VA = visual acuity.

Reprinted from Ewe SYP, Abell RG, Oakley CL, et al. A comparative cohort study of visual outcomes in femtosecond laser-assisted versus phacoemulsification cataract surgery. *Ophthalmology.* 2016;123:178-182, with permission from American Academy of Ophthalmology.

TABLE 4.—Perioperative Complications

Complication	Number (%) LCS (n = 988)	PCS (n = 888)	*P* Value
Incomplete capsulotomy	5 (0.5)	0 (0)	0.064 (NS)
Anterior capsulotomy tag	15 (1.52)	0 (0)	<0.0001
Anterior capsule tear	15 (1.52)	3 (0.34)	0.0087
Posterior capsule tear	11 (1.11)	2 (0.02)	0.024
Corneal haze	6 (0.61)	0 (0)	0.03
Corneal epithelial defect	7 (0.71)	0 (0)	0.02
Descemet's membrane trauma	3 (0.30)	0 (0)	NS
Zonular dialysis	1 (0.10)	2 (0.23)	NS

LCS = laser-assisted cataract surgery; NS = not significant; PCS = phacoemulsification cataract surgery.

Reprinted from Ewe SYP, Abell RG, Oakley CL, et al. A comparative cohort study of visual outcomes in femtosecond laser-assisted versus phacoemulsification cataract surgery. *Ophthalmology.* 2016;123:178-182, with permission from American Academy of Ophthalmology.

decision to pay (the out-of-pocket cost for LCS). Demographic and postoperative data were collected to determine differences between groups.

Main Outcome Measures.—Six-month postoperative visual and refractive outcomes. Masked subjective refractions were performed 2 to 6 months postoperatively.

Results.—There were 988 eyes in the LCS group and 888 eyes in the PCS group. Baseline best-corrected visual acuity (BCVA) was better in LCS compared with PCS (20/44.0 vs. 20/51.5; $P < 0.0003$). Preoperative surgical refractive aim differed significantly between groups (LCS −0.28 vs. PCS −0.23; $P < 0.0001$). More patients who received LCS had Toric lenses implanted compared with PCS (47.4% vs. 34.8%; $P < 0.0001$). Postoperative BCVA was better after LCS (20/24.5 vs. 20/26.4; $P = 0.0003$) with a greater proportion of LCS cases achieving BCVA >20/30 (LCS 89.7% vs. PCS 84.2%; $P = 0.0006$) and 20/40 (LCS 96.6% vs. PCS 93.9%; $P = 0.0077$). However, PCS cases had more letters gained compared with LCS cases (13.5 vs. 12.5 letters; $P = 0.0088$), reflecting baseline BCVA differences. Mean absolute error was higher in LCS compared with PCS (0.41 diopters [D] vs. 0.35 D; $P < 0.0011$). The percentage of eyes within 0.5 D of error from preoperative aim refraction was higher in the PCS group (LCS 72.2% vs. PCS 82.6%; $P < 0.0001$).

Conclusions.—Femtosecond LCS did not demonstrate clinically meaningful improvements in visual outcomes over conventional PCS (Tables 2 and 4).

▶ This is a prospective but nonrandomized and nonmatched study comparing outcomes in more than 1800 cases between femtosecond laser-assisted cataract surgery (LCS) and standard phacoemulsification cataract surgery (PCS). The results indicate a small but statistically significant advantage for LCS using best corrected visual acuity (BCVA) ≥20/25 (Table 2). The authors are experienced surgeons well past the initial learning curve for LCS. Still they found a somewhat greater incidence of intraoperative complications in the LCS group (Table 4), which deserves further investigation.

One problem is that they do not specify whether customized lens constants were used to account for potential differences in effective lens position (ELP) between LCS and PCS. If not, then uncorrected visual acuity assuming a goal of plano may not be a valid comparative measure. BCVA is more indicative of overall outcome, and LCS performed slightly better in this measure. The authors admit that selection bias based on ability to pay for LCS is a potentially significant confounding factor, and there is no way to adjust for this.

M. F. Pyfer, MD

Comparison of visual recovery and refractive stability between femtosecond laser–assisted cataract surgery and standard phacoemulsification: Six-month follow-up

Conrad-Hengerer I, Al Sheikh M, Hengerer FH, et al (Ruhr Univ Eye Clinic Bochum, Germany; Goethe Univ Eye Clinic, Frankfurt, Germany)

J Cataract Refract Surg 41:1356-1364, 2015

Purpose.—To compare visual recovery and refractive changes between femtosecond laser–assisted cataract surgery and standard cataract surgery.

Setting.—Center for Vision Science, Ruhr University Eye Clinic, Bochum, Germany.

Design.—Prospective randomized intraindividual cohort study.

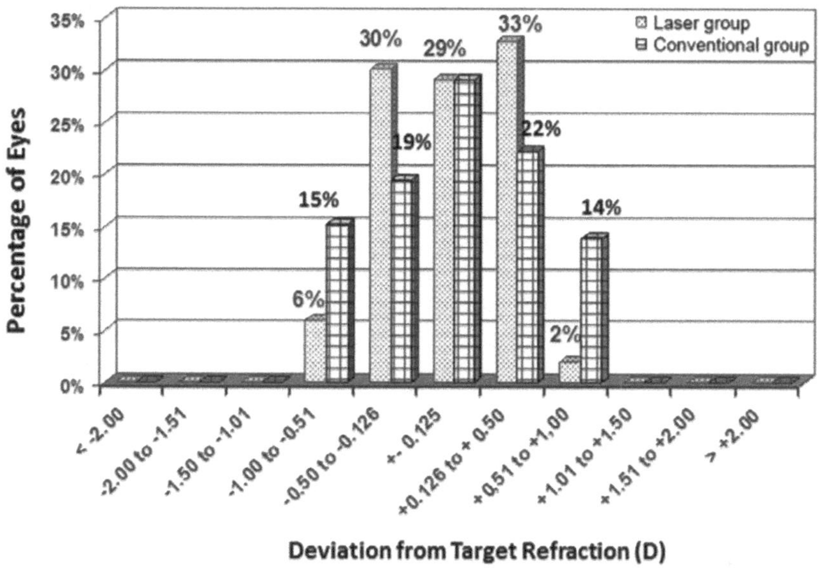

FIGURE 5.—Accuracy of SE refraction in the femtosecond laser—assisted group and the conventional group 6 months postoperatively. (Reprinted from Conrad-Hengerer I, Al Sheikh M, Hengerer FH, et al. Comparison of visual recovery and refractive stability between femtosecond laser—assisted cataract surgery and standard phacoemulsification: six-month follow-up. *J Cataract Refract Surg* 2015;41:1356-1364, with permission from ASCRS and ESCRS.)

Methods.—Eyes were treated with femtosecond laser—assisted cataract surgery or conventional phacoemulsification using pulsed ultrasound energy. Both groups had intraocular lens (IOL) implantation. The manifest refraction, corrected distance visual acuity, and anterior chamber depth were determined preoperatively and 2 hours, 3 to 4 days, 1 week, and 1, 2, 3, and 6 months postoperatively to determine the achieved deviation from target refraction, IOL position, and refractive stability.

Results.—One hundred eyes of 100 patients were treated with femtosecond laser—assisted cataract surgery; the fellow 100 eyes had conventional phacoemulsification. Six months postoperatively, 196 eyes were included and analyzed. At 6 months, 90 eyes (92%) in the femtosecond laser—assisted group and 70 eyes (71%) in the conventional group were within ±0.50 D of the target refractive outcome and 98 eyes (100%) in both groups were within ±1.00 D. The mean refractive spherical equivalent showed no significant change between 1 week and 1 month in the femtosecond laser—assisted group and between 1, 2, 3, and 6 months postoperatively in both groups.

Conclusion.—Femtosecond laser—assisted cataract surgery yielded faster visual recovery, less deviation from the target refraction, and earlier stabilization of refraction (Fig 5).

▶ This article should be evaluated together with another femtosecond laser-assisted cataract surgery (LCS) versus manual cataract surgery study,[1] also reviewed in this chapter. Despite using fewer cases, this is a stronger study because it is a randomized intraindividual cohort that eliminates selection bias. Also, here the authors evaluate deviation from predicted refraction in addition to best corrected vision. The intraocular lens type and prediction formula were the same in both eyes, which minimizes bias related to lens constant optimization.

The overall conclusion in this study is faster visual recovery and less deviation from target refraction for LCS (Fig 5). The authors' comment is similar,[1] noting that LCS has a small advantage that may not be sufficiently clinically relevant to justify the added expense at this time. However, the history of cataract surgery has demonstrated that technological advances resulting in small but measurable improvements eventually become more significant, as new surgical techniques or intraocular lens design changes are made that capitalize on those improvements. Also, the cost of new technology eventually comes down with marketplace competition and economies of scale. I believe this will ultimately prove to be true with LCS.

M. F. Pyfer, MD

Reference

1. Ewe SY, Abell RG, Oakley CL, et al. A comparative cohort study of visual outcomes in femtosecond laser-assisted versus phacoemulsification cataract surgery. *Ophthalmology*. 2016;123:178-182.

Postoperative IOL Axial Movements and Refractive Changes After Femtosecond Laser-assisted Cataract Surgery Versus Conventional Phacoemulsification

Toto L, Mastropasqua R, Mattei PA, et al (Ctr of Excellence on Aging, Chieti-Pescara, Italy; Univ of Verona, Italy; et al)
J Refract Surg 31:524-530, 2015

Purpose.—To evaluate intraocular lens (IOL) axial movements and refractive changes during a 6-month follow-up period after femtosecond laser-assisted cataract surgery and conventional cataract surgery, investigate the influence of capsulorhexis features on postoperative IOL axial changes, and assess the prediction error for both techniques.

Methods.—Eighty eyes of 80 candidates for cataract extraction were randomized into two groups: femtosecond laser (40 eyes) and manual (40 eyes).

Results.—The overall anterior chamber depth variation was significantly lower in the femtosecond laser group compared to the manual group during follow-up ($P < .001$). At 30 and 180 days postoperatively, the mean spherical equivalent showed a hyperopic shift (0.09 ± 0.28 diopters [D]) in the femtosecond laser group and a myopic shift in the manual group (-0.25 ± 0.18 D). Median absolute error was not significantly different between the two groups with standard formulas ranging between 0.29 and 0.64 (Hoffer Q) in the femtosecond laser group

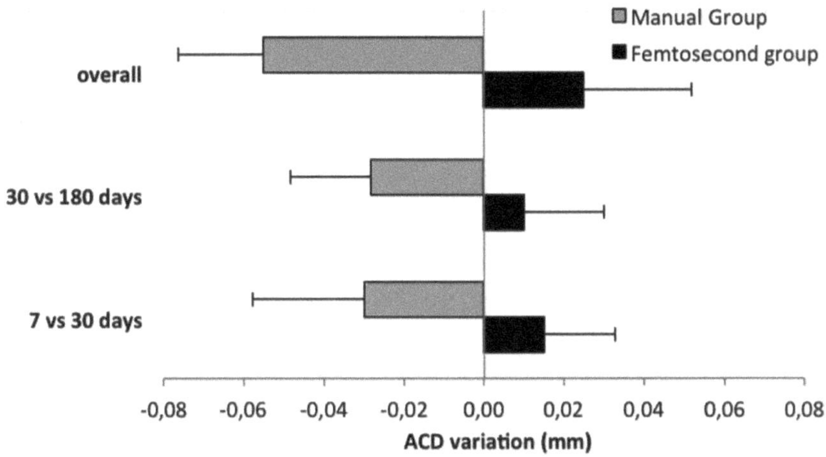

FIGURE 2.—Mean postoperative change of anterior chamber depth (ACD). The bars represent the standard error of the mean. Negative values indicate a decrease and positive values an increase in ACD. ACD was defined as the distance from the central corneal epithelium to the anterior intraocular lens surface. ****P* < .001 for the manual group. (Reprinted from Toto L, Mastropasqua R, Mattei PA, et al. Postoperative IOL axial movements and refractive changes after femtosecond laser-assisted cataract surgery versus conventional phacoemulsification. *J Refract Surg.* 2015;31:524-530, with permission from SLACK Incorporated.)

and between 0.24 (SRK-T) and 0.55 D (Hoffer Q) in the manual group. There was a significant lower deviation from intended versus achieved capsulotomy/capsulorhexis area in the femtosecond laser group (*P* < .001) compared to the manual group. The femtosecond laser group showed better IOL centration compared to the manual group at all time periods (*P* < .001).

Conclusions.—Femtosecond laser-assisted cataract surgery was related to a lower overall variability of anterior chamber depth compared to conventional cataract surgery with more stable postoperative refraction. The two techniques did not show significant differences of prediction error (Fig 2).

▶ In this prospective randomized study comparing femtosecond laser-assisted cataract surgery (FLACS) to manual conventional surgery, use of the laser resulted in a more stable postoperative refraction, due to lower variation in intraocular lens (IOL) position up to 6 months after surgery. Lens position was measured precisely by anterior chamber depth (ACD) using anterior segment optical coherence tomography at 1 week, 1 month, and 6 months after surgery (Fig 2). Lens centration was also better in the laser group; however, no significant difference was found in final refractive error.

Current monofocal IOL designs are somewhat forgiving in terms of centration and tilt and their effect on visual outcome. This is important for manual surgery, where small variations in capsulotomy size, shape, and implant position are unavoidable. However, given the added precision achievable with femtosecond laser-assisted cataract surgery as demonstrated in this study, new IOL designs that require more precise alignment to achieve superior outcomes can be developed. In the near future, I believe more widespread adoption of FLACS will spur development of new lens implants that improve on our current outcomes. History has shown that it is only a matter of time.

M. F. Pyfer, MD

Comparison of Outcomes of Primary Anterior Chamber Versus Secondary Scleral-Fixated Intraocular Lens Implantation in Complicated Cataract Surgeries

Chan TCY, Lam JKM, Jhanji V, et al (Hong Kong Eye Hosp, China; The Chinese Univ of Hong Kong, China)

Am J Ophthalmol 159:221-226, 2015

Purpose.—To compare the outcome of primary anterior chamber vs secondary scleral-fixated intraocular lens (IOL) implantation in complicated cataract surgeries.

Design.—Retrospective, comparative study.

Methods.—A consecutive series of complicated cataract surgeries with primary anterior chamber (ACIOL) or secondary scleral-fixated IOL implantation from January 1, 2004 to December 31, 2009 was analyzed. Main outcome measures included the postoperative best-corrected visual acuity (BCVA) and postoperative complications.

Results.—There were 89 eyes in the primary ACIOL group and 74 eyes in the secondary scleral-fixated IOL group. The mean follow-up duration was 64.1 ± 36.7 months. The mean postoperative logarithm of minimal angle of resolution (logMAR) BCVA at 1 year was 0.32 ± 0.54 and 0.34 ± 0.21 in the primary ACIOL group and the secondary scleral-fixated IOL group, respectively ($P = .734$). The mean latest logMAR BCVA was 0.68 ± 0.54 and 0.61 ± 0.47 in the primary ACIOL group and the secondary scleral-fixated IOL group, respectively ($P = .336$). The primary ACIOL group had more early postoperative complications ($P < .001$). No difference in late postoperative complications was observed between the 2 groups ($P = .100$). Regression analysis showed that primary ACIOL and secondary scleral-fixated IOL implantation had similar latest postoperative logMAR BCVA ($P = .927$), while the presence of late complications was associated with a worse final visual outcome ($P = .000$).

Conclusions.—This study shows that there are no long-term differences in the visual outcomes and complication profiles after primary ACIOL or secondary scleral-fixated IOL implantation in a complicated cataract operation when capsular support is inadequate.

▶ Anterior-chamber angle-supported intraocular lenses (ACIOLs) are an alternative to posterior chamber intraocular lenses (PCIOLs) in complicated cataract surgeries in which inadequate capsular support is present. Recently, ACIOLs have fallen out of favor, mainly due to potential vision-threatening complications, such as corneal endothelial cell loss, chronic uveitis, and elevated intraocular pressure. However, the literature supports the use of a properly sized and placed ACIOL without undue risk of complications.

This retrospective 5-year study at a single institution examines the outcomes of primary ACIOLs compared with secondary scleral-fixated IOLs in complicated cases without capsular support. With an average of 5 years of follow-up, no significant difference in best corrected vision between the 2 groups was found.

This study supports the use of an ACIOL in complicated cases, as long as adequate vitrectomy and proper lens placement can be achieved during the initial surgery. If a second procedure is required due to unavailable equipment or unforeseen complications during the primary surgery, then equivalent visual results can be obtained by placement of a secondary scleral fixated IOL at a later date.

M. F. Pyfer, MD

Visual function and reading speed after bilateral implantation of 2 types of diffractive multifocal intraocular lenses: Add-on versus capsular bag design

Liekfeld A, Ehmer A, Schröter U (Klinikum Ernst von Bergmann Gemeinnützige GmbH, Potsdam, Germany)

J Cataract Refract Surg 41:2107-2114, 2015

Purpose.—To compare the functional outcomes of primary implantation of a monofocal intraocular lens (IOL) in the capsular bag and an add-on multifocal IOL in the sulcus with the functional results of a conventional multifocal posterior chamber IOL and to evaluate the multifocal add-on IOL as an effective alternative to a conventional multifocal IOL.

Setting.—Ernst von Bergmann Eye Clinic, Potsdam, Germany.

Design.—Prospective nonrandomized case series.

Methods.—Cataract surgery patients were assigned to have bilateral implantation of a monofocal IOL (Aspira-aAY) in the capsular bag followed by a multifocal add-on IOL (Diff-sPB) in the sulcus (Group A) or with a conventional multifocal IOL (Diffractiva-s) in the capsular bag (Group B). The main study outcomes were assessed at the last follow-up visit (6 months postoperatively) and included refraction, intraocular pressure, visual acuity, reading speed, contrast sensitivity, defocus curve, and patient satisfaction.

Results.—The study comprised 26 patients (52 eyes) Cataract surgery was uneventful in all cases. No severe complications were observed 6 months postoperatively. Visual performance with a multifocal diffractive add-on IOL was equivalent to that achieved with a conventional multifocal diffractive posterior chamber IOL. Similarly, there were no significant differences in patient satisfaction and reading speed for any type of letter size between groups ($P > .05$).

Conclusion.—Implanting a multifocal add-on IOL in the sulcus in addition to a monofocal IOL in the capsular bag produced outcomes similar to

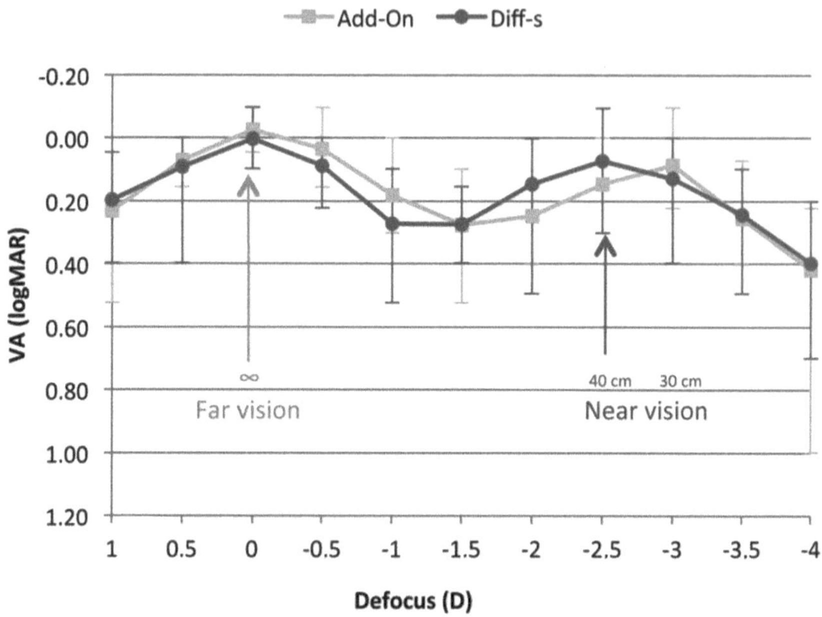

FIGURE 1.—Median binocular defocus curves. Error bars represent the range associated with each median value (VA = visual acuity). (Reprinted from Liekfeld A, Ehmer A, Schröter U. Visual function and reading speed after bilateral implantation of 2 types of diffractive multifocal intraocular lenses: add-on versus capsular bag design. *J Cataract Refract Surg*. 2015;41:2107-2114, with permission from ASCRS and ESCRS.)

those of single implantation of a standard multifocal IOL in the capsular bag (Fig 1).

▶ This prospective nonrandomized study compares the visual results for bilateral implantation of a sulcus fixated add-on diffractive multifocal intraocular lens (IOL) versus a single capsular bag fixated multifocal IOL of similar optical design. The rather remarkable conclusion is that the measured outcomes are equivalent between the 2 groups. Uncorrected visual acuity at distance, intermediate, and near; contrast sensitivity; reading speed; and subjective patient satisfaction were all similar (Fig 1). No complications from the sulcus add on design occurred up to 6 months postoperatively, except 1 lens had to be explanted due to decentration.

Add-on multifocal IOLs are not currently available in the United States but they are, for several reasons, an intriguing option for the future once approved by the Food and Drug Administration. Secondary sulcus fixated lenses are easily implanted even years after primary cataract and IOL surgery, and they are removable with low risk. Also, add-on IOLs provide the opportunity to correct small amounts of residual ametropia. I feel there is a large potential market for an add-on multifocal IOL in patients who already have monofocal implants but now desire greater spectacle independence. We look forward to having this option to add to our arsenal for refractive cataract surgery.

M. F. Pyfer, MD

Incidence, Risk Factors, and Impact of Age on Retinal Detachment after Cataract Surgery in France: A National Population Study

Daien V, Le Pape A, Heve D, et al (Inserm 1061, Montpellier, France; Regional Agency of Health, Montpellier, France; et al)

Ophthalmology 122:2179-2185, 2015

Purpose.—To assess the incidence, risk factors, and impact of age on retinal detachment (RD) after cataract surgery.

Design.—Cohort study.

Participants.—All patients older than 40 years of age who underwent a primary cataract surgery in France between January 2009 and December 2012.

Methods.—A Cox proportional-hazard regression model was used to analyze risk factors of RD after cataract surgery.

Main Outcome Measures.—Risk factors of RD after cataract surgery.

Results.—Over 4 years, 2 680 167 eyes in 1 787 021 patients (59.4% women; mean age, 73.9 ± 9.5 years) underwent cataract surgery. A total of 11 424 patients experienced RD after cataract surgery, with an estimated risk of 0.99% at 4 years after surgery. The odds ratio associated with increased risk of RD was 3.87 (95% confidence interval [CI], 3.79–3.95) for cataract surgery itself. The multiadjusted hazard ratio (HR) associated with increased risk of RD was 5.22 (95% CI, 5.05–5.39) for patients 40 to 54 years of age, 3.69 (95% CI, 3.60–3.79) for those 55 to 64 years of age, and 1.98 (95% CI, 1.93–2.03) for those 65 to 74 years of age as compared with those 75 years of age or older. Retinal detachment was associated with high myopia (HR, 6.12; 95% CI, 5.84–6.41), vitrectomy for perioperative capsular rupture (HR, 4.36; 95% CI, 4.07–4.68), history of eye trauma (HR, 3.98; 95% CI, 3.69–4.30), extracapsular extraction (HR, 3.11; 95% CI, 2.94–3.30), male gender (HR, 2.39; 95% CI, 2.35–2.44), and history of diabetes (HR, 1.18; 95% CI, 1.15–1.21). In myopic patients, the multiadjusted HR associated with increased risk of RD was 25.02 (95% CI, 24.76–25.18) for patients 40 to 54 years of age, 20.37 (95% CI, 20.21–20.53) for those 55 to 64 years of age, and 17.05 (95% CI, 16.85–17.25) for those 65 to 74 years of age as compared with nonmyopic patients 75 years of age or older.

Conclusions.—We provide a hierarchy of risk factors for RD onset: high myopia, young age, capsular rupture, history of eye trauma, extracapsular extraction technique, male gender, and diabetes. Young age was an additional risk factor in myopic patients (Table 3).

► Retinal detachment (RD) is a serious vision-threatening late complication associated with cataract surgery, with about a 50% chance of final visual outcome

TABLE 3.—Stratified Analysis of the Multiadjusted Hazard Ratio of Retinal Detachment after Cataract Extraction among Myopic and Nonmyopic Patients

	Myopic Patients		Nonmyopic Patients	
Age (yrs)	Adjusted Hazard Ratio*	95% Confidence Interval	Adjusted Hazard Ratio*	95% Confidence Interval
≥75	13.45	13.19–13.71	1.00	
65–74	17.05	16.85–17.25	1.98	1.92–2.04
55–64	20.37	20.21–20.53	3.76	3.70–3.82
40–54	25.02	24.76–25.18	5.46	5.40–5.52

*As compared with nonmyopic patients 75 years of age or older, adjusted for gender, history of diabetes, eye trauma, and anterior vitrectomy for perioperative capsular rupture and surgical technique (extracapsular cataract extraction vs. phacoemulsification).

below 20/40 after surgical RD repair.[1] Reported incidence of retinal detachment after cataract surgery varies widely, but recent literature estimates it is about 0.7% lifetime. This is at least 4 times higher than the roughly 1 in 1500 incidence rate of rhegmatogenous retinal detachment in the general population.[2]

This report examines more than 2.6 million cataract extractions from the French national medical database over a 4-year period to determine the incidence and risk factors for RD after cataract surgery. The database is derived from hospital discharge reports, which are required for payment under the national health insurance system, so it should miss very few cases. Also, because RD is fairly common, unlike rare complications such as endophthalmitis, a small number of missing reports would not change the overall statistics. The study looks only at a 4-year window, so it likely underestimates the lifetime cumulative incidence of pseudophakic RD.

Myopia and younger age are both established risk factors for retinal detachment after cataract surgery. This study agrees, showing that for myopic patients under 55 years old, RD is 25 times more likely than for a nonmyopic patient over 75 (see Table 3). Also, it found that men are about twice as likely as women to have RD after cataract surgery, so for a myopic male under 55 the incidence of RD after cataract surgery may be as high as 10%. For me, this is an unacceptable risk in an elective refractive procedure, so I do not recommend clear lens extraction in myopes (axial length > 26 mm).

In summary, this article provides numerical estimates for surgeons to use in counseling patients about RD risk after cataract surgery. It also helps identify higher risk groups, so greater surveillance, prophylactic treatment, or deferral of surgery can be recommended appropriately.

M. F. Pyfer, MD

References

1. Haddad WM, Monin C, Morel C, et al. Retinal detachment after phacoemulsification: a study of 114 cases. *Am J Ophthalmol.* 2002;133:630-638.
2. Haug SJ, Bhisitkul RB. Risk factors for retinal detachment following cataract surgery. *Curr Opin Ophthalmol.* 2012;23:7-11.

Prevention of Cystoid Macular Edema After Cataract Surgery in Nondiabetic and Diabetic Patients: A Systematic Review and Meta-Analysis

Wielders LHP, Lambermont VA, Schouten JSAG, et al (Maastricht Univ Med Ctr+, Netherlands; et al)

Am J Ophthalmol 160:968-981, 2015

Purpose.—To evaluate the optimum medical strategy to prevent cystoid macular edema (CME) after cataract surgery.

Design.—Systematic review and meta-analysis.

Methods.—Setting: Cochrane, MEDLINE, and EMBASE databases were searched to identify eligible randomized controlled trials (RCTs).

Study Population.—RCTs comparing medical strategies to prevent CME after uncomplicated cataract surgery in nondiabetic and diabetic patients.

Observation Procedures.—Data were extracted by 2 authors independently. Quality of individual RCTs was assessed using the Cochrane Collaboration's tool for assessing risk of bias and Delphi criteria.

Main Outcome Measures.—Odds of developing CME within 3 months postoperatively and foveal thickness, macular volume and corrected distance visual acuity change within 3 months postoperatively, as compared to baseline.

Results.—Seventeen trials reported incidence rates. Topical nonsteroidal anti-inflammatory drugs (NSAIDs) significantly reduced the odds of developing CME as compared to topical corticosteroids in nondiabetic (odds ratio [OR] 0.11; 95% confidence interval [95% CI] 0.03–0.37) and mixed populations (OR 0.05; 95% CI 0.02–0.11). A combination of topical corticosteroids and NSAIDs significantly reduced the odds of developing CME as compared to topical corticosteroids in nondiabetic (OR 0.21; 95% CI 0.10–0.44) and diabetic patients (OR 0.17; 95% CI 0.05–0.50). Intravitreal corticosteroid or anti–vascular endothelial growth factor injections did not show any additional benefit in diabetic subjects.

Conclusions.—Topical NSAIDs significantly reduced the odds of developing CME, as compared to topical corticosteroids, in nondiabetic and mixed populations. A combination of topical NSAIDs and corticosteroids reduced the odds of developing CME in nondiabetic and diabetic patients, as compared to topical corticosteroids (Table 4).

▶ This is a detailed meta-analysis using validated scientific methods to investigate strategies for cystoid macular edema (CME) prevention after cataract surgery. The medical literature from 1947 to 2014 was searched, and 17 eligible randomized controlled clinical trials were identified. The results (see Table 4) are strongly conclusive for both diabetic and nondiabetic patients: topical nonsteroidal anti-inflammatory drugs (NSAIDs) are the best way to prevent vision-threatening CME after cataract surgery. Using NSAIDs with topical corticosteroids, as most cataract surgeons do currently, yields the lowest incidence of CME. There was no added benefit to intravitreal or sub-Tenon steroid

TABLE 4.—Efficacy of Various Treatment Strategies to Prevent the Occurrence of Cystoid Macular Edema After Uncomplicated Cataract Surgery in Nondiabetic, Diabetic, and Mixed Populations

			Population Studied (No. of Studies)	OR (95% CI)
Topical NSAID	>	Topical CS	Nondiabetic (3)	0.11 (0.03–0.37)
			Mixed population (3)	0.05 (0.02–0.11)
Topical NSAID	≈[a]	Topical CS & topical NSAID	Nondiabetic (n.a.)	0.54 (0.13–2.20)
Topical NSAID & topical CS	>	Topical CS	Nondiabetic (4)	0.21 (0.10–0.44)
			Diabetic (1)	0.17 (0.05–0.50)
Topical CS & intravitreal anti-VEGF	≈	Topical CS	Diabetic (1)	0.13 (0.02–1.21)
Topical CS & intravitreal anti-VEGF	≈[a]	Topical CS & intravitreal CS	Diabetic (n.a.)	0.71 (0.02–28.76)
Topical CS & intravitreal CS	≈	Topical CS	Diabetic (1)	0.09 (0.00–1.89)
Subconjunctival CS	≈	Topical CS	Nondiabetic (1)	1.18 (0.53–2.62)
Subconjunctival CS & sub-Tenon CS & oral AZ	≈	Topical CS & subconjunctival CS & oral AZ	Nondiabetic (1)	0.31 (0.03–3.16)
Topical NSAID & oral CS	≈	Topical CS & oral CS	Nondiabetic (1)	0.06 (0.00–1.10)

AZ = acetozolamide; CME = cystoid macular cdema; CS = corticosteroid; n.a. = not applicable; no. = number; NSAID = nonsteroidal anti-inflammatory drug; OR = odds ratio; VEGF = vascular endothelial growth factor; 95% CI = 95% confidence interval.

[a]Indirect treatment comparison using the Bucher method.

Reprinted from Wielders LHP, Lambermont VA, Schouten JSAG, et al. Prevention of cystoid macular edema after cataract surgery in nondiabetic and diabetic patients: a systematic review and meta-analysis. *Am J Ophthalmol.* 2015;160:968-981, with permission from Elsevier Inc.

injection or intravitreal anti–vascular endothelial growth factor (VEGF) injection for CME prevention in diabetic patients. The study did not examine other risk factors for CME, such as epiretinal membrane or prior history of CME. It also did not measure the incidence of diabetic macular edema or worsening of diabetic retinopathy after cataract surgery. These conditions may still benefit from anti-VEGF injection in the preoperative period, which has been demonstrated in other studies.[1]

Despite recent claims by some that the addition of topical NSAIDs to the postcataract surgical regimen is unnecessary and costly, resulting mainly from effective drug company marketing efforts, this analysis shows a clear and conclusive benefit. Left untreated or identified late, postoperative CME is truly a vision-threatening complication of cataract surgery that should be largely preventable. Prophylactic treatment with NSAIDs in all patients for 4 to 6 weeks after surgery, and for 3 months in high-risk patients is strongly advised. The incidence of CME and the loss of vision attributable to it is almost 2 orders of magnitude greater than postoperative endophthalmitis, which has dominated the literature and discussions at meetings recently. Even if using the new "dropless" techniques involving transzonular or intravitreal antibiotic and steroid injection during surgery, I would strongly advise adding a topical NSAID for CME prophylaxis in light of this article, especially in higher risk patients.

M. F. Pyfer, MD

Reference

1. Brown DM, Schmidt-Erfurth U, Do DV, et al. Intravitreal aflibercept for diabetic macular edema: 100-week results from the VISTA and VIVID studies. *Ophthalmology.* 2015;122:2044-2052.

Oxygen therapy for corneal edema after cataract surgery

Sharifipour F, Panahi-Bazaz M, Idani E, et al (Ahvaz Jundishapur Univ of Med Sciences, Ahvaz, Iran)

J Cataract Refract Surg 41:1370-1375, 2015

Purpose.—To evaluate the effects of oxygen therapy on corneal edema after cataract surgery.

Setting.—Imam Khomeini Hospital, Ahvaz, Iran.

Design.—Randomized controlled trial.

Methods.—Patients with severe corneal edema were randomized into 3 groups. Group 1 (control) received conventional therapy including topical sodium chloride, timolol, and betamethasone. Group 2 received the same therapy in addition to systemic normobaric oxygen at a flow rate of 10 L/min for 1 hour twice daily for 3 weeks. Group 3 received conventional therapy and transcorneal oxygen at a flow rate of 5 L/min for 1 hour twice daily for 3 weeks. Preoperative pachymetry and specular microscopy were performed. Pachymetry was performed 1, 3, 5, 7, 10, and 14 days

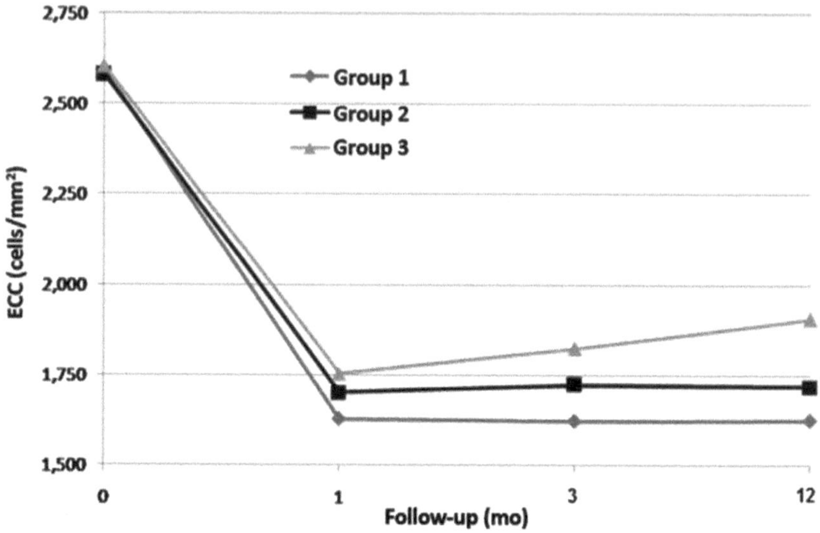

FIGURE 2.—Endothelial cell count after cataract surgery (ECC = endothelial cell count). (Reprinted from Sharifipour F, Panahi-Bazaz M, Idani E, et al. Oxygen therapy for corneal edema after cataract surgery. *J Cataract Refract Surg.* 2015;41:1370-1375, with permission from ASCRS and ESCRS.)

postoperatively. At 1, 3 and 12 months, pachymetry and specular microscopy were performed.

Results.—The study enrolled 45 patients. Preoperatively, there was no significant difference between the groups. Pachymetry was more than 1000 μm 1 day postoperatively in all patients. The preoperative pachymetry was restored in 14 days in Group 3 only. After 1 year, the endothelial cell count (ECC) was 1603 cells/mm^2, 1693 cells/mm^2, and 1911 cells/mm^2 with a loss of 37%, 32%, and 25% in Group 1, Group 2, and Group 3, respectively (P =.034, Groups 1 and 3). Group 3 had a higher ECC than the control group at 3 months (P =.037) and 1 year (P =.025). One patient in Group 1 and 1 patient in Group 2 developed bullous keratopathy.

Conclusion.—Transcorneal oxygen decreased corneal edema more rapidly than conventional and systemic oxygen therapies and preserved more endothelial cells than conventional therapy (Fig 2).

▶ This is a fascinating study of a relatively small group of patients with corneal edema after cataract surgery. It shows that intensive oxygen treatment directly to the cornea for 3 weeks postoperatively can hasten the clearing of edema and lead to a higher endothelial cell count up to 1 year after surgery (Fig 2). The mechanism of this effect is not tested, but speculated that hyperbaric oxygen helps preserve injured endothelial cells.

I have long noticed that patients on home oxygen therapy for respiratory disease have clearer corneas immediately after cataract surgery. Now with the results of this study, perhaps oxygen treatment specifically for endothelial cell rescue could become a standard treatment option, along with corticosteroids and control of intraocular pressure. This technique may speed visual recovery and help avoid endothelial keratoplasty for patients with compromised corneal endothelium after cataract surgery. This is the first article on this subject, so further study on dosing and delivery methods is warranted to verify the results.

M. F. Pyfer, MD

Comparison of Methods to Predict Residual Astigmatism After Intraocular Lens Implantation

Abulafia A, Hill WE, Franchina M, et al (Sir Charles Gairdner Hosp, Nedlands, Western Australia, Australia; East Valley Ophthalmology, Mesa, AZ; et al)
J Refract Surg 31:699-706, 2015

Purpose.—To evaluate and compare the accuracy of three toric intraocular lens (IOL) calculators using keratometry measurements derived from the anterior corneal curvature and direct measurements of the posterior corneal curvature.

Methods.—Postoperative corneal astigmatism was measured by the IOLMaster (Carl Zeiss Meditec, Jena, Germany) and Pentacam (Oculus Optikgeräte, Wetzlar, Germany). The data were processed by the Alcon, Holladay, and Barrett toric IOL calculators. The error in predicted residual astigmatism (PredRA) was calculated by subtracting the PredRA from the postoperative subjective refraction by vector analysis.

Results.—The centroid errors in PredRA were against-the-rule (ATR) with the Alcon (0.56 diopters [D]) and Holladay (0.55 D) toric calculators using the IOLMaster (Carl Zeiss Meditec, Jena, Germany) measurements.

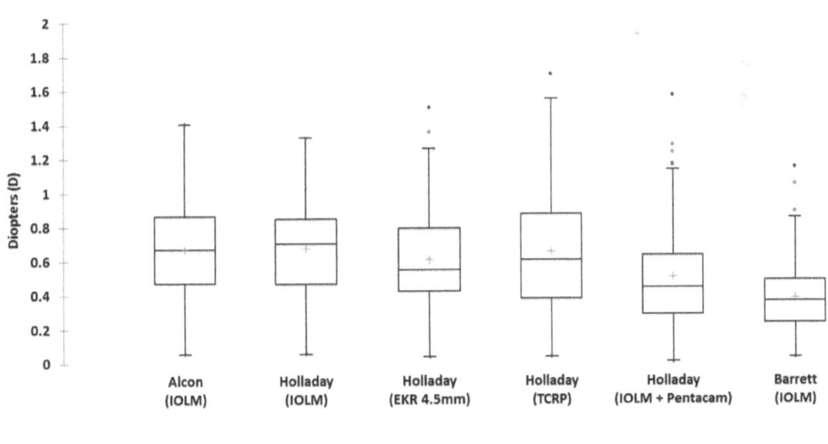

FIGURE 1.—Absolute error in predicted residual astigmatism by measuring device and method of calculation. IOLM = IOLMaster; EKR = equivalent keratometry reading; TCRP = total corneal refractive power. The IOLMaster is manufactured by Carl Zeiss Meditec, Jena, Germany, and the Pentacam by Oculus Optikgeräte, Wetzlar, Germany. (Reprinted from Abulafia A, Hill WE, Franchina M, et al. Comparison of methods to predict residual astigmatism after intraocular lens implantation. *J Refract Surg.* 2015;31:699-706, with permission from SLACK Incorporated.)

The centroid errors in PredRA were lower when Pentacam (Oculus Optikgeräte, Wetzlar, Germany) measurements were used (0.38 D, ATR). The Barrett toric calculator using the IOLMaster measurements had the lowest centroid errors in PredRA (0.02 D, $P < .001$) and achieved the most accurate results: 75.8% and 92.9% of eyes were within 0.50 and 0.75 D of the PredRA, respectively.

Conclusions.—The prediction of the postoperative astigmatic outcome can be improved by using appropriate methods of adjustment for posterior corneal astigmatism (Fig 1).

▶ Toric intraocular lenses (IOLs) have dramatically improved the management of corneal astigmatism in patients undergoing cataract surgery. However, limitations or errors in measurement, especially concerning the effect of the posterior cornea, affect the accuracy of final refractive results with these IOLs. The Barrett toric IOL calculator is a new alternative method for determining the appropriate power and axis for toric IOLs to minimize postoperative refractive error. Compared with other popular toric IOL calculators, even including measurement of posterior corneal astigmatism using the Pentacam, the Barrett toric calculator yielded the best overall results in this retrospective analysis (Fig 1).

Significantly, the Barrett toric calculator does not require a measurement of the posterior cornea to achieve this increased accuracy. It was used here simply with the IOL Master keratometry data. This is an impressive result. Any cataract surgeon who implants toric IOLs should give strong consideration to using the Barrett calculator, now available online on the American Society of Cataract and Refractive Surgery and Asia-Pacific Association of Cataract and Refractive Surgeons websites.

M. F. Pyfer, MD

Corneal Diameter as a Factor Influencing Corneal Astigmatism After Cataract Surgery

Theodoulidou S, Asproudis I, Kalogeropoulos C, et al (Univ of Ioannina, Greece; et al)

Cornea 35:132-136, 2016

Purpose.—To evaluate the corneal horizontal diameter [white-towhite (WTW) distance] as a factor influencing surgically induced astigmatism (SIA) and postoperative astigmatism.

Methods.—A total of 330 eyes with corneal astigmatism ≤1.5 D underwent cataract surgery with phacoemulsification. A 3-step, superotemporal for the right eye and superonasal for the left eye, clear corneal incision of 3.0 mm was made. Four groups were created according to WTW distance: group A ≤11.6 mm, group B 11.7 to 11.9 mm, group C 12.0 to 12.2 mm, and group D ≤12.3 mm. SIA was calculated by vector analysis using the Alpins method. We noted all cases, in which a change greater than 0.5 diopters (D) in astigmatism took place and a change greater than 20

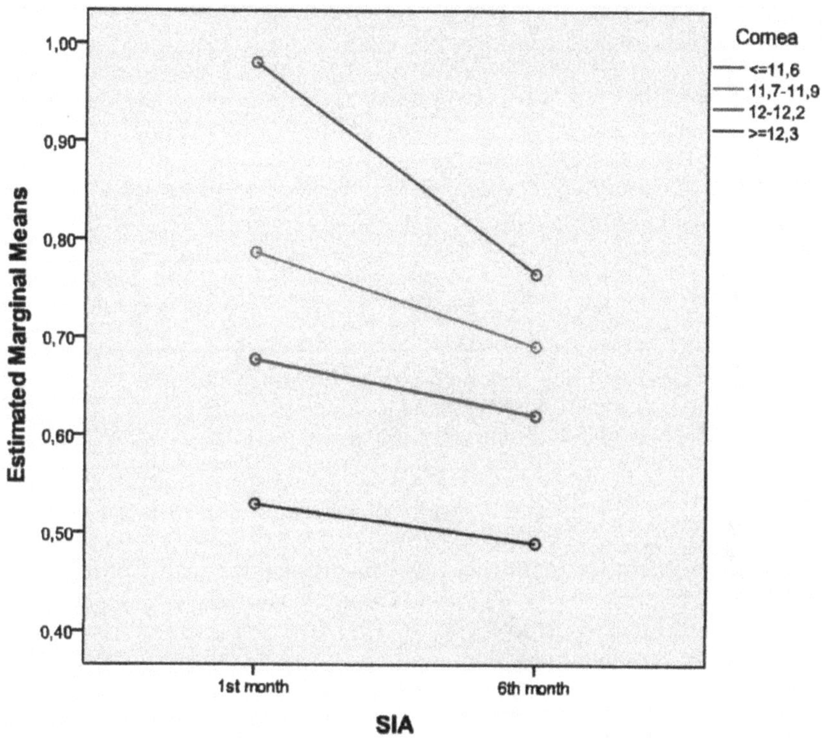

FIGURE 1.—Changes in SIA from the first to sixth postoperative months. (Reprinted from Theodoulidou S, Asproudis I, Kalogeropoulos C, et al. Corneal diameter as a factor influencing corneal astigmatism after cataract surgery. *Cornea.* 2015;35:132-136, with permission from Wolters Kluwer Health, Inc.)

degrees in axis torque, despite axis direction, on the first and sixth postoperative months.

Results.—SIA was found in group A 0.98 D ± 0.6 (SD), B 0.79 D ± 0.43 (SD), C 0.68 D ± 0.45 (SD), and D 0.53 D ± 0.32 (SD) at the first postoperative month. At the sixth postoperative month, SIA was 0.77 D ± 0.43 (SD), 0.69 D ± 0.34 (SD), 0.62 ± 0.36 (SD), and 0.49 D ± 0.27 (SD), respectively. A change greater than 0.5 D in corneal astigmatic power at the first and sixth months postoperatively was significantly lower in eyes with WTW distance 12.0 to 12.2 mm and ≥12.3 mm in comparison with eyes with WTW distance ≤11.6 mm and 11.7 to 11.9 mm ($P < 0.05$). Changes greater than 20 degrees in astigmatic axis at the first and sixth postoperative months were not significantly different according to the horizontal corneal diameter.

Conclusions.—WTW distance should always be measured preoperatively when planning cataract surgery and should be accounted for in cases of large and small corneas (Fig 1).

▶ This is an interesting study, the first I am aware of to propose adjusting estimated surgically induced astigmatism (SIA) for corneal diameter. The conclusion is intuitively appealing because we know that arcuate keratotomy incisions have increased effect as distance from the corneal apex decreases. The same is true for limbal clear corneal surgical incisions, as the authors demonstrate (Fig 1). It is important to account for SIA in refractive cataract surgery, especially for toric intraocular lens cases. It also makes sense to adjust limbal relaxing incisions (LRIs) for corneal diameter, but I am not aware of any published LRI nomogram that takes horizontal white-to-white into account. I have made the adjustment to my personal SIA and LRI nomograms after reading this article.

M. F. Pyfer, MD

Capacity of straylight and disk halo size to diagnose cataract

Palomo-Álvarez C, Puell MC (Complutense Univ of Madrid, Spain)
J Cataract Refract Surg 41:2069-2074, 2015

Purpose.—To examine the capacity of straylight and disk halo size to diagnose cataract.

Setting.—Faculty of Optics and Optometry, Universidad Complutense de Madrid, Spain.

Design.—Prospective study.

Methods.—Straylight, disk halo radius, and high-contrast corrected distance visual acuity (CDVA) measurements were compared between patients with age-related cataract and age-matched normal-sighted control subjects by calculating the area under the curve (AUC) receiver operating characteristic.

Results.—Measurements were made in 53 eyes of 53 patients with a mean age of 67.94 years ± 7.11 (SD) and 31 eyes of 31 controls with a mean age 66.06 ± 5.43 years. Significantly worse ($P < .001$) mean straylight (1.38 ± 0.24 log[s]), mean disk halo radius (2.40 ± 0.18 log minutes of arc [arcmin]), and mean CDVA (0.17 ± 0.11 logMAR) were recorded in the cataract group than in the control group (1.17 ± 0.11 log[s], 2.10G 0.16 log arcmin, and 0.08 ± 0.08 logMAR). Significant differences in AUCs were observed for disk halo radius (0.89 ± 0.04) versus straylight (0.77 ± 0.05) ($P = .03$) and disk halo radius versus CDVA (0.72 ± 0.05) ($P = .001$). The comparison of disk halo radius versus the discriminant function with input from CDVA and straylight (0.80 ± 0.05) was at the limit of significance only (0.091 ± 0.05, $P = .051$).

Conclusion.—Although all 3 variables discriminated well between normal eyes and eyes with cataract, the disk halo radius showed the best diagnostic capacity (Fig 1).

► A simple objective measurement that correlates to cataract density would allow better systematic determination of eligibility for cataract surgery. Surgeons are well aware of the limitations of Snellen acuity reduction as a measure of cataract significance, but this metric is universal and difficult to change.

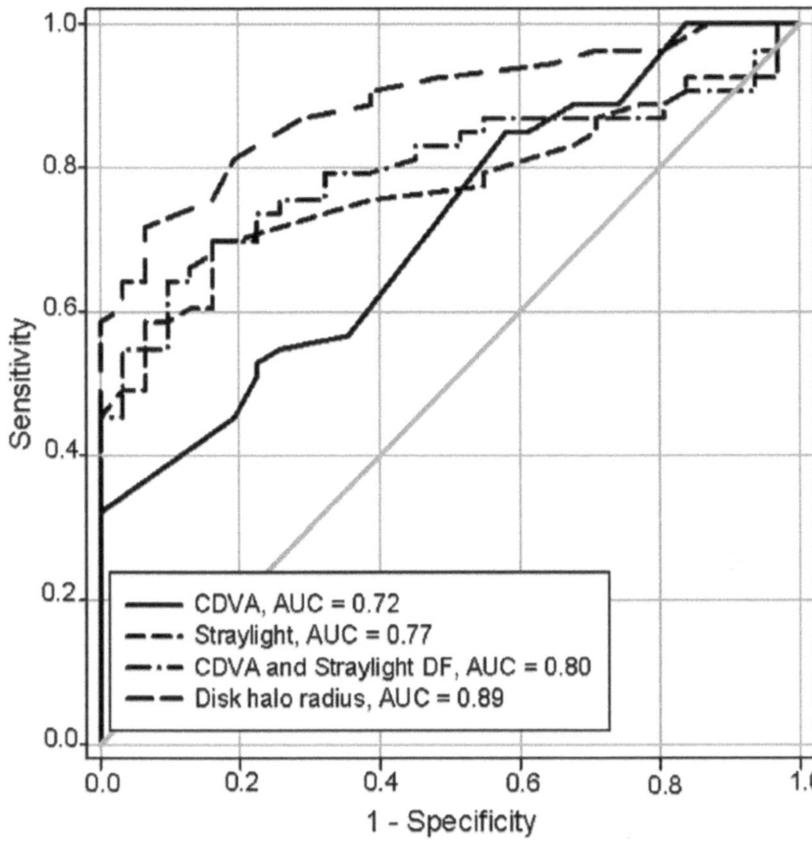

FIGURE 1.—Areas under the ROC curves for CDVA, straylight, disk halo radius, and the discriminant function CDVA plus straylight (AUC = area under the receiving operating characteristic; CDVA = corrected distance visual acuity). (Reprinted from Palomo-Álvarez C, Puell MC. Capacity of straylight and disk halo size to diagnose cataract. *J Cataract Refract Surg*. 2015;41:2069-2074, with permission from ASCRS and ESCRS.)

Here, several methods were tested to differentiate normal from cataract eyes, and it turns out that disk halo radius was superior to the others (Fig 1). This could lead to a simple practical office test to supplement standard Snellen acuity in the preoperative cataract evaluation. Most other supplemental metrics that have been recommended, including contrast sensitivity, glare acuity, and vision-related quality of life metrics, are more difficult to measure in a brief office visit.

M. F. Pyfer, MD

Efficacy and safety of combined cataract surgery with 2 trabecular microbypass stents versus ab interno trabeculotomy

Khan M, Saheb H, Neelakantan A, et al (Univ of Toronto, Ontario, Canada; McGill Univ Health Centre, Montreal, Quebec, Canada; the Glaucoma Ctr of Texas, Dallas; et al)

J Cataract Refract Surg 41:1716-1724, 2015

Purpose.—To compare the outcomes of combined cataract surgery with trabecular microbypass stents and ab interno trabeculotomy in patients with open-angle glaucoma.

Setting.—University of Toronto, Toronto, Ontario, and University of Montreal, Montreal, Quebec, Canada, and Glaucoma Associates of Texas, Dallas, Texas, USA.

Design.—Retrospective case series.

Methods.—Patients with primary open-angle, pseudoexfoliative, or pigmentary dispersion glaucoma were included. Primary outcome measures were intraocular pressure (IOP), postoperative medications, success (IOP ≤18 mm Hg, no glaucoma medications or reoperations), and postoperative adverse events.

Results.—The average patient age was 76.5 years ± 12 [SD]. Forty-nine eyes had phacoemulsification and 2 had stent implantations; 52 eyes had phacoemulsification and trabeculotomy surgery with a 12-month postoperative follow-up. The analysis of variance indicated a significant reduction in mean IOP from baseline to 12 months for stent (19.6 ± 5.3 mm Hg to 14.3 ± 3.1 mm Hg; $P < .001$) and trabeculotomy (20.6 ± 6.8 mm Hg to 17.3 ± 6.5 mm Hg; $P < .001$) and lower mean IOP at 12 months in the stent group ($P = .01$). The median number of glaucoma medications decreased from baseline to 12 months in both groups and was lower in the stent group at 3, 6, and 12 months. Thirty-nine percent (19 eyes) in the stent group and 14% (7 eyes) in the trabeculotomy group achieved success at 12 months ($P = .006$). The incidence of hyphema was lower in the stent group ($P = .008$).

Conclusions.—Both types of surgery achieved a significant reduction in IOP and medication use at 12 months, with the stent group achieving higher success and a reduced incidence of postoperative hyphema (Fig 3).

▶ Microinvasive glaucoma surgery (MIGS) combined with cataract surgery is an appealing option compared with the traditional glaucoma triple procedure of combined cataract extraction, lens implantation, and trabeculectomy/guarded filtration procedure. Lower risk of complications and faster recovery are the main advantages of MIGS. Implantation of Glaukos iStent and ab interno trabeculotomy using the Trabectome are 2 increasingly common MIGS options for patients with open-angle glaucoma. These procedures are well within the skill set of the cataract/anterior segment surgeon in most cases.

This retrospective study comparing iStent to trabeculotomy along with cataract surgery found both procedures to be effective; however, the stent resulted in lower intraocular pressure (IOP) and less glaucoma medication use up to

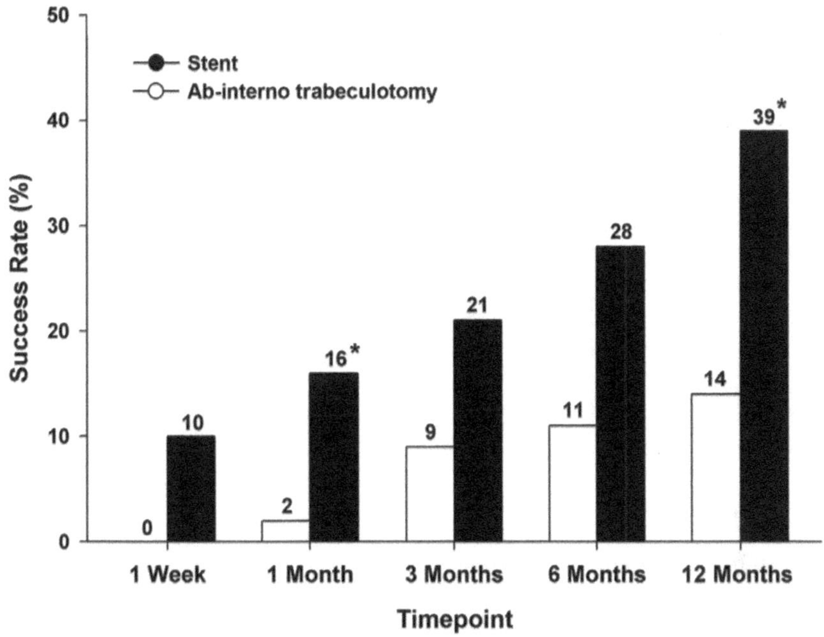

FIGURE 3.—Percentage of patients achieving success (IOP ≤ 18 mm Hg, no medications, no loss of light perception, and no need for glaucoma reoperation) in both study groups over 12 months. (Reprinted from Khan M, Saheb H, Neelakantan A, et al. Efficacy and safety of combined cataract surgery with 2 trabecular microbypass stents versus ab interno trabeculotomy. *J Cataract Refract Surg.* 2015;41:1716-1724, with permission from ASCRS and ESCRS.)

12 months after surgery (Fig 3). The usual limitations of a retrospective study apply, including selection bias. The stent group had more patients with pseudoexfoliation glaucoma, which could also bias the results. The authors addressed this showing that subgroup analysis without these patients did not change the outcome. There was also no control group for cataract surgery alone without MIGS; however, other studies have shown both techniques to yield lower IOP compared with cataract surgery alone.[1,2]

Overall, this study provides compelling evidence in favor of the stent when combined with cataract surgery. The major barrier in the United States is cost because only 1 device is reimbursed currently, while this study from Canada and others have used 2 devices with greater efficacy.[3] This limitation will be addressed soon by a modified design containing 2 stents on 1 injector, which is currently under Food and Drug Administration review and should be available in the United States by next year.

M. F. Pyfer, MD

References

1. Fea AM, Consolandi G, Zola M, et al. Micro-bypass implantation for primary open-angle glaucoma combined with phacoemulsification: 4-year follow-up. *J Ophthalmol.* 2015;2015:795357.

2. Kaplowitz K, Bussel II, Honkanen R, Schuman JS, Loewen NA. Review and meta-analysis of ab-interno trabeculectomy outcomes. *Br J Ophthalmol.* 2016 [Epub ahead of print].
3. Katz LJ, Erb C, Carceller GA, et al. Prospective, randomized study of one, two, or three trabecular bypass stents in open-angle glaucoma subjects on topical hypotensive medication. *Clin Ophthalmol.* 2015;9:2313-2320.

Sustained-release dexamethasone for the treatment of ocular inflammation and pain after cataract surgery

Walters T, Endl M, Elmer TR, et al (Texan Eye Care, Austin, TX; Fichte, Endl & Elmer Eyecare, Niagara Falls, NY; et al)
J Cataract Refract Surg 41:2049-2059, 2015

Purpose.—To evaluate the safety and efficacy of dexamethasone as a sustained-release drug depot when placed in the canaliculus for the treatment of ocular inflammation and pain in cataract surgery patients.

Setting.—Four private practice sites in the United States.

Design.—Multicenter randomized double-masked clinical trial.

Methods.—Patients were randomized (1:1) to receive either the sustained-release dexamethasone or a placebo vehicle punctum plug inserted into the inferior distal canaliculus of the operated eye intraoperatively during cataract surgery. The primary endpoints were the proportions of patients with absence of cells or pain in the anterior chamber at 8 days. Secondary endpoints included cells, flare, pain, and the presence of the device at various timepoints through 30 days.

Results.—Approximately one fifth (20.7%) of patients in the sustained-release dexamethasone group had an absence of anterior chamber cells at 8 days compared with 10.0% in the placebo group ($P = .1495$). A higher proportion of patients in the sustained-release dexamethasone group (79.3%) than in the placebo group (30.0%) had an absence of ocular pain at 8 days ($P < .0001$) and at all other timepoints ($P < .0002$). There were significantly higher proportions of patients in the sustained-release dexamethasone group than in the placebo group with an absence of anterior chamber cells, anterior chamber flare, and pain at several timepoints through 30 days ($P \leq .0251$).

Conclusion.—Sustained-release dexamethasone provided elution of drug for up to 1 month after cataract surgery, providing clinically significant reductions in inflammation and pain.

▶ Methods to eliminate the need for postoperative eyedrop medications after cataract surgery are getting more attention recently. This is due mainly to commercially available compounded medications for intraocular injection during surgery. With the rapid improvement in visual acuity and comfort made possible by modern cataract surgical techniques, patients are now more noticeably inconvenienced by the need for prolonged postoperative topical medication regimens. This is the most common complaint I receive from patients after surgery. In addition, older patients often have difficulty self-administering eyedrops, and multiple bottles of medications may be misidentified, creating a compliance problem.

I believe sustained-release steroid-eluting inserts, whether in the canaliculus as in this article or intraocular, will replace the topical steroid eyedrops after cataract surgery within the next 3 to 5 years. This study supports the effectiveness of an intracanalicular dexamethasone implant for reducing inflammation and pain after cataract surgery. However, this device still did not suppress all inflammation in 80% of patients at 1 week postop, so a higher concentration insert, multiple inserts, or supplemental topical medication will be required in most patients for a few weeks.

M. F. Pyfer, MD

Cataract surgery in the small eye

Hoffman RS, for the ASCRS Cataract Clinical Committee, Challenging/Complicated Cataract Surgery Subcommittee (Oregon Health and Science Univ, Portland; et al)

J Cataract Refract Surg 41:2565-2575, 2015

The surgical management of cataract in the small eye presents the ophthalmic surgeon with numerous challenges. An understanding of the anatomic classification in addition to a thorough preoperative assessment will help individualize each case and enable the surgeon to better prepare for the obstacles that might be encountered during surgery. Small eyes are especially challenging in terms of intraocular lens (IOL) calculations and possible current limitations of available IOL powers, which could necessitate alternative means of achieving emmetropia. Surgical strategies for minimizing complications and maximizing good outcomes can be developed from knowledge of the anatomic differences between various small-eye conditions and the pathologies that may be associated with each. A thorough understanding of the challenges inherent in these cases and the management of intraoperative and postoperative complications will ensure that surgeons approaching the correction of these eyes will achieve the best possible surgical results.

▶ This is a consensus viewpoint and detailed outline of current recommendations for cataract surgery in nanophthalmic and microphthalmic eyes. It is an excellent guideline for achieving good visual results and avoiding complications in these challenging cases. All details, including preoperative evaluation, biometry, surgical technique, and postoperative management, are covered, and there is nothing that I can add to this complete review. This article should be required reading for all cataract surgeons.

M. F. Pyfer, MD

Laser iridotomy to treat uveitis-glaucoma-hyphema syndrome secondary to reverse pupillary block in sulcus-placed intraocular lenses: Case series

Singh H, Modabber M, Safran SG, et al (Univ of Toronto, Ontario, Canada; McGill Univ, Montreal, Quebec, Canada; Capital Health System, Pennington, NJ)

J Cataract Refract Surg 41:2215-2223, 2015

Purpose.—To present cases of uveitis-glaucoma-hyphema (UGH) syndrome due to reverse pupillary block in sulcus-placed posterior chamber intraocular lenses (PC IOLs) that were managed with laser peripheral iridotomy (LPI).

Setting.—Community-based subspecialty clinics.

Design.—Retrospective interventional case series.

Methods.—A chart review of patients with a sulcus-placed PC IOLs presenting with UGH syndrome and reverse pupillary block with posterior iris bowing as diagnosed by gonioscopy and anterior segment optical coherence tomography was carried out. Laser peripheral iridotomy was performed in the eyes included in the study. The main outcome measure was clinical resolution of UGH syndrome.

Results.—The study included 6 eyes of 6 patients with a mean age of 59.8 years (range 43.0 to 66.0 years) who presented with unilateral UGH syndrome a mean of 28.7 months (range 0.3 to 84.0 months) after PC IOL implantation. All patients were previously myopic, with 5 (83.3%) having a history of vitrectomy. The mean axial length was 27.0 mm ± 1.4 (SD). An LPI was used to treat the reverse pupillary block with resultant improvement in iris profile and resolution of UGH syndrome in all eyes. The mean intraocular pressure decreased from 30.5 ± 10.0 mm Hg on 0.5 ± 0.8 glaucoma medications to 15.5 ± 3.2 mm Hg postoperatively on 0.7 ± 1.2 medications.

Conclusions.—The UGH syndrome due to reverse pupillary block occurred after sulcus-placed PC IOLs in susceptible patients, those with axial myopia, and post-vitrectomized eyes. The cases were managed with LPIs (Fig 7).

▶ Uveitis-glaucoma-hyphema (UGH) syndrome is a potential late complication of cataract surgery with an intraocular lens (IOL) implant. It has been reported with all types of IOLs: anterior chamber, iris-supported, 1-piece, and 3-piece posterior chamber lenses.[1] It may occur when a posterior chamber lens is fully or partially contained in the capsular bag or in the iridociliary sulcus. Lenses that are poorly fixated, mobile, or in contact with uveal tissue are more likely to cause UGH syndrome. Certain conditions also increase the risk for UGH syndrome, including pseudoexfoliation syndrome, longer axial length, significant iridodonesis, and prior vitrectomy.

This article reports on a series of patients who had UGH syndrome associated with reverse pupillary block and sulcus fixated IOLs. Laser peripheral iridotomy (LPI) was successful both in relieving the pupillary block and the UGH syndrome. Most cases of UGH syndrome eventually require surgical intervention

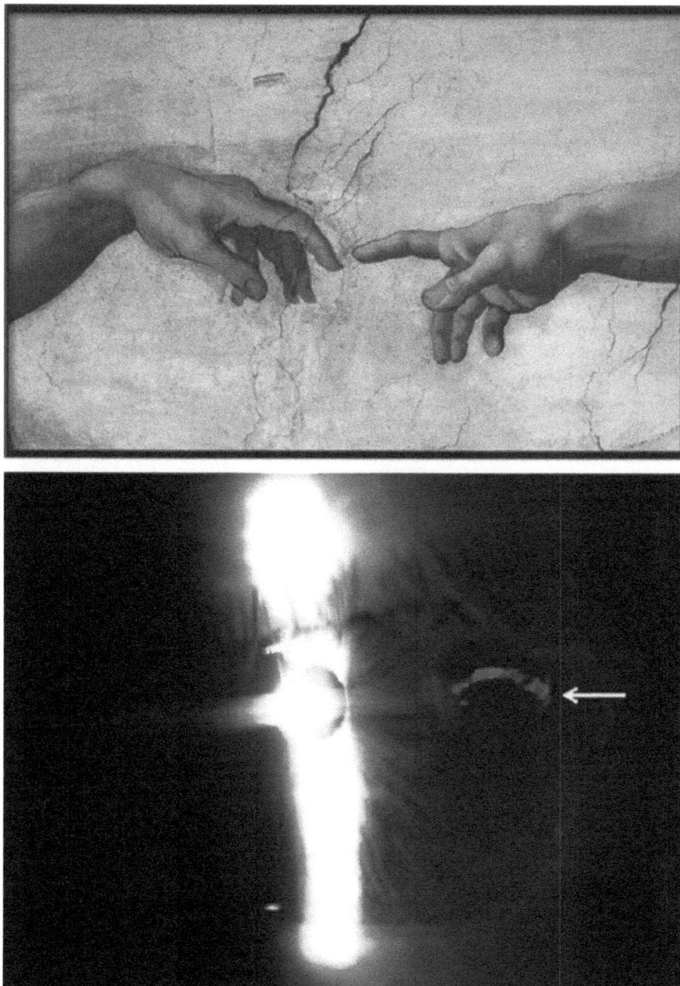

FIGURE 7.—Finger of God sign, reflecting the fingerlike transillumination defects commonly observed in reverse pupillary block. (Reprinted from Singh H, Modabber M, Safran SG, et al. Laser iridotomy to treat uveitis-glaucoma-hyphema syndrome secondary to reverse pupillary block in sulcus-placed intraocular lenses: case series. *J Cataract Refract Surg*. 2015;41:2215-2223, with permission from ASCRS and ESCRS.)

to relieve the uveal irritation by the IOL, through repositioning, suture, or intrascleral fixation or through IOL exchange. In this series of 6 patients, there was no recurrence of UGH syndrome after LPI with followup of 1 to 4 years.

It is reasonable to try LPI in any patient with a posterior chamber IOL and UGH syndrome, in whom there is a possibility of reverse pupillary block. Signs of reverse pupillary block include posterior iris bowing and characteristic iris transillumination defects (see Fig 7). This conservative low-risk intervention may eliminate the need for more complex intraocular surgery.

M. F. Pyfer, MD

Reference

1. Zhang L, Hood CT, Vrabec JP, Cullen AL, Parrish EA, Moroi SE. Mechanisms for in-the-bag uveitis-glaucoma-hyphema syndrome. *J Cataract Refract Surg.* 2014; 40:490-492.

Suture-guided capsular tension ring insertion to reduce risk for iatrogenic zonular damage

Page TP (Oakland Univ William Beaumont School of Medicine, Royal Oak, MI)
J Cataract Refract Surg 41:1564-1567, 2015

The capsular tension ring (CTR) is a useful device for managing a zonular dialysis. However, insertion of the CTR has potential complications.

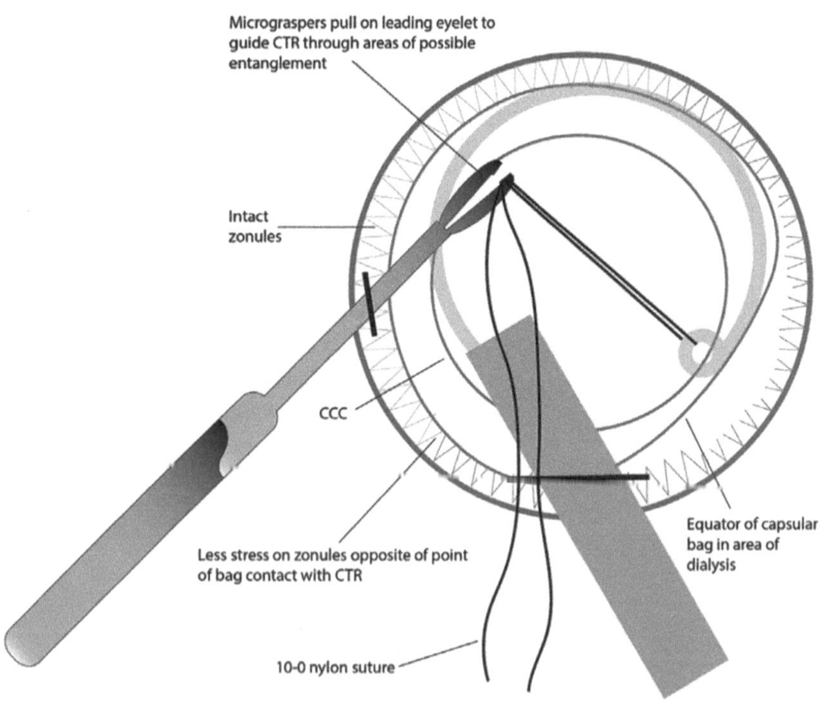

FIGURE 4.—Suture-guided CTR insertion to prevent entanglement of the leading eyelet and iatrogenic damage to zonular fibers (iris omitted for illustration purposes) (CTR = capsular tension ring; CCC = continuous curvilinear capsulorhexis). (Reprinted from Page TP. Suture-guided capsular tension ring insertion to reduce risk for iatrogenic zonular damage. *J Cataract Refract Surg.* 2015;41:1564-1567, with permission from ASCRS and ESCRS.)

TABLE 1.—Comparison of CTR Insertion Techniques

Technique*	Technique and Potential Advantage	Potential Disadvantage
Standard CTR insertion Hara 1991[1]	Simple technique can be used with inserter or forceps to rotate the CTR into the capsular bag.	Displacement of the capsular bag may occur.[7] Leading eyelet may become entangled in capsular fornix during insertion, causing further zonular damage.
Fishtail technique Angunawela 2007[9]	Bending the CTR in half and then inserting the apex through the incision eliminates rotation of the CTR, minimizing entanglement and bag displacement.	Significant bending and potential damage to the CTR.[9] Precision control of the leading eyelet during insertion is lost.
Fishtail on a Line technique Rixen 2014[10]	Suture placed in leading eyelet to achieve fishtail configuration places less torque on CTR.	Significant bending of CTR inside the anterior chamber. Precision control of the leading eyelet during insertion is lost.
Suture-guided CTR technique Page 2015	Suture in leading eyelet guided by a microforceps enables surgeon to dial in the CTR, mitigating torque and entanglement. Allows precision control with intended CTR shape and direction of insertion.	Requires an inserter and second micro instrument in the anterior chamber to guide the suture in the leading eyelet.

Editor's Note: Please refer to original journal article for full references.
CTR = capsular tension ring
*First author
Reprinted from Page TP. Suture-guided capsular tension ring insertion to reduce risk for iatrogenic zonular damage. *J Cataract Refract Surg*. 2015;41:1564-1567, with permission from ASCRS and ESCRS.

The CTR can damage zonular fibers during deployment into the capsular bag. Also, the angle and point of initial contact of the CTR with the capsular bag relative to the orientation of the dialysis must be considered to avoid damage to the zonular fibers. Adequate fill of the capsular bag with an ophthalmic viscosurgical device is important to minimize the risk for capsule entanglement with the leading eyelet of the CTR. A simple technique is described to prevent these complications. The technique can be used with both standard and modified CTRs (Fig 4, Table 1).

▶ This article describes a novel technique for decreasing the potential capsule and zonule trauma during capsule tension ring (CTR) insertion. It is a surgical technique article, which is usually not selected for inclusion here. However, the author provides excellent diagrams of the procedure (Fig 4), and an online video that help the cataract surgeon understand and perform this maneuver successfully. He also includes a review of other techniques for CTR insertion that have been published (Table 1). The technique described here is the best I have seen for this purpose.

One other popular technique that is not mentioned in the article, is using a second instrument such as a Sinskey hook, through a paracentesis, to guide the ring into the capsule fornix and relieve some of the force applied to the end of the ring. However, this technique is not as effective once the ring has been inserted more than 180 degrees into the capsular bag. The maneuver described here involves looping a suture through the leading eyelet of the

CTR, then grasping the suture within the anterior chamber using a microforceps when countertraction is needed. The surgeon must have microforceps available in the operating room, ready to use, and have sufficient manual dexterity with the nondominant hand to perform this 2-handed maneuver. I feel that most anterior-segment surgeons today should be able to master this maneuver, which is important when encountering difficulty with the standard CTR insertion procedure.

M. F. Pyfer, MD

2 Refractive Surgery

Three-Year Results of Small Incision Lenticule Extraction for High Myopia: Refractive Outcomes and Aberrations

Pedersen IB, Ivarsen A, Hjortdal J (Aarhus Univ Hosp, Aarhus C, Denmark)

J Refract Surg 31:719-724, 2015

Purpose.—To assess the 3-year refractive and visual outcomes after small incision lenticule extraction (SMILE) in patients with high myopia and to evaluate the optical changes from 3 months to 3 years after surgery.

Methods.—A total of 87 eyes (87 patients) undergoing SMILE for high myopia were included. Preoperative and 3-month and 3-year postoperative follow-up examinations included manifest refraction and uncorrected and corrected distance visual acuities. Pentacam HR (Oculus Optikgeräte, Wetzlar, Germany) was used to evaluate the total corneal refractive power and the root mean square of spherical aberration, coma, and total higher-order aberrations. The paired *t* test and Wilcoxon signed rank test were used.

Results.—The preoperative spherical equivalent averaged -7.30 ± 1.40 diopters (D); no significant changes occurred between 3 months and 3 years after surgery (-0.30 ± 0.50 vs -0.40 ± 0.60 D, $P = .071$). Uncorrected distance visual acuity was stable from 3 months to 3 years after SMILE (0.04 ± 0.17 vs 0.03 ± 0.19 logMAR; $P = .28$), whereas corrected distance visual acuity improved from -0.05 ± 0.15 to -0.08 ± 0.11 logMAR ($P < .001$). At 3 months, 82% and 93% of eyes were within ±0.50 and ±1.00 D, respectively. At 3 years, 78% and 90% were within ±1.00 D of the attempted refraction, respectively. Spherical and higher-order aberrations significantly decreased from 3 months to 3 years, whereas coma remained stable. A significant regression of 0.36 ± 0.29 D was seen in total corneal refractive power ($P < .001$).

Conclusions.—The refractive and visual outcomes seemed stable years after SMILE. A minor myopic regression was observed in total corneal refractive power but not in subjective refraction. There seems to be a significant long-term improvement in higher-order aberrations after surgery (Fig 1).

► This is the longest follow-up study on small incision lenticule extraction (SMILE) that I know of, and it is in high myopes (−6 to −10 diopters). Although not a particularly large study (87 eyes of 87 patients), it does demonstrate good stability of the results from 3 months to 3 years (Fig 1).

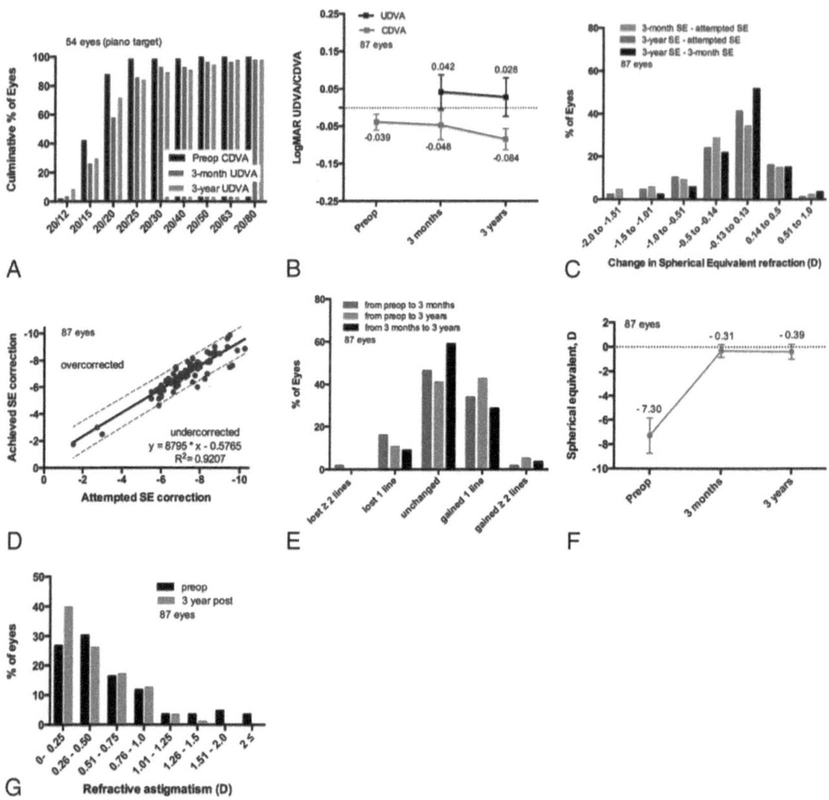

FIGURE 1.—(A) Cumulative percentage of preoperative corrected distance visual acuity (CDVA) and postoperative uncorrected distance visual acuity (UDVA) at the 3-month and 3-year follow-up. Only eyes with emmetropia as target were included (n = 57). (B) LogMAR UDVA and CDVA with 95% confidence intervals from preoperative to 3 months and 3 years postoperatively. Preoperative logMAR UDVA is not illustrated. (C) Distribution of the difference in attempted versus achieved spherical equivalent (SE) refractive correction 3 months and 3 years after small incision lenticule extraction, and change in achieved SE from 3 months to 3 years. All eyes were included. D = diopters. (D) Achieved (3 years postoperatively) versus attempted change in SE refraction. (E) Change in logMAR of CDVA from 3 months to 3 years, and from preoperative to 3 months and 3 years after small incision lenticule extraction. (F) Mean preoperative and 3-month and 3-year postoperative SE with standard deviation. (G) Percentage of patients reaching specified levels of refractive astigmatism preoperative and 3 postoperatively. (Reprinted from Pedersen IB, Ivarsen A, Hjortdal J. Three-year results of small incision lenticule extraction for high myopia: refractive outcomes and aberrations. *J Refract Surg.* 2015;31:719-724, with permission from SLACK Incorporated.)

There were small improvements in uncorrected and best corrected vision and also a decrease in higher order aberrations and spherical aberration's from 3 months to 3 years, along with a tiny myopic shift. Given that these were relatively early SMILE cases, these data are quite encouraging.

C. J. Rapuano, MD

Vision-related quality of life and visual outcomes after small-incision lenticule extraction and laser in situ keratomileusis

Ang M, Ho H, Fenwick E, et al (Singapore Natl Eye Centre; Univ of Melbourne, Australia; et al)

J Cataract Refract Surg 41:2136-2144, 2015

Purpose.—To compare vision-related quality of life (VRQoL) scores and clinical outcomes between small-incision lenticule extraction and laser in situ keratomileusis (LASIK).

Setting.—Singapore National Eye Centre, Singapore.

Design.—Prospective study.

Methods.—Patients had small-incision lenticule extraction using the Visumax 500 kHz femtosecond laser; or LASIK excimer ablation with the Wavelight Allegretto 400 Hz laser. Primary outcomes were 3-month predictability, efficacy, and safety. Secondary outcomes were intraoperative experience, visual symptoms, and VRQoL (validated Quality of Life Impact of Refractive Correction [QIRC] questionnaire) in 25 a subgroup of patients in each group. Following Rasch analysis, "Functional" and "Emotional," QIRC dimensions were analysed separately.

Results.—At 3 months, predictability (82.5% versus 85.3%, ±0.5 diopters attempted correction, $P = .453$), safety index (1.13 ± 0.19 [SD] versus 1.07 ± 0.16, $P = .158$), and efficacy index (0.91 ± 0.21 versus 0.97 ± 0.19; $P = .002$) were found when comparing small-incision lenticule extraction (172 eyes) and LASIK (matched 688 eyes). Intraoperative experience between groups was not statistically different; visual fluctuations ($P = .020$) and episodes of visual blurring ($P = .008$) were greater after small-incision lenticule extraction than after LASIK at 1 month but not at 3 months. There was no difference in "functional" (66.7 ± 15.7 versus 55.3 ± 22.2, $P = .064$) and "emotional" (42.7 ± 23.2 versus 37.9 ± 23.8, $P = .394$) QIRC dimensions between the 2 groups (25 patients in each group) at 3 months.

Conclusion.—The study, 3-month predictability, safety, and VRQL scores were not statistically different between small-incision lenticule extraction and LASIK.

▶ Potential advantages of small-incision lenticule extraction (SMILE) compared with laser in situ keratomileusis (LASIK) include the use of a single laser for the procedure, reduced laser energy and a much smaller superficial incision (flapless surgery), with less postoperative discomfort, neurotrophy, and dry eye. Although the technique is relatively new compared with LASIK (and not currently Food and Drug Administration approved), early visual acuity and refractive outcome experience demonstrate it to be comparable to LASIK.

The authors performed a prospective study involving patients who chose to have LASIK (688 eyes) or SMILE (172 eyes). The primary outcomes were efficacy, predictability, and safety at 3 months. Although the safety and predictability results were the same in the 2 groups, the mean efficacy and percent of eyes that saw 20/20 or better uncorrected was statistically significantly better in the LASIK eyes. The authors do go on to state that the efficacy results of the SMILE eyes at 6 months were comparable to the LASIK eyes at 3 months.

For the vision-related quality-of-life aspect of this study, the authors randomly selected 25 patients from each group to answer questionnaires. On the one hand, LASIK patients were "more fearful" of the flap creation stage of the surgery. On the other hand, LASIK patients had statistically significantly fewer complaints of visual fluctuation and occasional blurring of vision at 1 month but not at 3 months. Similarly, LASIK patients reported significantly greater vision-related functional and emotional well-being than the SMILE patients at 1 month, but not at 3 months.

The primary outcomes of this study were at 3 months, so it is hard to fault the authors for glossing over the better "functional" and "emotional" results of LASIK compared with SMILE at 1 month. However, only 64% of SMILE eyes were 20/20 uncorrected compared with 80% of LASIK eyes at 3 months ($P = .001$). I think this is important to know. We do need to keep in mind that this study was performed between 2010 and 2012, in the relatively early days of SMILE. I would expect better results now, 4 to 6 years later.

C. J. Rapuano, MD

Dry Eye Disease after Refractive Surgery: Comparative Outcomes of Small Incision Lenticule Extraction versus LASIK

Denoyer A, Landman E, Trinh L, et al (Quinze-Vingts Natl Ophthalmology Hosp, Paris, France; et al)

Ophthalmology 122:669-676, 2015

Purpose.—To compare small incision lenticule extraction (SMILE) versus LASIK for post-refractive dry eye disease.

Design.—Prospective, comparative, nonrandomized clinical study.

Participants.—Thirty patients scheduled for bilateral myopic SMILE and 30 age-, sex-, and refraction-matched patients scheduled for bilateral myopic LASIK were enrolled and followed for 6 months after the surgery.

Methods.—Complete evaluation of dry eye disease was performed at 1 and 6 months postoperatively, which included vision related quality of life (Ocular Surface Disease Index [OSDI]), clinical examinations (tear film breakup time [TBUT], Schirmer I test, corneal staining), and tear osmolarity measurements, together with an overall severity score. Function and morphology of the corneal innervation were evaluated by corneal esthesiometry and subbasal nerve imaging using in vivo confocal microscopy (IVCM).

Main Outcome Measures.—Overall analysis of dry eye disease and corneal innervation.

Results.—High incidence of mild to moderate dry eye disease was observed in both groups 1 month postoperatively, which remained significantly higher in the LASIK group than in the SMILE group 6 months after

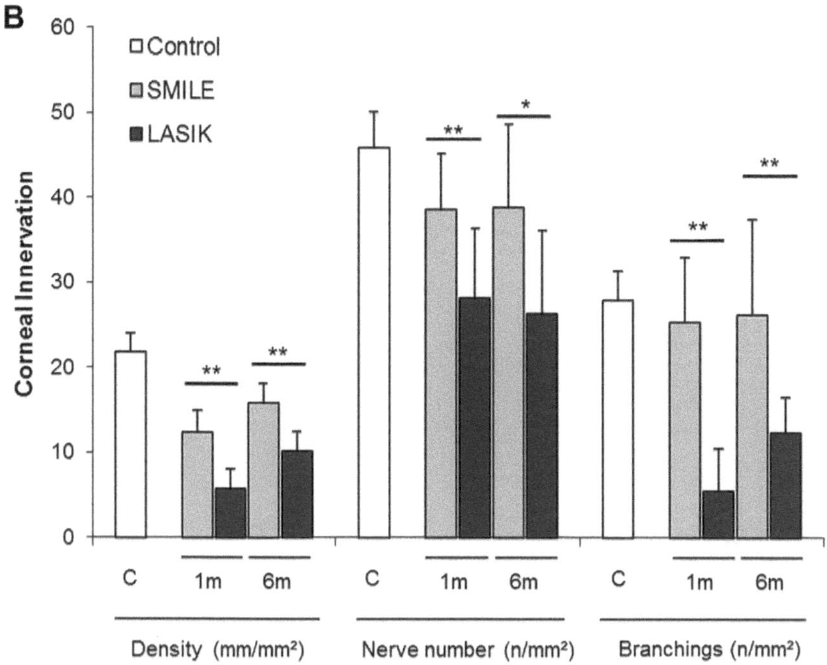

FIGURE 3.—Morphologic and functional assessment of corneal innervation 1 month and 6 months after small incision lenticule extraction (SMILE) versus LASIK. **B**, Corneal innervation as assessed using in vivo confocal microscopy. Nerve density, number of long fibers, and secondary branchings were higher in SMILE than in LASIK eyes (*$P < 0.05$; **$P < 0.01$). Control group is presented for illustrative purposes, which is taken from a previous study conducted by our team (n = 15). (Reprinted from Denoyer A, Landman E, Trinh L, et al. Dry eye disease after refractive surgery: comparative outcomes of small incision lenticule extraction versus LASIK. *Ophthalmology.* 2015;122:669-676, with permission from American Academy of Ophthalmology.)

surgery (overall severity score [0–4]: 1.2 ± 1.1 vs. 0.2 ± 0.4, respectively, $P < 0.01$), leading to more frequent use of tear substitutes over the long term. Corneal sensitivity was better in SMILE than in LASIK eyes 1 month postoperatively (3.5 ± 1.79 vs. 2.45 ± 2.48, respectively, $P < 0.01$) and then recovered to statistically similar values at 6 months. Corneal nerve density, number of long fibers, and branchings as assessed by IVCM were significantly higher in the SMILE group compared with the LASIK group 1 and 6 months after surgery. Corneal sensitivity was negatively correlated with dry eye-related corneal damage ($R^2 = 0.48$, $P < 0.01$), and the long fiber nerve density was independently correlated with the OSDI score ($R^2 = 0.50$, $P < 0.01$) and the Schirmer test ($R^2 = 0.21$, $P < 0.01$) 6 months postoperatively.

Conclusions.—The SMILE procedure has a less pronounced impact on the ocular surface and corneal innervation compared with LASIK, further

TABLE 2.—Dry Eye Disease 1 and 6 Months after Refractive Surgery

	1 Month			6 Months		
	SMILE	LASIK	*P*	SMILE	LASIK	*P*
OSDI (0–100)	19.7 ± 12.7	23.9 ± 14.8	0.09	**7.5 ± 4.5**	**20.6 ± 20.8**	**<0.01**
TBUT (s)	5.9 ± 1.7	5.1 ± 1.9	0.16	**7 ± 1.8**	**5.2 ± 1.8**	**0.01**
Schirmer I test (mm/5′)	13.2 ± 6.1	19.9 ± 10.5	0.08	17.3 ± 8.2	16.9 ± 7.8	0.85
Oxford score (0–5)	0.08 ± 0.28	0.27 ± 0.55	0.16	0	0.4 ± 0.6	0.06
Tear osmolarity (mOsm)	**305.1 ± 12.5**	**316.3 ± 11.6**	**<0.01**	**300.3 ± 11.4**	**315.0 ± 11.9**	**<0.01**
Dry eye severity score (0–4)	1.0 ± 0.8	1.5 ± 0.9	0.06	**0.2 ± 0.4**	**1.2 ± 1.1**	**<0.01**

Editor's Note: Please refer to original journal article for full references.

OSDI = Ocular Surface Disease Index; SMILE = small incision lenticule extraction; TBUT = tear film breakup time. The dry eye severity score was calculated according to the modified Delphi approach.[3,10] Data are reported as mean ± standard deviation. Boldface indicates statistical significance ($P < 0.01$).

reducing the incidence of dry eye disease and subsequent degradation in quality of life after refractive surgery (Fig 3B, Table 2).

▶ We have known for years that laser-assisted in situ keratomileusis (LASIK) (and photorefractive keratectomy, perhaps to a somewhat lesser degree) induces dry eye symptoms in a large percentage of patients. In fact, dry eye symptoms are one, if not the leading, cause of complaints after refractive surgery. Damage to the corneal nerves is thought to be an important factor in causing these dry eye symptoms. The LASIK flap severs ~300° of anterior corneal nerves, whereas in the small incision lenticule extraction (SMILE) technique, only ~40 to 60° of anterior corneal nerves are severed in the location of the tunnel through which the lenticule is removed. One would suspect that severing fewer anterior corneal nerves would yield fewer dry eye symptoms, but is that really the case?

The authors looked at just that question. Although they only included 30 patients in each group, patients were matched for age, gender, and refraction. Additionally, they performed extensive evaluations for dry eye and ocular surface disease, including in vivo confocal microscopy of the corneal nerves at 1 month and 6 months postoperatively. They found a similar high degree of dry eye signs and symptoms in both groups at 1 month (although tear osmolarity was statistically significantly lower [less dryness] in the SMILE eyes than the LASIK eyes) but statistically significantly fewer signs and symptoms in the SMILE eyes than LASIK eyes at 6 months (Table 2). Corneal nerve density and branching were statistically significant lower in the LASIK eyes compared with the SMILE eyes at 1 and 6 months, which correlated with worse dry eye symptoms and corneal staining (Fig 3B).

This article supports the concept that SMILE damages fewer corneal nerves than LASIK and is associated with fewer dry eye signs and symptoms. This finding is another potential benefit of SMILE over LASIK, but we in the United

States are still waiting Food and Drug Administration approval to test it for ourselves.

C. J. Rapuano, MD

SMILE Procedures With Four Different Cap Thicknesses for the Correction of Myopia and Myopic Astigmatism

Güell JL, Verdaguer P, Mateu-Figueras G, et al (Instituto Microcirugia Ocular, Barcelona, Spain; Universitat de Girona, Spain; et al)

J Refract Surg 31:580-585, 2015

Purpose.—To study the feasibility of performing myopic femtosecond small incision lenticule extraction (SMILE) with four different cap thicknesses (130, 140, 150, and 160 μm).

Methods.—In this retrospective, comparative, nonrandomized clinical trial, a refractive lenticule of intrastromal corneal tissue was cut with the VisuMax femtosecond laser system (Carl Zeiss Meditec AG, Jena, Germany) using different depths of the nonrefractive lenticule cut. Manifest refraction, uncorrected distance visual acuity (UDVA), corrected distance visual acuity (CDVA), and Objective Scattering Index (OSI) were evaluated. Minimum followup time was 1 year.

Results.—Ninety-four eyes of 47 patients with myopia with (14 patients) and without (33 patients) astigmatism were treated. One year after the surgery, mean log-MAR UDVA, logMAR CDVA, SE, and OSI were 0.07 ± 0.12, 0.01 ± 0.37, 0.07 ± 0.57, and 0.88 ± 0.17, respectively ($P < .05$). There were no significant statistical differences in logMAR UDVA, logMAR CDVA, SE, or OSI ($P > .05$) variables when the different groups were compared for the same periods of time.

Conclusions.—No differences in visual acuity, refractive outcomes in optical visual quality, or complications were observed when using SMILE at four different depths.

▶ It is my understanding that the optimal depth of the refractive lenticule in small incision lenticule extraction has not been determined. In fact, there may not be an optimal depth for all eyes. Moreover, I think it would depend on individual corneal thickness, refractive error, and perhaps other factors, such as age. Given the equivalent refractive results with the 4 lenticule depths found in this study, I predict that with more experience, we will have a nomogram optimizing the lenticule depth based on multiple parameters.

Potential advantages to a more superficial refractive lenticule include a thicker, stronger unaltered stromal bed and perhaps less damage to the corneal endothelium. Potential advantages to a deeper refractive lenticule include less damage to the superficial corneal nerves and greater mechanical strength of the cap. More experience with larger number of eyes will certainly help us determine the optimal lenticule depth.

I was struck by one aspect of this study. The authors increased the spherical equivalent attempted correction by 3% for every 10-μm thicker cap over

130 μm. So eyes with a 160-μm cap had their spherical equivalent refractive treatment increased by 10%. This alteration was done to "overcome potential energy loss" for thicker caps. This would make perfect sense to me if the laser were ablating tissue, as in excimer laser surgery, but it makes less sense to me when the femtosecond laser is cutting tissue at a predetermined depth. Does "energy loss" change the depth at which the femtosecond laser is focusing to cut tissue? If so, this is an extremely important concept that requires further investigation.

C. J. Rapuano, MD

Diffuse lamellar keratitis after small-incision lenticule extraction

Zhao J, He L, Yao P, et al (Eye and ENT Hosp of Fudan Univ, Shanghai, China)

J Cataract Refract Surg 41: 400-407, 2015

Purpose.—To determine the incidence and clinical features of diffuse lamellar keratitis (DLK) after small-incision lenticule extraction (SMILE).

Setting.—Department of Ophthalmology, Eye and ENT Hospital of Fudan University, Shanghai, China.

Design.—Retrospective case control study.

Methods.—Small-incision lenticule extraction for myopia was performed from September 1, 2011, to October 31, 2013. Preoperative clinical characteristics; treatment parameters; and intraoperative and postoperative complications, including the incidence, severity, clinical outcome, and resolution of DLK, were recorded. The independent *t* test, chi-square test, univariate repeated measures, and multivariate linear regression analysis were used to make statistical comparisons between eyes that developed DLK and those that did not.

Results.—The study enrolled 1112 eyes (590 patients). Eighteen eyes (1.6%) (11 patients) developed DLK. These patients presented 1 to 3 days postoperatively with mild to moderate inflammation. Thirteen eyes (72.2%) had stage 1 DLK, 4 (22.2%) had stage 2, and 1 (5.6%) had stage 3. After intensive treatment with topical corticosteroids, the stage 1 and stage 2 cases resolved within 3 weeks and the stage 3 case resolved in 1 month. The postoperative corrected distance visual acuity was the same or better than preoperatively in all eyes. There was a statistically significant increase in the incidence of DLK with thinner lenticules ($P = .02$) and larger diameter lenticules ($P = .01$), although multifactorial analysis showed lenticule thickness to be the only factor ($P = .03$).

Conclusions.—Diffuse lamellar keratitis is a potential complication after small-incision lenticule extraction, although it had a low incidence. The risk factors for DLK must be further elucidated.

▶ Although small-incision lenticule extraction (SMILE) has significant potential advantages over laser-assisted in situ keratomileusis including using 1 laser, no traumatic flap displacements, better biomechanical stability, and less dry eye, it does not appear that eliminating diffuse lamellar keratitis (DLK) is one of these advantages. After performing SMILE in more than 1000 eyes, these authors noted a 1.6% incidence of DLK, most with stage 1, some with stage 2, and 1 eye with stage 3. All responded well to treatment. The main risk factor identified was thinner lenticule thickness. The authors recommend that patients with smaller refractive errors should be informed about their slight increased risk for DLK.

I found interesting that 42% of all treated eyes were in male patients, but 64% of all eyes that developed DLK were in men, which was a statistically significant difference (*P* = .02). I found it even more interesting that the authors did not comment on this difference in their Discussion section.

C. J. Rapuano, MD

Flap lift and photorefractive keratectomy enhancements after primary laser in situ keratomileusis using a wavefront-guided ablation profile: Refractive and visual outcomes

Schallhorn SC, Venter JA, Hannan SJ, et al (Univ of California, San Francisco; Optical Express, Glasgow, United Kingdom)

J Cataract Refract Surg 41:2501-2512, 2015

Purpose.—To analyze results of wavefront-guided laser vision correction retreatments performed either by lifting the original flap or by surface ablation over the flap.

Setting.—Optical Express, Glasgow, United Kingdom.

Design.—Retrospective case series.

Methods.—This retrospective study included patients grouped according to whether they had flap lift enhancement or photorefractive keratectomy (PRK) performed over the LASIK flap. All retreatment procedures were performed with the Visx Star S4 IR excimer laser with wavefront-guided ablation profile derived from the iDesign aberrometer. Visual acuities, refractive outcomes, vector analysis of refractive cylinder and complications were analyzed in this study. The results of the last available clinical visit are presented.

Results.—This retrospective study included 290 eyes of 202 patients divided into 2 groups: 119 eyes that had flap lift enhancement (Group A), and 171 eyes in which photorefractive keratectomy (PRK) was performed over the LASIK flap (Group B). The mean follow-up was 4.0 ± 1.9 months in Group A and 4.2 ± 1.6 in Group B. The mean postoperative manifest spherical equivalent was −0.01 ± 0.35 D and +0.06 ± 0.39 D in Groups A and B, respectively. The percentage of eyes with postenhancement UDVA 20/20 or better was 87.4% in Group A and 79.5% in Group B (*P* = .09). In Group A, 22 eyes (18.5%) developed epithelial ingrowth, of which surgical intervention was required in 2 eyes (1.7%). Grade 1 or less haze was noted in 9 (5.3%) eyes in Group B, and resolved in all cases within the first 6 postoperative months.

Conclusion.—Both retreatment techniques were considered to be effective, predictable, and safe.

► Although the authors clearly state that this is a retrospective case series, the reader's natural tendency is to compare the results of the 2 groups as if they were equivalent. But they were not. The operating surgeon decided on the type of enhancement procedure and the Methods section states that the surgeon generally preferred flap lift enhancements in patients who were within 12 to 18 months of their primary procedures and PRK if they were beyond 12 months of their primary procedures. This is clearly reflected in the Results section where the time from primary procedure to enhancement was 14 months in the flap lift group and 35 months in the PRK group.

It is nice to know that both types of enhancements were successful. To me the biggest issue with flap lift enhancement is epithelial ingrowth, which in fact was seen in 18.5% of eyes. Only 2 eyes (1.7%) required surgery. One resulted in no recurrent ingrowth, whereas the other developed recurrent ingrowth that is being followed. Given that the mean follow-up time after the flat lift enhancement was 4 months, I am not convinced this represents all the cases of epithelial ingrowth that can occasionally occur late and may be difficult to treat.

My biggest concern with photorefractive keratectomy (PRK) after laser in situ keratomileusis (LASIK) is corneal haze. The use of mitomycin C (MMC) has helped dramatically to mitigate this issue. The authors found 1+ haze in 5.3% of eyes, all of which resolved by 6 months. Of course, late haze can rarely occur, which would not have been captured in the mean 4.5-month follow-up in the PRK eyes.

Surgeons who have attempted to lift LASIK flaps over the years have most likely found, as did the authors of this study, that femtosecond LASIK flaps are more difficult to lift than microkeratome flaps, which may also influence the decision regarding which enhancement technique to perform. Interestingly the authors note that they were able to lift a flap 65 months after femtosecond laser LASIK. I think I would have done PRK with MMC in that eye.

C. J. Rapuano, MD

Effect of postoperative keratometry on quality of vision in the postoperative period after myopic wavefront-guided laser in situ keratomileusis

Schallhorn SC, Venter JA, Hannan SJ, et al (Univ of California San Francisco; Optical Express, Glasgow, United Kingdom)

J Cataract Refract Surg 41:2715-2723, 2015

Purpose.—To determine whether postoperative keratometry is a predictor of patient-reported satisfaction and night-vision phenomena after wavefront-guided myopic laser in situ keratomileusis (LASIK).

Setting.—Optical Express, Glasgow, United Kingdom.

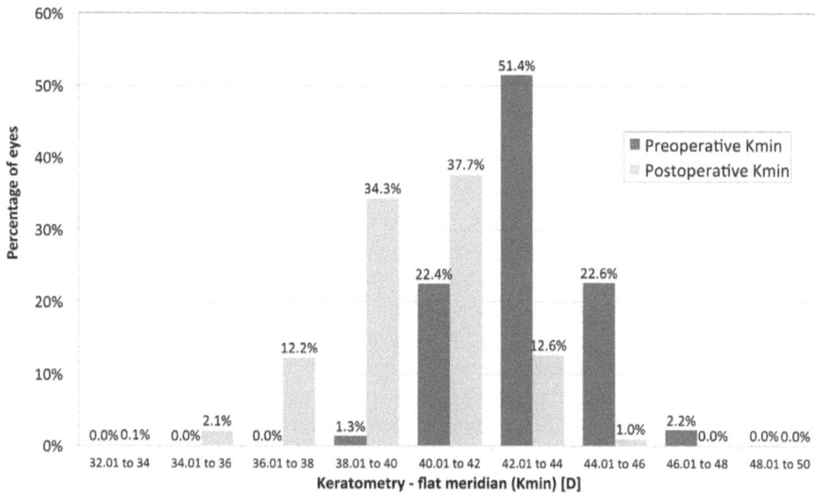

FIGURE 1.—Distribution of pre-operative and postoperative keratometry (Kmin Z flat corneal meridian). (Reprinted from Schallhorn SC, Venter JA, Hannan SJ, et al. Effect of postoperative keratometry on quality of vision in the postoperative period after myopic wavefront-guided laser in situ keratomileusis. *J Cataract Refract Surg.* 2015;41:2715-2723, with permission from ASCRS and ESCRS.)

Design.—Retrospective case series.

Methods.—Myopic eyes treated with wavefront-guided LASIK were analyzed in this study. All patients completed pre-operative and 1-month postoperative questionnaires, in which the satisfaction with visual outcomes and pre-operative and postoperative night-vision symptoms (glare, halos, starburst, ghosting/double-vision) were rated. Multivariate regression analysis was performed to determine factors associated with questionnaire outcomes.

Results.—This study evaluated 8672 myopic eyes of 4602 patients. The mean pre-operative manifest spherical equivalent was −3.72 diopters (D) ± 2.00 (SD) (range −0.50 to −11.00 D) and the mean pre-operative keratometry (K) value was 43.64 ± 1.43 D (38.38 to 49.00). At 1 month after surgery, 93.7% and 99.1% of eyes were within 0.50 D and 1.00 D of emmetropia, and 94.6% and 98.3% of eyes achieved monocular and binocular uncorrected-distance visual acuity(UDVA) of 20/20 or better, respectively. There were 48.7% of eyes that had the flat corneal meridian (minimum K) of 40.0 D or less. Although postoperative keratometry was a significant predictor of patient-reported satisfaction and the change in halo reports in the regression analysis, its relative contribution was very low and accounted for less than 0.50% of the variance explained by either model. Postoperative keratometry was not a significant predictor of a change in reports of glare, starburst, and ghosting or double vision.

Conclusion.—In this large cohort of patients, postoperative keratometry played a minimal and clinically insignificant role in predicting post-LASIK halo visual phenomena and patient-reported satisfaction (Fig 1).

▶ Dr Schallhorn and his colleagues have provided us with terrific data on many aspects of refractive surgery over the past 2 decades, first with the US Navy and now with the huge database of refractive surgery performed at Optical Express in the United Kingdom. This study looked at the age-old question of whether postoperative LASIK keratometry readings affect refractive surgery outcomes, especially quality of vision. As the authors state, "It has been generally accepted that excessive flattening should be avoided." The exact amount of flattening that is considered "excessive" has been debated but is commonly considered (albeit without much data) to be ~34 diopters.

Using a large number of eyes (>8600) and preoperative and 1-month postoperative questionnaires, they determined that postoperative keratometry readings accounted for a tiny degree (<0.50%) of patient satisfaction results. This does not really surprise me, given that the vast majority of postoperative keratometry readings are above 34 D (Fig 1), which would likely mask any deleterious effects at the low end. What did surprise me was that they had 7 patients with postoperative keratometry readings flatter than 34 D, and they were all "very satisfied" or "satisfied" with their visual outcomes; none expressed severe difficulty with glare, halos, starburst, and ghosting. Given this a small number of patients, I am not convinced that going below 34 D is a great idea, but it may not be terrible either.

C. J. Rapuano, MD

Role of Percent Tissue Altered on Ectasia After LASIK in Eyes With Suspicious Topography

Santhiago MR, Smadja D, Wilson SE, et al (Univ of São Paulo, Brazil; Univ Ctr Hosp of Bordeaux, France; Cleveland Clinic, OH; et al)

J Refract Surg 31:258-265, 2015

Purpose.—To investigate the association of the percent tissue altered (PTA) with the occurrence of ectasia after LASIK in eyes with suspicious preoperative corneal topography.

Methods.—This retrospective comparative case–control study compared associations of reported ectasia risk factors in 129 eyes, including 57 eyes with suspicious preoperative Placido-based corneal topography that developed ectasia after LASIK (suspect ectasia group), 32 eyes with suspicious topography that remained stable for at least 3 years after LASIK (suspect control group), and 30 eyes that developed ectasia with bilateral normal topography (normal topography ectasia group). Groups were subdivided based on topographic asymmetry into high- or low-suspect groups. The PTA, preoperative central corneal thickness (CCT), residual stromal bed (RSB), and age (years) were evaluated in univariate and multivariate analyses.

Results.—Average PTA values for normal topography ectasia (45), low-suspect ectasia (39), high-suspect ectasia (36), low-suspect control (32), and high-suspect control (29) were significantly different from one another in all comparisons ($P < .003$) except high- and low-suspect ectasia groups ($P = .033$), and presented the highest discriminative capability of all variables evaluated. Age was only significantly different between the high-suspect ectasia and normal topography ectasia groups, and CCT was not significantly different between any groups. Stepwise logistic regression revealed the PTA as the most significant independent variable ($P < .0001$), with RSB the next most significant parameter.

Conclusions.—There remains a significant correlation between PTA values and ectasia risk after LASIK, even in eyes with suspicious corneal topography. Less tissue alteration, or a lower PTA value, was necessary to induce ectasia in eyes with more remarkable signs of topographic abnormality, and PTA provided better discriminative capabilities than RSB for all study populations (Tables 1 and 2).

▶ The concept that the "safe" residual stromal bed thickness to avoid corneal ectasia after refractive surgery might be different between eyes depending on the preoperative corneal thickness sounds reasonable. In fact, this idea is not new at all. The first edition of the American Academy of Ophthalmology's *Refractive Surgery Basic Clinical Science Course* (BCSC) textbook, published in 2004, stated that some surgeons believe the residual stromal bed thickness should be at least 50% of the central corneal thickness, and this might be a better metric than an arbitrary absolute value of 250-, 275-, or 300-μm residual stromal bed thickness for all eyes. Last year in the Year Book Of Ophthalmology, I commented on an article, also by Santhiago and colleagues, that demonstrated that the percent tissue altered (PTA) value of >40% with the single best predictor of developing ectasia after laser in situ keratomileusis (LASIK) and photorefractive keratectomy in eyes with normal preoperative corneal topography. In my commentary, I suggested that some sort of PTA calculation be incorporated in refractive surgeons preoperative evaluations.

In this article, the authors wanted to learn whether the PTA value was also associated with ectasia in eyes with abnormal preoperative topography. It is presumed that ectasia after refractive surgery generally develops in 2 situations: (1) the eye was "weak" preoperatively and had a high risk of developing ectasia (eg, keratoconus) without of surgery; and (2) the eye was "weakened" to such a degree with surgery that it becomes ectatic. Of course both can occur in the same eye.

The authors determined that in eyes with a normal preoperative topography, the PTA was rather high (mean 45%) in eyes that developed ectasia. In eyes with mildly to moderately abnormal preoperative topography that developed ectasia after LASIK, the PTA was lower (mean 36%-39%). In eyes with mild to moderately abnormal preoperative topography that did not develop ectasia over a minimum of 3 years, the PTA was much lower (mean 27%-30%) (Tables

TABLE 1.—Patient Risk Factor Demographics by Suspect Group[a]

	Mean ± SD (95% CI; Range)				
Parameter	High-Suspect Controls (n = 17)	Low-Suspect Controls (n = 15)	High-Suspect Ectasia (n = 40)	Low-Suspect Ectasia (n = 17)	Normal Topography Ectasia (n = 30)
PTA	29.2 ± 4.7 (26.9 to 31.7; 24 to 39)	31.6 ± 3.0 (29.9 to 33.2; 28 to 39)	35.9 ± 6.3 (33.9 to 37.9; 18 to 54)	39.3 ± 5.2 (36.4 to 42.0; 29 to 48)	45.1 ± 3.9 (43.6 to 46.6; 35 to 54)
RSB (μm)	385.17 ± 28.3 (370.6 to 399.7; 325 to 42[illegible])	361.33 ± 16.9 (351.9 to 370.7; 315 to 383)	337.35 ± 49.1 (323.0 to 351.7; 231 to 506)	325.2 ± 33.5 (307.1 to 342.5; 265 to 375)	293.4 ± 24.8 (284.0 to 302.7; 239 to 337)
CCT (μm)	544.8 ± 18.2 (535.5 to 554.2; 520 to 58[illegible])	526.3 ± 14.2 (518.4 to 534.1; 507 to 552)	525.3 ± 24.2 (514.3 to 536.2; 473 to 619)	536.7 ± 36.4 (518.1 to 555.4; 458 to 595)	534.6 ± 26.9 (524.6 to 544.7; 480 to 594)
Age (years)	34.5 ± 12.1 (28.3 to 40.7; 21 to 61)	31.8 ± 7.1 (27.9 to 35.7; 23 to 52)	34.7 ± 9.4 (31.6 to 37.7; 20 to 56)	34.5 ± 8.5 (30.1 to 38.9; 23 to 47)	29.3 ± 6.9 (26.7 to 31.9; 21 to 50)

SD = standard deviation; CI = confidence interval; PTA = percent tissue altered; RSB = residual stromal bed; CCT = central corneal thickness

[a]high-suspect control = eyes that underwent uneventful LASIK despite high-suspect preoperative topography; low-suspect control = eyes that underwent uneventful LASIK despite low-suspect preoperative topography; high-suspect ectasia = eyes developing ectasia after LASIK with high-suspect preoperative topography; low-suspect ectasia = eyes developing ectasia after LASIK with low-suspect preoperative topography; normal topography ectasia = eyes developing ectasia after LASIK with normal preoperative topography

Reprinted from Santhiago MR, Smadja D, Wilson SE, et al. Role of percent tissue altered on ectasia after LASIK in eyes with suspicious topography. *J Refract Surg*. 2015;31:258-265, with permission from SLACK Incorporated.

TABLE 2.—Statistical Analyses (*P*) and Specific Comparison of Eyes Included in the Study

Parameter	High-Suspect Control vs High-Suspect Ectasia	High-Suspect Control vs Low-Suspect Ectasia	Low-Suspect Control vs High-Suspect Ectasia	Low-Suspect Control vs Low-Suspect Ectasia	High-Suspect Ectasia vs Low-Suspect Ectasia	High-Suspect Ectasia vs Normal Topography Ectasia	Low-Suspect Ectasia vs Normal Topography Ectasia
PTA	.0001[a]	< .0001[a]	.002[a]	< .0001[a]	.033	< .0001[a]	.0001[a]
RSB	.0004[a]	< .0001[a]	.004	.003[a]	.491	< .0001[a]	.001[a]
Age	.967	.999	.302	.347	.964	.002[a]	.026
CCT	.029	.413	.912	.305	.191	.217	.827

high-suspect control = eyes that underwent uneventful LASIK despite high-suspect preoperative topography; low-suspect control = eyes that underwent uneventful LASIK despite low-suspect preoperative topography; high-suspect ectasia = eyes developing ectasia after LASIK with high-suspect preoperative topography; low-suspect ectasia = eyes developing ectasia after LASIK with low-suspect preoperative topography; normal topography ectasia = eyes developing ectasia after LASIK with normal preoperative topography; PTA = percent tissue altered; RSB = residual stromal bed; CCT = central corneal thickness

[a]Statistically significant.

Reprinted from Santhiago MR, Smadja D, Wilson SE, et al. Role of percent tissue altered on ectasia after LASIK in eyes with suspicious topography. *J Refract Surg*. 2015;31:258-265, with permission from SLACK Incorporated.

1 and 2). These results support the idea that "weaker" and "less biomechanically stable" corneas require less surgical "destabilization" to develop ectasia. This is not to say that it is perfectly safe to perform low degrees of refractive surgery in eyes with abnormal topography, but just that the risk of ectasia will be lower with less ablation.

The authors also state that the PTA metric may not apply to small incision lenticule extraction (SMILE), when there is less disruption to the anterior corneal fibers, which are more important than the posterior corneal fibers in maintaining a stable corneal curvature. They note that they know of no cases of ectasia after SMILE, but I am pretty sure they will eventually be reported as more patients undergo that procedure.

C. J. Rapuano, MD

Contralateral Eye-to-Eye Comparison of Wavefront-Guided and Wavefront-Optimized Photorefractive Keratectomy: A Randomized Clinical Trial

He L, Manche EE (Byers Eye Inst at Stanford, Palo Alto, CA)

JAMA Ophthalmol 133: 51-59, 2015

Importance.—Wavefront-guided (WFG) and wavefront-optimized (WFO) platforms for refractive surgery are designed for improved visual outcomes. It is unclear which treatment profile is superior for patients undergoing photorefractive keratectomy (PRK).

Objective.—To compare the safety, efficacy, predictability, stability, and higher-order aberrations in eyes undergoing WFG and WFO PRK.

Design, Setting, and Participants.—A prospective, randomized, fellow-eye–controlled clinical trial was conducted at the Byers Eye Institute at Stanford with enrollment between April 2009 and March 2011; 1 year of follow-up was included. Of 90 patients screened, 71 patients (142 eyes) with less than 12.00 diopters (D) of spherical myopia and less than 3.00 D of astigmatism were enrolled consecutively.

Interventions.—One eye was randomized to undergo WFG PRK treatment (Visx CustomVue Star S4 IR excimer laser system; Abbott Medical Optics), and the fellow eye received WFO PRK treatment (WaveLight Allegretto Wave Eye-Q 400 Hz excimer laser system; Alcon Surgical).

Main Outcomes and Measures.—Data on the manifest refraction, uncorrected visual acuity, best-corrected visual acuity, 5% and 25% contrast best-corrected visual acuity, and higher-order aberrations were collected preoperatively and at the 1-, 3-, 6-, and 12-month follow-up visits.

Results.—Eyes undergoing both treatments had improved best-corrected visual acuity (WFG: mean, 0.05 [95% CI, 0.03-0.07];WFO: mean, 0.04 [95% CI, 0.02-0.06]) and less sphere (WFG: mean, −4.79 [95% CI, −5.31 to −4.26]; WFO: mean, −4.61 [95% CI, −5.18 to −4.03]), cylinder (WFG: mean, 0.66 [95% CI, 0.49-0.82]; WFO: mean, 0.52 [95% CI, 0.35-0.69]), and spherical equivalents (WFG: mean, −4.45 [95% CI, −4.99 to −3.91]; WFO: mean, −4.34 [95% CI, −4.92 to −3.76]) ($P < .001$) but higher levels of spherical aberration (WFG:

mean, −0.11 [95% CI, −0.15 to −0.06]; WFO: mean, −0.11 [95% CI, −0.14 to −0.07]) ($P < .001$) and higher-order root-mean-square aberrations (WFG: mean, −0.07 [95% CI, −0.12 to −0.02]; WFO: mean, −0.12 [95% CI, −0.17 to −0.07]) ($P = .005$ in WFG eyes and $P < .001$ in WFO eyes) at 12 months compared with preoperative measurements. A total of 93.0% of the eyes in the WFG group and 94.4% in the WFO had an uncorrected visual acuity of 20/20 or better at 12 months, with 56.3% in the WFG group and 43.7% in the WFO group gaining 1 or more lines of best-corrected visual acuity. The stability of the refractive correction was excellent for both groups.

Conclusions and Relevance.—A difference in uncorrected visual acuity or contrast acuity between eyes undergoing WFG or WFO treatment at 3 months and beyond could not be identified. This lack of difference suggests that both systems can be used to provide excellent improvement in vision for persons with myopia.

Trial Registration.—clinicaltrials.gov Identifier: NCT01135719.

▶ The term "wavefront" seems ubiquitous in the refractive surgery literature these days. Wavefront analysis allows measurement of lower order aberrations (LOAs) such as sphere and cylinder and also higher order aberrations (HOAs) such as spherical aberration, coma, and trefoil. HOAs are thought to be at least partly responsible for degradation in quality of vision, even in eyes with 20/20 high contrast Snellen visual acuity. "Wavefront" treatments attempt to minimize HOAs, in addition to LOAs.

There are 2 main types of wavefront treatments: wavefront guided and wavefront optimized. Wavefront-guided treatments require that aberrometry measurements be obtained before surgery and input into the laser unit; the information is used to generate an individualized laser treatment pattern for that particular eye. Wavefront-optimized treatments, in contrast, do not require individual aberrometry measurements but rather use mathematical formulas to decrease HOAs. But which is better? The answer in the literature for laser-assisted in situ keratomileusis is inconclusive. There is minimal literature regarding this question for photorefractive keratectomy (PRK).

These authors performed an excellent randomized contralateral eye study to address this exact question. One eye received a VISX STAR S4 IR wavefront-guided PRK treatment and the fellow eye received a Wavelight Allegretto Wave Eye Q 400 Hz wavefront-optimized PRK treatment. No eye received topical mitomycin C, and all eyes received a tapering dose of fluorometholone drops for 4 weeks. Preoperatively, the 2 groups were similar except the wavefront-guided eyes had more sphere ($P = .04$) and more cylinder ($P = .01$) than the wavefront-optimized eyes, but there was no statistically significant difference in spherical equivalence ($P = .16$). Postoperatively, the high-contrast and low-contrast acuity measurements were similar in the 2 groups from 3 to 12 months. The wavefront-guided eyes had less coma, trefoil, and higher order root-mean-square aberrations, although the clinical significance of these findings is not known. The bottom line for me is that both these systems work incredibly well to treat high degrees of myopic astigmatism.

C. J. Rapuano, MD

Photorefractive keratectomy in 22 adult eyes with infantile nystagmus syndrome

Fresina M, Giannaccare G, Gizzi C, et al (Univ of Bologna, Italy)

J Cataract Refract Surg 41:1448-1453, 2015

Purpose.—To analyze visual and refractive outcomes of photorefractive keratectomy (PRK) in adult patients with infantile nystagmus syndrome.

Setting.—Ophthalmology Unit, Department of Experimental Diagnostic and Specialty Medicine, Saint Orsola-Malpighi Hospital, University of Bologna, Bologna, Italy.

Design.—Retrospective case series.

Methods.—Photorefractive keratectomy was performed in both eyes of patients with infantile nystagmus syndrome under topical anesthesia using an eye-tracking excimer laser. Patient satisfaction was tested using a questionnaire. The main outcomes were a decrease in refractive error, an improvement in postoperative corrected distance visual acuity (CDVA), and an uncorrected distance visual acuity (UDVA) equal to or better than the preoperative UDVA.

Results.—Twenty-two eyes of 11 patients with infantile nystagmus syndrome were evaluated. The mean patient age was 30.82 years (range 22 to 42 years). All eyes had simple, compound, or mixed astigmatism (mean −3.40 D; range −0.75 to −6.00 diopters [D]). The mean postoperative astigmatism (−0.70 D ± 0.81 [SD]) and spherical equivalent (−0.420 ± 0.652 D) were statistically significantly better than the preoperative values (−3.40 ± 1.31 D and −3.426 ± 3.343 D, respectively ($P < .0001$ and $P = .0002$, respectively). The mean monocular postoperative CDVA (0.24 ± 0.19 logMAR) and UDVA (0.25 ± 0.18 logMAR) were better than the mean preoperative CDVA (0.32 ± 0.28 logMAR) ($P = .0045$ and $P = .0338$, respectively). The mean binocular postoperative UDVA was better than the mean preoperative CDVA (0.15 ± 0.14 logMAR versus 0.23 ± 0.23 logMAR) ($P = .05$). No patient required repeat surgery.

Conclusions.—Nystagmus patients are eligible for PRK. The results were promising; gaining a few Snellen lines in visual acuity can be very important to these patients for their daily life.

▶ Glasses are not ideal for patients with nystagmus for numerous reasons. Although perhaps obvious, contact lenses are not great in patients with nystagmus either because of the increased risk of eye damage during contact lens insertion and removal. Laser-assisted in situ keratomileusis, whether performed with a mechanical microkeratome or a femtosecond laser, has increased risks of flap complications in eyes with nystagmus. Photorefractive keratectomy (PRK) would seem to be a reasonable surgical option for these eyes.

I feel one of the main issues with any form of laser vision correction (LVC) in eyes with nystagmus is keeping the ablation centered on the pupil during the laser treatment. Consequently laser tracking is absolutely key when considering LVC in these eyes. Given the higher degree of astigmatism in patients with infantile nystagmus than in the general population, correct laser alignment to optimally treat the astigmatism is also important in these eyes. For the VISX laser used in these patients, a good-quality CustomView wavefront analysis needs to be obtained to have a chance to use the iris registration, which corrects for cyclotorsion.

All eyes reportedly had adequate CustomView wavefront scans and engagement of iris registration, which is likely at least partly responsible for their excellent results. Interestingly, the authors did note in their discussion that engaging the iris registration at the beginning of the procedures was more difficult than average, but once engaged, it was not an issue during the actual LVC procedure. It should be noted that the VISX iris registration is static, meaning that it corrects for cyclotortion at the beginning of the procedure, but does not compensate for ocular rotation changes during the actual laser ablation. The authors also mentioned that they only treated patients who had a rest position (least amount of nystagmus) in primary position. I have been hesitant to treat patients with nystagmus in general. However, I, too, have had good results with PRK in several patients with nystagmus but have only treated patients when (1) I get a good CustomView wavefront map and (2) I am able to engage iris registration under the laser.

C. J. Rapuano, MD

Comparison of Three Epithelial Removal Techniques in PRK: Mechanical, Alcohol-assisted, and Transepithelial Laser

Shapira Y, Mimouni M, Levartovsky S, et al

J Refract Surg 31:760-766, 2015

Purpose.—To compare the visual and refractive results obtained after photorefractive keratectomy (PRK) in patients who underwent one of three different epithelial removal techniques.

Methods.—The authors reviewed the medical files of consecutive eyes with myopia and myopic astigmatism that were treated during a 10-year period by mechanical PRK, alcohol-assisted PRK, or transepithelial PRK (in the phototherapeutic keratectomy mode), and observed for more than 1 year.

Results.—A total of 3,417 patients (3,417 eyes) were included in this study. At 3 and 6 months postoperatively, the outcome of alcohol-assisted PRK was superior both in efficacy ($P < .01$) and safety ($P < .001$) to those of both mechanical PRK and transepithelial PRK, which were similar. At more than 1 year postoperatively, the mean efficacy index was still high for alcohol-assisted PRK, but low for the transepithelial PRK, corresponding to a mean uncorrected visual acuity of more than one Snellen line lower than those of the other two techniques ($P < .0001$). All three techniques showed a regression toward myopia more than 1 year postoperatively, with significant undercorrection obtained in eyes treated with transepithelial PRK ($P < .0001$).

Conclusions.—Significant differences were detected in both the visual outcomes and the refractive results of the three epithelial removal techniques. The long-term outcomes were best for alcohol-assisted PRK.

▶ I started performing photorefractive keratectomy (PRK) in the early 1990s as part of the VISX Food and Drug Administration trials. At that time, only mechanical epithelial removal was performed. Over the years, I have tried numerous other epithelial removal techniques including laser epithelial keratomileusis with alcohol, epithelium-on and epithelium-off epi–laser-assisted in situ keratomileusis, and alcohol-assisted PRK. I never tried transepithelial laser removal because I did not feel the supposed benefits were worth the uncertainty and imprecision of the technique. I was never sure how deep to treat, 40 or 45 or 50 μm (this study used 50 μm), because, as we know, epithelial thickness varies between patients. We also know epithelial thickness varies between the central and peripheral cornea, which laser epithelial removal does not account for. In general, additional epithelial "scraping" was always needed. The purported advantage (possibly mainly for marketing purposes) of "all-laser PRK" was not really true. Plus, the VISX laser that I use only goes out to 6.5 mm for the epithelial removal, whereas most PRK ablation zones go out to approximately 8 mm, so peripheral mechanical epithelial removal was needed anyway.

I found the results of the study quite interesting. The exact reasons transepithelial PRK fared worse than both mechanical and alcohol-assisted epithelial removal are not known and are probably multifactorial, but the differences in this article are striking.

I must admit, I was a bit hesitant to routinely use alcohol-assisted PRK, especially in combination with mitomycin C because I was concerned about the untoward effects of the alcohol on the cornea. However, having done it for a while now with excellent results, I am much less concerned. I agree with the authors, who state, "It seems that the suspected toxic effects of alcohol on epithelium and the potential inhibition of stromal recovery ... do not affect long-term outcomes."

C. J. Rapuano, MD

Analgesic effect of preoperative topical nonsteroidal antiinflammatory drugs on postoperative pain after laser-assisted subepithelial keratectomy

Kim SK, Hong JP, Nam SM, et al (Yonsei Univ College of Medicine, Seoul, South Korea; et al)

J Cataract Refract Surg 41:749-755, 2015

Purpose.—To assess the effect of preoperative topical nonsteroidal anti-inflammatory drugs (NSAIDs) on postoperative pain after laser-assisted subepithelial keratectomy (LASEK) and to investigate their mechanism.

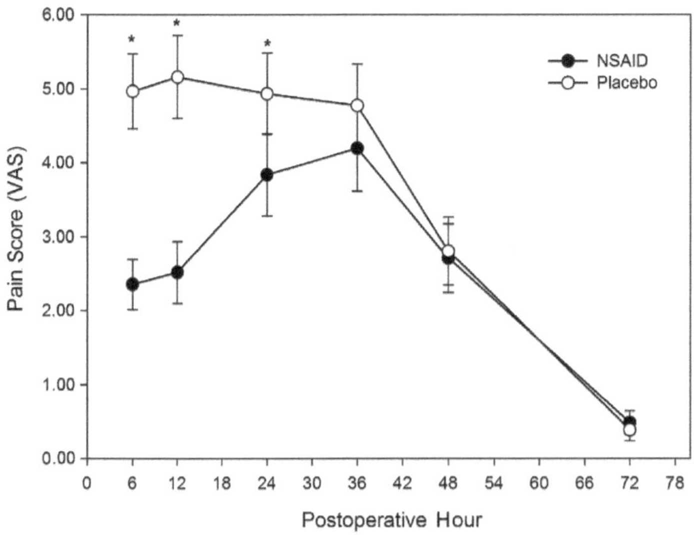

FIGURE 1.—Pain score at each postoperative hour (* = $P < .05$) (NSAID = nonsteroidal antiinflammatory drug; VAS = visual analog scale). (Reprinted from Kim SK, Hong JP, Nam SM, et al. Analgesic effect of preoperative topical nonsteroidal antiinflammatory drugs on postoperative pain after laser-assisted subepithelial keratectomy. *J Cataract Refract Surg*. 2015;41:749-755, with permission from ASCRS and ESCRS.)

Setting.—Severance Eye Hospital and Saeyan Eye Clinic, Seoul, South Korea.

Design.—Prospective randomized clinical trial.

Methods.—Participants in 2 related studies were assessed. Study 1 comprised patients scheduled for bilateral LASEK (Group 1) who were randomized to receive an NSAID in 1 eye and a placebo in the fellow eye 30, 20, and 10 minutes before LASEK. Postoperative pain, glare, tearing, and irritation were assessed using a visual analog scale. Study 2 comprised healthy subjects (Group 2) who were randomly divided into subgroups. The participants in these subgroups were randomized to receive ketorolac tromethamine 0.5% in 1 eye and placebo (ofloxacin 0.3%) in the fellow eye (Group 2A), proparacaine hydrochloride 0.5% in 1 eye and placebo in the fellow eye (Group 2B), or ketorolac tromethamine 0.5% in 1 eye and placebo in the fellow eye, followed 10 minutes later by 1 drop of proparacaine hydrochloride 0.5% in both eyes (Group 2C). In all 3 groups, corneal sensitivity was measured after 1, 2, and 6 hours.

Results.—The mean postoperative pain score in the NSAID-pretreated eye was statistically significantly lower than in the placebo-pretreated eye 6, 12, and 24 hours postoperatively ($P < .05$). The mean corneal sensitivity was statistically significantly lower in the NSAID-treated eye than in the placebo-treated eye at 1 and 2 hours in Groups 2A and 2C ($P < .05$).

Conclusion.—Preoperative administration of topical NSAIDs before LASEK effectively reduces postoperative pain (Fig 1).

▶ This article discusses 2 totally separate but related studies. One was in a group of patients undergoing laser epithelial keratomileusis who received nonsteroidal antiinflammatory (NSAID) drops in 1 eye and placebo in the fellow eye. No eyes received any postoperative NSAID drops. The results of this first study were statistically significantly less pain in the NSAID eyes for the first 24 hours, but not at 36 hours (Fig 1). Having said that, the NSAID group did have substantial pain at 24 hours, although it was less than the placebo group. Both groups reported substantial pain at 24, 36, and 48 hours but minimal pain at 72 hours.

Study 2 tested corneal sensitivity in normal subjects after an NSAID drop, anesthetic drop, or both drops in 1 eye and placebo in the fellow eye. They found similar statistically significantly decreased corneal sensation at 2 hours but not at 6 hours in the NSAID alone and NSAID plus anesthetic drop groups, but there was no decreased corneal sensation after 1 hour in the anesthetic alone eyes.

None of these results are particularly surprising to me. It is interesting that the authors of this article seem to advocate preoperative but not postoperative NSAID drops to decrease the pain after surface ablation, due to the rare complications related to postoperative NSAID drops. However, their results demonstrate that the preoperative drops only worked well for about 12 hours postoperatively in this study. As we all know, the pain after surface ablation generally lasts about 3 to 4 days in most patients. Consequently, my standard protocol is NSAID drops in the preoperative area and also for the next 3 days and then stopping it. I think this regimen gives me the best combination of pain control and safety.

C. J. Rapuano, MD

Mitomycin-C in Corneal Surface Excimer Laser Ablation Techniques: A Report by the American Academy of Ophthalmology

Majmudar PA, Schallhorn SC, Cason JB, et al (Rush Univ Med Ctr, Chicago, IL; Univ of California, San Francisco; Naval Med Ctr, San Diego, CA; et al)
Ophthalmology 122:1085-1095, 2015

Objective.—To review the published literature assessing the efficacy and safety of mitomycin-C (MMC) as an adjunctive treatment in corneal surface excimer laser ablation procedures.

Methods.—Literature searches of the PubMed and Cochrane Library databases were last conducted on August 19, 2014, without language or date limitations. The searches retrieved a total of 239 references. Of these, members of the Ophthalmic Technology Assessment Committee Refractive Management/Intervention Panel selected 26 articles that were considered to be of high or medium clinical relevance, and the panel methodologist rated each article according to the strength of evidence. Ten studies were rated as level I evidence, 5 studies were rated as level II evidence, and the remaining 11 studies were rated as level III evidence.

Results.—The majority of the articles surveyed in this report support the role of MMC as an adjunctive treatment in surface ablation procedures. When MMC is applied in the appropriate concentration and confined to the central cornea, the incidence of post-surface ablation haze is decreased. Although a minority of studies that evaluated endothelial cell density (ECD) reported an MMC-related decrease in ECD, no clinical adverse outcomes were reported.

Conclusions.—Over the past 15 years, the use of MMC during surgery in surface ablation has become widespread. There is good evidence of the effectiveness of MMC when used intraoperatively as prophylaxis against haze in higher myopic ablations. Although there are reports of decreased endothelial counts after the administration of MMC during surgery, the clinical significance of this finding remains uncertain, because no adverse outcomes were reported with as much as 5 years of follow-up. Optimal dosage, effectiveness as prophylaxis in lower myopic and hyperopic ablations, and long-term safety, particularly in eyes with reduced corneal endothelial cell counts from prior intraocular surgery, have yet to be established.

▶ The American Academy of Ophthalmology's Ophthalmic Technology Assessments (OTA) take an evidence-based look at new and evolving technologies. They are consistently excellent documents—well researched, well written, well documented, with conclusions supported by the literature but with clinically applicable discussion and conclusions.

The OTA on the safety and effectiveness of mitomycin C (MMC) in corneal surface excimer laser ablation culled 25 of the best and most relevant articles from the literature for extensive review by the methodologist and other authors. They conclude that the literature supports the use of MMC to decrease the risk of corneal haze after surface ablation in higher myopes. How high is "higher" is not established. They also conclude that optimal dosage (concentration and duration of application) has not been established nor its use in hyperopic and lower myopic eyes. They do stress the need to apply the MMC just to the central cornea (eg, using a sponge), so it does not contact the limbal stem cells or conjunctiva.

I personally use MMC 0.02% on an 8-mm sponge for 12 seconds in most of my surface ablation cases with spherical equivalents over approximately −3 diopters or with significant degrees of astigmatism. I also use it in a similar manner but for 30 seconds in eyes that have had radial keratotomy or LASIK surgery because I believe they are at higher risk for postoperative corneal haze.

C. J. Rapuano, MD

Longitudinal Evaluation of Posterior Corneal Elevation after Laser Refractive Surgery Using Swept-Source Optical Coherence Tomography

Chan TCY, Liu D, Yu M, et al (The Chinese Univ of Hong Kong, China; Hang Seng Management College, Hong Kong, China; et al)

Ophthalmology 122:687-692, 2015

Purpose.—To investigate the change in posterior corneal elevation up to 1 year after myopic femtosecond-assisted LASIK and photorefractive keratectomy (PRK).

Design.—Prospective, longitudinal, comparative study.

Participants.—Patients undergoing femtosecond-assisted LASIK or PRK.

Methods.—Corneal imaging was performed using swept-source optical coherence tomography at baseline and at each postoperative follow-up. A 2-way analysis of variance model with repeated measures and a linear mixed effect model were used to compare the differences in posterior corneal elevation between LASIK and PRK at different points after adjusting for the preoperative spherical equivalent (SEQ), central corneal thickness (CCT), thinnest corneal thickness (TCT), residual bed thickness (RST), and ablation depth (AD).

Main Outcome Measures.—The changes in posterior corneal elevation 1 month, 3 months, 6 months, and 12 months after surgery.

Results.—Ninety-eight eyes of 49 patients (mean age 35.2 ± 8.5 years) (62 LASIK, 36 PRK) were included. The mean change in posterior corneal elevation values after LASIK and PRK were 4.88 ± 0.47 μm versus 3.67 ± 0.48 μm (B-1), 2.42 ± 0.56 μm versus 3.00 ± 0.47 μm (B-3), 3.76 ± 0.46 μm versus 2.76 ± 0.46 μm (B-6), and 2.92 ± 0.46 μm versus 2.72 ± 0.46 μm (B-12), respectively. Significant differences in posterior corneal elevation after LASIK were found from month 1, to month 3, to month 6, to month 12 ($P \leq 0.001$), whereas posterior corneal elevation did not change significantly from month 3, to month 6, to month 12 ($P \geq 0.373$) after PRK. LASIK and PRK eyes showed significant differences at months 3 and 12 ($P \leq 0.023$). A similar pattern was observed for the changes in posterior corneal elevation after LASIK and PRK after adjusting for the effect of SEQ, CCT, TCT, RST, and AD. The adjusted forward displacements of the posterior corneal surface were statistically significant throughout the study period after both refractive surgeries ($P < 0.05$).

Conclusions.—The findings of our study suggested that there was a mild but significant forward protrusion of the posterior cornea after femtosecond laser-assisted LASIK and PRK. The posterior cornea fluctuated during the first postoperative year after LASIK, whereas it stabilized as early as 3 months after PRK (Fig 1, Table 1).

▶ I chose to comment on this study for a few reasons. One of the reasons was *not* because I am convinced a 2- to 5-μm change in posterior corneal elevation over a year after laser in situ keratomileusis (LASIK) and photorefractive

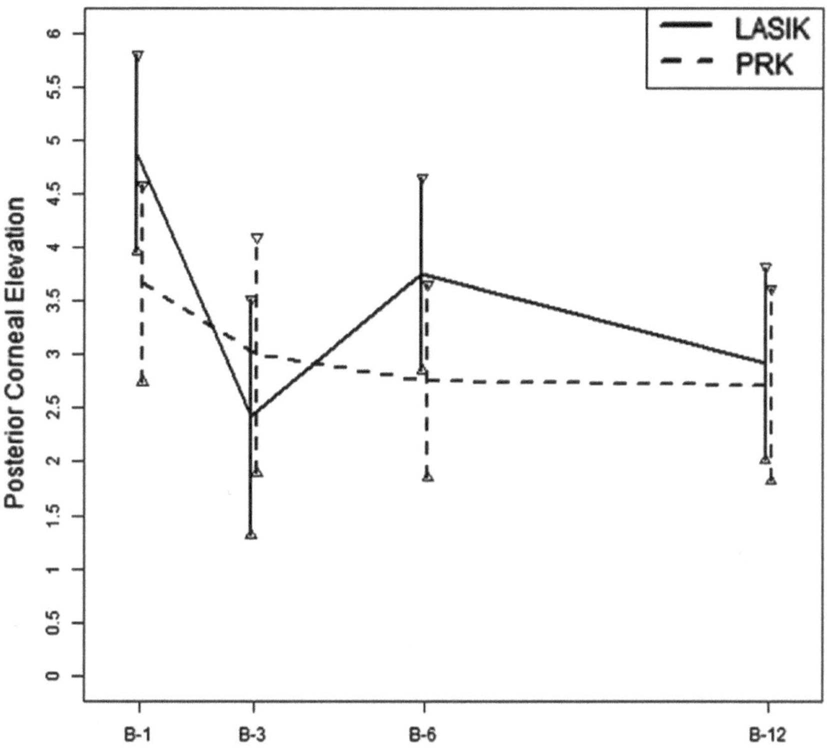

FIGURE 1.—Graph showing the mean change and standard deviation in posterior corneal elevation values after femtosecond laser-assisted LASIK and photorefractive keratectomy (PRK). B-1 = difference between baseline and 1 month; B-3 = difference between baseline and 3 months; B-6 = difference between baseline and 6 months; B-12 = difference between baseline and 12 months. (Reprinted from Chan TCY, Liu D, Yu M, et al. Longitudinal evaluation of posterior corneal elevation after laser refractive surgery using swept-source optical coherence tomography. *Ophthalmology.* 2015;122:687-692, with permission from American Academy of Ophthalmology.)

TABLE 1.—Demographic Characteristics of Patients Who Underwent Femtosecond Laser-Assisted LASIK and Phototherapeutic Keratectomy in the Current Study

	LASIK		Phototherapeutic Keratectomy		
	Mean	*Standard Deviation*	*Mean*	*Standard Deviation*	*P* Value
Age (yrs)	35.1	1.1	34.9	1.7	0.957
Spherical equivalent refraction (diopters)	5.80	0.24	7.22	0.57	0.021
Central corneal thickness (μm)	549.9	4.1	516.1	4.8	0.000
Thinnest corneal thickness (μm)	545.8	4.2	513.1	5.0	0.000
Residual bed thickness (μm)	360.2	5.9	353.0	9.1	0.505
Ablation depth (μm)	87.98	3.63	111.60	8.00	0.007

Reprinted from Chan TCY, Liu D, Yu M, et al. Longitudinal evaluation of posterior corneal elevation after laser refractive surgery using swept-source optical coherence tomography. *Ophthalmology.* 2015;122:687-692, with permission from American Academy of Ophthalmology.

keratectomy (PRK) is anything to be concerned about. One of the reasons *is* to remind us all that we have no "gold standard, absolutely correct" measurement of posterior corneal elevation. Our data are only as good as our technology. For example, as noted in this article, previous reports with scanning slit tomography reported a forward shift of posterior elevation in the 40- to 50-μm range after LASIK. These values were quite concerning but did not match with our other clinical data. Scheimpflug imaging tomography later contradicted these results, reporting minimal to no increase in posterior elevation after LASIK and PRK. Only then did we realize that scanning slit tomography did not accurately image the posterior cornea after PRK and LASIK: "Garbage in, garbage out." As our technology is generating our data, we need to make sure it is measuring what we think it is measuring and as accurately as we need it to.

The second reason is we need to look at the accuracy/reliability of the technology we are using. The authors claim that the swept-source optical coherence tomography used for this study is better at imaging the posterior cornea than Scheimpflug photography because of its shorter scanning time and less light scatter, which I have every reason to believe. However, they also state that "The axial and transverse resolution of the device is <10 μm and <30 μm respectively." It is hard for me to understand how 10-micron accuracy in the measurement of the anterior cornea and 10-micron accuracy of the measurement of the posterior cornea can give reliable posterior elevation data in the 2-to 5-micron range (Fig 1). A large number of study eyes can partially compensate for this issue, but it is for the statisticians to decide how many eyes would be needed.

Finally, it is difficult to compare the LASIK and PRK eyes in this study because they were so different. The PRK eyes were ~1.4 diopters more myopic, had a >20-micron deeper ablation, and started off ~35 microns thinner than the LASIK eyes (Table 1). I do agree with the authors that future studies are needed to investigate the reliability of these techniques and to evaluate their clinical significance.

C. J. Rapuano, MD

Implantable Collamer Lens for Myopia: Assessment 12 Years After Implantation

Moya T, Javaloy J, Montés-Micó R, et al (Clínica Baviera, Valencia, Spain; Miguel Hernández Univ, Alicante, Spain; Universidad de Valencia, Spain; et al)
J Refract Surg 31:548-556, 2015

Purpose.—To evaluate the long-term refractive and visual stability and the risks related to the implantation of Implantable Collamer Lens (ICL; STAAR Surgical, Monrovia, CA) phakic intraocular lens (PIOL) for myopia.

Methods.—This retrospective, consecutive, cumulative clinical study was performed in a group of 144 eyes implanted with ICL PIOL for myopia. Only the cases with clinical data available 12 years after the implantation were included in the series. Corrected distance visual acuity (CDVA), uncorrected distance visual acuity, spherical equivalent,

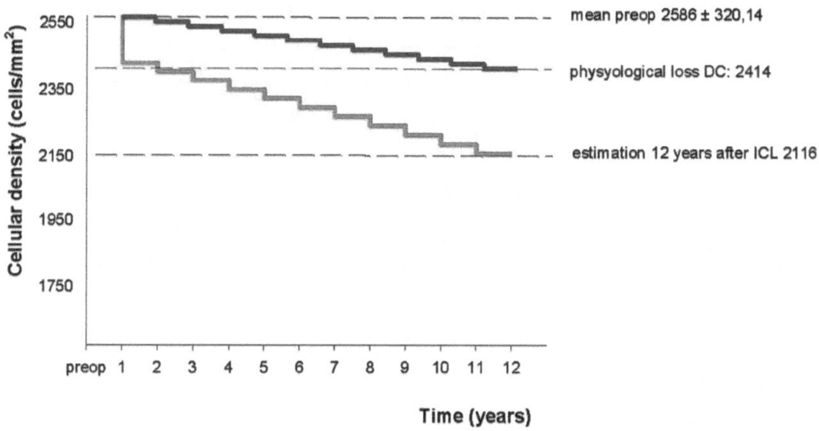

FIGURE 2.—Life analysis graphs showing the evolution of endothelial cell density (ECD) expressed in percent of loss and comparing the theoretical and physiological drop in ECD for a healthy unoperated eye (blue line) and the observed reduction in the eyes included in the series (red line). The first step represents the estimation of endothelial cell loss, which could be attributed to the surgical act (12 months after the implants). The following 11 stages have been calculated by distributing the final ECD drop between the remaining clinical controls. (For interpretation of the references to color in this figure legend, the reader is referred to web version of this article) (Reprinted from Moya T, Javaloy J, Montés-Micó R, et al. Implantable collamer lens for myopia: assessment 12 years after implantation. *J Refract Surg*. 2015;31:548-556, with permission from SLACK Incorporated.)

refractive astigmatism, endothelial cell density, ICL vaulting, and postoperative complications were analyzed.

Results.—Mean spherical equivalent refraction was -16.90 ± 4.26 diopters (D) preoperatively and -1.77 ± 1.93 D 12 years postoperatively. Mean CDVA at the first and last visit were 0.31 ± 0.19 logMAR and 0.22 ± 0.22 logMAR, respectively (Mann–Whitney *U* test, $P < .001$). Twelve years postoperatively, 8.9% of eyes had lost more than two lines of CDVA. The incidence of clinically relevant cataracts (13.88%) was significantly linked to the use of the V3 model ICL (chi-square test, $P = .007$). During the follow-up period, a significant reduction in PIOL vaulting was observed (Kruskal–Wallis test, $P < .05$), and the mean endothelial cell density decreased by 19.75%.

Conclusions.—The ICL PIOL provided good refractive outcomes and stability in the long term. The incidence of cataracts is low when the latest models of this PIOL are used (Fig 2).

▶ Overall, these authors report pretty good refractive and safety results 12 years after Implantable Collamer Lens (ICL) implantation. Of the 144 eyes that had ICL surgery more than 12 years ago, 112 (78%) were included in the study. About one-third of those excluded (11 eyes) had undergone ICL removal combined with cataract surgery, and two-thirds (21 eyes) were lost to follow-up. Mean preoperative spherical equivalent was quite myopic at −16.9 D, which is higher than most other studies using the ICL, and certainly higher than the US Food and Drug Administration studies. Consequently, many eyes also underwent excimer laser vision correction treatment approximately 3 months after ICL implantation.

Interestingly, 75% of eyes were within 1 D of emmetropia at 1 year but only 34% at 12 years. Twenty of the 144 eyes (14%) developed significant lens opacity (defined as 2 or more lines of decreased best corrected visual acuity). Most of these eyes had the V3 ICL model, which has a lower vault than the V4 model used in the rest of the eyes in this study. Five eyes (3.5%) developed a retinal detachment, 1 after trauma and 4 spontaneous, all successfully treated with pars plana vitrectomy. Several other eyes developed choroidal neovascular membranes and macular hemorrhage. Given the small numbers in this study and high-risk population, it is difficult to know whether ICL surgery increased the risk of these untoward retinal events. The authors also do not comment on whether the retinal detachments occurred in patients who had undergone cataract surgery or whether the cataracts occurred after pars plana vitrectomy. Even so, I remain concerned about cataract development in these relatively young patients with high myopia. I am hopeful that the newer ICL models have significantly decreased the incidence of cataract formation.

Lastly, the other major long-term concern with ICLs is corneal endothelial cell loss. We know there is significant endothelial cell loss in the first year after ICL implantation (3.7%–12%) due to the surgical procedure. This study found that the endothelial cell loss leveled off after 1 year to about 1.2% per year, which is still double the physiologic rate of cell loss of 0.6% per year (Fig 2). Even so, the authors note that for an average 30-year-old patient with an average endothelial cell density of 2586 cells/mm^2, it would take 92 years to reach the "critical level" of 800 cells/mm^2. Of course that does not take into account cataract surgery or retinal surgery.

C. J. Rapuano, MD

Iris-fixated phakic intraocular lens implantation to correct myopia and a predictive model of endothelial cell loss

Bouheraoua N, Bonnet C, Labbé A, et al (Sorbonne Universités, Paris, France; Institut de la Vision, Paris, France; et al)

J Cataract Refract Surg 41:2450-2457, 2015

Purpose.—To report long-term results of Artisan phakic intraocular lens (pIOL) to correct myopia and to propose a model predicting endothelial cell loss after pIOL implantation.

Setting.—Quinze-Vingts National Ophthalmology Hospital, Paris, France.

Design.—Retrospective, interventional case series.

Methods.—Uncorrected distance visual acuity (UDVA), corrected distance visual acuity (CDVA), and central endothelial cell count (ECC) were determined before and at yearly intervals up to 5 years after pIOL implantation. Linear model analysis was performed to present a model

TABLE 3.—Minimal Preoperative Endothelial Cell Density (ECD) to Have a Density of ≥1500 cells/mm² at the Mean Cataract Age of 70 Years

Age, y	20	25	30	35	40	45	50	55	60	65
Minimal ECD (cells/mm²)	>3620	>3322	>3049	>2800	>2569	>2358	>2164	>1986	>1823	>1673

Initial loss: 3.9%; annual loss: 1.7%.
Reprinted from Bouheraoua N, Bonnet C, Labbé A, et al. Iris-fixated phakic intraocular implantation to correct myopia and a predictive model of endothelial cell loss. *J Cataract Refract Surg*. 2015;41:2450-2457, with permission from ASCRS and ESCRS.

that describes endothelial cell loss as a linear decrease and an additional decrease depending on postoperative loss.

Results.—A total of 49 patients (68 eyes) implanted with pIOLs from January 2000 to January 2009 were evaluated. The mean preoperative and final spherical equivalent (SE) were -13 ± 4.10 and -0.75 ± 0.74 diopters (D), respectively. The mean preoperative and final central ECC were 2629 ± 366 and 2250 ± 454 cells/mm², respectively. There were no intraoperative complications for any of the eyes. One eye required surgery for repositioning the pIOL, and 1 eye required pIOL exchange for postoperative refractive error. The model predicted that for patients with preoperative ECC of 3000, 2500, and 2000 cells/mm², a critical ECC of 1500 cells/mm² will be reached at 39, 28, and 15 years after implantation, respectively.

Conclusions.—Implantation of the pIOL was an effective and stable procedure after 5 years of follow-up. The presented model predicted EC loss after pIOL implantation, which can assist ophthalmologists in patient selection and follow-up (Table 3).

► Not to beat a dead horse, but this is another study looking at corneal endothelial cell loss with the Artisan iris-clip phakic anterior chamber intraocular lens (ACIOL). Although not a huge study (only 68 eyes), the authors did have 5-year follow-up in all patients. Endothelial cell loss was 6.27% at 1 year and 15.15% at 5 years, far above natural physiologic endothelial cell loss (~0.6% per year). To help determine in which patients it is safe to implant these lenses, the authors calculated a minimal preoperative endothelial cell density at a given age that would result in a >1500 cells/mm² at the "mean cataract age of 70 years" given an initial endothelial cell density of 2629 cells/mm² (mean of their population) in Table 3. Surgeons should keep these numbers in mind when considering implantation of an Artisan phakic ACIOL.

In the Discussion, the authors conclude, "Complications are uncommon and rarely cause loss of corrected distance visual acuity. However, the ongoing endothelial cell loss demonstrated herein is concerning and raises some safety concerns for long-term use," which is a rather different tone from the conclusion in the abstract. This is just another example of why it is often not adequate to read only the abstract of an article.

C. J. Rapuano, MD

Phakic intraocular lens: Two-year results and comparison of endothelial cell loss with iris-fixated intraocular lenses

Aerts AAS, Jonker SMR, Wielders LHP, et al (Maastricht Univ Med Ctr, the Netherlands)

J Cataract Refract Surg 41:2258-2265, 2015

Purpose.—To evaluate the efficacy, safety, and stability of a foldable angle-supported Acrysof Cachet phakic intraocular lens (pIOL) to correct moderate to high myopia and compare endothelial cell loss after iris-fixated Artisan and Artiflex pIOL implantation.

Setting.—University Eye Clinic Maastricht, the Netherlands.

Design.—Retrospective observational study.

Methods.—Foldable angle-supported pIOL implantation for myopia ranging from −6.0 to −16.5 diopters (D) was done. Uncorrected (UDVA) and corrected (CDVA) distance visual acuity, spherical equivalent (SE), and adverse events were documented preoperatively and 6 months and 1 and 2 years postoperatively. Endothelial cell loss after implantation of the foldable anglesupported pIOL and iris-fixated pIOLs was compared 6 months and 1 and 2 years postoperatively.

Results.—There were 158 eyes. The UDVA was equal to or more than 20/25 in 95% of eyes at 1 and 2 years postoperatively. The mean SE was −0.17 D ± 0.43 (SD) 2 years postoperatively. One patient developed pupil ovalization, resulting in explantation of the pIOL from both eyes. Acute endothelial cell loss in the foldable angle-supported pIOL group was −3.2% ± 0.7%, significantly higher than after iris-fixated pIOL implantation. Chronic endothelial cell loss from 6 to 24 months after surgery was −3.8% ± 0.7%. At the 2-year follow-up, the chronic endothelial cell loss in the foldable angle-supported pIOL group was not different than with iris-fixated pIOLs ($P > .05$).

Conclusions.—The foldable angle-supported pIOL effectively corrected moderate to high myopia. However, acute surgical endothelial cell loss was significantly higher than with iris-fixated pIOLs (Fig 9).

▶ It sure would be nice to have a phakic intraocular lens (IOL) that could be slipped into the anterior chamber angle through a small incision, avoiding the issues with lens damage during (or after) IOL insertion or problems securing (enclavating) an iris clip phakic anterior chamber IOL (ACIOL). However, just as pseudophakic ACIOLs have issues with corneal endothelial cell damage and pupil ovalization, so do phakic ACIOLs.

The authors looked at their results of a foldable angle-supported phakic IOL and compared them with results of several iris-fixated phakic IOLs. Keep in mind, of the 158 angle-supported phakic IOLs, only 124 were seen at

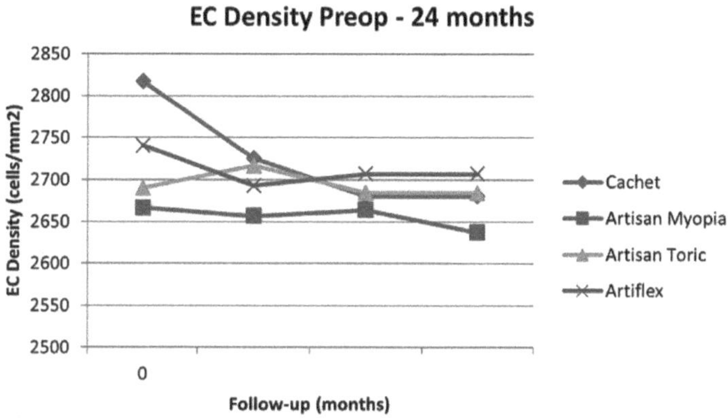

FIGURE 9.—The ECD after implantation of pIOLs. (Reprinted from Aerts AAS, Jonker SMR, Wielders LHP, et al. Phakic intraocular lens: two-year results and comparison of endothelial cell loss with iris-fixated intraocular lenses. *J Cataract Refract Surg.* 2015;41:2258-2265, with permission from ASCRS and ESCRS.)

1 year and 79 at 2 years. Acute (defined as preoperative to 6 months postoperative) corneal endothelial cell loss was 3.2%. From preoperatively to 1 year postoperatively, endothelial cell loss was 6.9%. Chronic endothelial cell loss (from 6 months to 2 years postoperatively) was 3.8%. These are all higher than physiologic endothelial cell loss (~0.6% per year) and also higher than the other iris-fixated phakic IOLs (Fig 9). Four eyes had additional refractive surgery with laser epithelial keratomileusis, 2 eyes required repositioning of the angle supported phakic IOL, and 1 eye had the angle supported phakic IOL exchanged for an iris-fixated phakic IOL due to residual refractive error. Two eyes developed pupil ovalization and had the angle-supported phakic IOL exchanged for an iris-fixated phakic IOL. Larger (and longer) studies are needed before I am ready to use an angle-supported phakic IOL.

C. J. Rapuano, MD

Retinal Complications After Anterior Versus Posterior Chamber Phakic Intraocular Lens Implantation in a Myopic Cohort

Al-Abdullah AA, Al-Falah MA, Al-Rasheed SA, et al (King Khaled Eye Specialist Hosp, Riyadh, Saudi Arabia; King Faisal Univ, Al-Ahsa, Saudi Arabia; et al)

J Refract Surg 31:814-819, 2015

Purpose.—To compare the incidence and characteristics of retinal complications following implantation of two types of phakic intraocular lenses (PIOLs) in patients with myopia.

Methods.—In this comparative, retrospective study, 603 eyes of 344 patients with myopia underwent implantation of either an Artisan iris-fixated phakic intraocular lens IOL (Artisan; Ophtec, Groningen,

TABLE 1.—Patient Demographics[a]

Characteristic	Artisan (n = 185 Eyes)	ICL (n = 418 Eyes)	LASIK (n = 418 Eyes)
Age (y)	28.7 ± 6.32	27.22 ± 6.48	31.05 ± 8.71
Male/female (%)	39/61	46/54	67/33
Preoperative mean spherical equivalent refraction (D)	-13.80 ± 3.80	-11.80 ± 4.50	-16.28 ± 4.92
Follow-up (months)	42.8 ± 27.6	19.8 ± 14.1	48 ± 33

D = diopters

The Artisan IOL is manufactured by Ophtec, Groningen, Netherlands, and the Visian Implantable Collamer Lens (ICL) is manufactured by STAAR Surgical Company, Monrovia, CA.

[a]Values are mean ± standard deviation.

Reprinted from Al-Abdullah AA, Al-Falah MA, Al-Rasheed SA, et al. Retinal complications after anterior versus posterior chamber phakic intraocular lens implantation in a myopic cohort. *J Refract Surg*. 2015;31:814-819, with permission from SLACK Incorporated.

Netherlands) (Artisan group) or a Visian implantable collamer lens (ICL; STAAR Surgical Company, Monrovia, CA) (ICL group) between June 2005 and December 2013. Preoperative, operative, and postoperative clinical data were collected on the incidence of retinal complications, including rhegmatogenous retinal detachment (RRD) or choroidal neovascular membrane (CNVM).

Results.—The Artisan lens was implanted in 185 (30.68%) eyes and 418 (69.32%) eyes underwent ICL implantation. Mean follow-up was 26.78 months (range: 9 days to 98 months). Mean preoperative spherical equivalent (SE) was -12.44 ± 4.43 D (range: -1.13 to -31.00 D). The overall rate of retinal complications was 1%. Postoperatively, 3 (0.7%) eyes developed RRD in the ICL group, and no eyes developed RRD in the Artisan group. Submacular hemorrhage was observed in 1 (0.24%) eye in the ICL group. Two (1%) eyes developed CNVM in the Artisan group. The mean time from PIOL implantation to retinal complications was 15.6 months (range: 0.03 to 43 months).

Conclusions.—Implantation of ICL or Artisan phakic IOL demonstrated comparable rates of retinal complications. Anterior chamber PIOL does not increase the risk of retinal detachment or CNVM in patients with myopia (Table 1).

► This study tries to answer the question of whether phakic intraocular lenses (IOLs) increase the risk of retinal complications such as rhegmatogenous retinal detachment and choroidal neovascular membrane formation. We know the high myopic patient population getting phakic IOLs is at a higher baseline risk of retinal complications than emmetropes or even low myopes. It is reasonable to think that ocular trauma (in this case, surgical trauma) might increase the risk of retinal problems.

Although this study is retrospective, it has a reasonable number of eyes with reasonable mean follow-up time (Table 1). Note that the laser-assisted in situ keratomileusis (LASIK) eyes had a much higher level of myopia than the phakic IOL eyes, so it is not a perfect "control" group. All in all, they found that both the Artisan iris clip phakic anterior chamber IOL and Intraocular Collamer Lens phakic posterior chamber IOL had comparable rates of retinal complications in highly myopic eyes after LASIK and also to published rates of retinal complications in unoperated high myopes. It is nice to know that it does not appear as if these surgical treatments are increasing the risk of retinal issues, at least in the relatively short term (given the young age of most of their patients as seen Table 1).

C. J. Rapuano, MD

Phakic Intraocular Lens Explantation: Causes in 240 Cases

Alió JL, Toffaha BT, Peña-Garcia P, et al (Vissum Corporation, Alicante, Spain; Universidad Miguel Hernández, Alicante, Spain; et al)

J Refract Surg 31:30-35, 2015

Purpose.—To describe the main causes of explantation of phakic intraocular lenses (PIOLs) according to the anatomical site of implantation (angle supported, iris fixated, or posterior chamber).

Methods.—This multicentric, retrospective, and consecutive study sponsored by the Spanish Ministry of Health comprised a total of 240 eyes (226 patients) explanted due to PIOL complications. Clinical data of 144 angle-supported lenses, 24 iris-fixated lenses, and 72 posterior chamber lenses explanted were recorded preoperatively and postoperatively.

Results.—Mean age of the patients at explantation was 46.30 ± 11.84 years (range: 25 to 80 years). The mean time between implantation and explantation was 381.14 ± 293.55 weeks (range: 0.00 to 1,551.17 weeks). It was 422.33 ± 287.81 weeks for the angle-supported group, 488.03 ± 351.95 weeks for the iris-fixated group, and 234.11 ± 4,221.60 weeks for the posterior chamber group. It was 8.10 ± 5.52 years for the angle-supported group, 9.36 ± 6.75 years for the iris-fixated group, and 4.49 ± 4.25 years for the posterior chamber group. This period of time was significantly shorter in the posterior chamber group ($P < .001$). Overall, the main causes of explantation were cataract formation (132 eyes, 55%), endothelial cell loss (26 eyes, 10.83%), corneal decompensation (22 eyes, 9.17%), PIOL dislocation/decentration (16 eyes, 6.67%), inadequate PIOL size or power (12 eyes, 5%), and pupil ovalization (10 cases, 4.17%). Cataract development was the cause of explantation in 51.39% of angle-supported cases, 45.83% of iris-fixated cases, and 65.28% of posterior chamber cases. Endothelial cell loss was the cause of explantation in 15.97% of angle-supported PIOLs, 8.33% of iris-fixated PIOLs, and 1.39% of posterior chamber PIOLs.

TABLE 1.—Causes of Explantation per Anatomical Site of Explantation and Type of Procedure Performed

Cause of Explantation	No. of Cases in All Groups	No. of Cases in Angle-Supported Group	No. of Cases in Iris-Fixated Group	No. of Cases in Posterior Chamber Group	No. of Procedures
Cataract	132 (55%)	74 (51.39%)	11 (45.83%)	47 (65.28%)	132 coaxial phacoemulsification; bilensectomy
Endothelial cell loss	26 (10.83%)	23 (15.97%)	2 (8.33%)	1 (1.39%)	13 MICS bilensectomy; 8 simple PIOL explantation; 5 PIOL exchange
Corneal decompensation	22 (9.17%)	15 (10.42%)	5 (20.83%)	2 (2.78%)	12 coaxial phacoemulsification bilensectomy; 7 bilensectomy and penetrating keratoplasty; 3 simple PIOL explantation
PIOL dislocation	16 (6.67%)	11(7.64%)	1 (4.17%)	4 (5.56%)	13 PIOL exchange; 2 simple PIOL explantation; 1 coaxial phacoemulsification; bilensectomy
High IOP	12 (5%)	5 (3.47%)	1 (4.17%)	6 (8.33%)	7 PIOL exchange; 3 coaxial phacoemulsification bilensectomy; 2 simple PIOL explantation
Inadequate PIOL size or power	12 (5%)	3 (2.08%)	1 (4.17%)	8(11.11%)	3 PIOL exchange; 3 simple PIOL explantation; 6 coaxial phacoemulsification; bilensectomy
Oval pupil	10 (4.17%)	9 (6.25%)	1 (4.17%)	0 (0%)	6 PIOL exchange; 4 coaxial phacoemulsification; bilensectomy
Retinal detachment	7 (2.92%)	2 (1.39%)	2 (8.33%)	3 (4.17%)	3 coaxial phacoemulsification bilensectomy; 4 coaxial phacoemulsification; bilensectomy + vitrectomy
Halos and glare	3 (1.25%)	2 (1.39%)	0 (0%)	1 (1.39%)	1 PIOL exchange; 2 simple PIOL explantation
Total	240	144	24	72	240

MICS = microincision cataract surgery; PIOL = phakic intraocular lens; PIOL exchange = change of the IOL, phakic, for another PIOL; IOP = intraocular pressure

Reprinted from Alió JL, Toffaha BT, Peña-Garcia P, et al. Phakic intraocular lens explantation: causes in 240 cases. *J Refract Surg*. 2015;31:30-35, with permission from SLACK Incorporated.

Conclusions.—Cataract is the main cause of PIOL explantation, especially in posterior chamber PIOLs. In the angle-supported group, endothelial cell loss was the second cause of explantation (Table 1).

▶ This is the largest study (I believe) looking at the reasons for phakic intraocular lens (PIOL) explantation. The authors included 240 eyes over an approximately 6.5-year time period. Most explanted lenses were angle supported PIOLs, which are not currently Food and Drug Administration approved; however, 40% were iris fixated or posterior chamber PIOLs.

Although some PIOLs in all groups were explanted for inadequate size or power, most were explanted because of visually significant cataracts or progressive endothelial cell loss. Table 1 details the exact causes for explantation. I was somewhat surprised by a couple of findings. I expected posterior chamber PIOLs to have more explantations for cataract and fewer for progressive endothelial cell loss, which was the case. I was not expecting around half of the explantations in the angle-supported and iris-fixated groups to be due to cataract. (Not surprisingly, they were mostly nuclear cataracts in the angle supported PIOL eyes and mostly anterior subcapsular cataracts in the posterior chamber PIOL eyes.) I had expected most of the explantations in the angle supported and iris fixated groups to be due to progressive endothelial cell loss or corneal decompensation, but it was the reason for explantation in only approximately 30% of the eyes in these 2 groups. I would have expected the PIOL dislocation rate to be much higher in the iris fixated group than the 2 other groups, but it was similar in all 3 groups at approximately 4% to 7%.

Although not the goal of this article, I would have been interested in the authors' sense of incidence of the PIOL explantation for each of these lenses, perhaps based on the numbers of each of these implants performed at their centers, or perhaps national statistics. Such data might help explain why the Food and Drug Administration has not approved angle-supported PIOLs and also the relatively low uptake of these lenses in general in the United States.

C. J. Rapuano, MD

Safety and efficacy of a hydrogel inlay with laser in situ keratomileusis to improve vision in myopic presbyopic patients: One-year results

Garza EB, Chayet A (Laser Ocular Hidalgo, Monterrey, Nuevo Leon, Mexico; Codet Vision Inst, Tijuana, Baja California, Mexico)

J Cataract Refract Surg 41:306-312, 2015

Purpose.—To study the safety and efficacy of implanting a hydrogel corneal inlay (Raindrop Near Vision Inlay) concurrently with performing laser in situ keratomileusis (LASIK) to treat myopic presbyopia and to compare the results with results of the same treatment in emmetropic and hyperopic patients.

Setting.—Two private clinics, Tijuana and Monterrey, Mexico.

Design.—Prospective nonrandomized clinical trial.

Near	Intermediate	Distance
Read medicine instructions	Find items on kitchen shelf	Read street signs
Read newspaper article	Read a computer screen	Identify people across room
Examine fingernails	Use a bathroom mirror	Judge car distances
Dial cell phone	Use a wall calendar	Read house numbers
Read magazine	Recognize photo portraits	Tell time from wall clock

FIGURE 2.—Common visual tasks used to rate near, intermediate, and distance vision.(Reprinted from Garza EB, Chayet A. Safety and efficacy of a hydrogel inlay with laser in situ keratomileusis to improve vision in myopic presbyopic patients: one-year results. *J Cataract Refract Surg.* 2015;41:306-312, with permission from ASCRS and ESCRS.)

Methods.—Bilateral myopic LASIK was performed and a corneal inlay was concurrently implanted in the nondominant eye under a flap created using a femtosecond laser. Primary safety outcomes were the retention of corrected distance (CDVA) and near (CNVA) visual acuities. Efficacy was evaluated on the basis of uncorrected near (UNVA), intermediate (UIVA), and distance (UDVA) visual acuities. A patient questionnaire was used to assess the preoperative and postoperative incidence of visual symptoms, the ability to perform common tasks with no correction, and patient satisfaction with vision.

Results.—Thirty eyes were enrolled. At each postoperative visit, the mean CDVA and CNVA were within one half line of preoperative measurements and no eye lost 2 or more lines of CDVA. The mean binocular UDVA, UIVA, and UNVA were better than 20/25 Snellen at all postoperative visits. By 6 months, 93% of patients had a binocular Snellen acuity of 20/25 or better across all visual ranges. According to patient questionnaires, 1 year after surgery, visual symptoms were at preoperative levels, 98% of all visual tasks could be easily performed without correction, and 90% of patients were satisfied or very satisfied with their overall vision.

Conclusion.—A hydrogel corneal inlay with concurrent LASIK was safe and effective for treating myopic presbyopia (Fig 2).

▶ The benefits of corneal inlays to improve uncorrected near vision for hyperopes and presbyopic emmetropes is pretty obvious. However, for myopes, who often have excellent uncorrected near vision (and have had it for years), correcting their distance visual acuity with refractive surgery compromises their near vision as they reach around age 40 years and beyond. In fact, in my experience, poor uncorrected near vision is one of the most important reasons for dissatisfaction after refractive surgery in patients in the presbyopic age group. Unless some type of correction for near vision (eg, monovision or a corneal inlay) is being performed, patients in the pre-presbyopic and presbyopic age range need significant counseling on the fact that although their uncorrected distance vision will (it is hoped) improve significantly after refractive surgery, their near vision will become worse right away or in the near future.

This article looked at the results of a hydrogel inlay (Raindrop inlay) in myopic presbyopes undergoing LASIK, a group of patients that otherwise would have noted a significant worsening in uncorrected near vision postoperatively. The inlay is 30 μm thick at the center and 2 mm in diameter, which induces central corneal steepening to correct near vision in the nondominant eye. 1-year results were excellent for uncorrected distance and near vision (Fig 2). The authors note that patient satisfaction with near vision after the Raindrop inlay was 95% to 100% in their previous studies in emmetropic and hyperopic patients. This makes sense because these patients had poor uncorrected near vision preoperatively. However, only 72% of myopic presbyopes in this study reported being satisfied or very satisfied with near vision postoperatively, and 21% were neutral, even though their uncorrected near vision was excellent. This should not surprise anyone because these patients likely had pretty good uncorrected near vision preoperatively.

As in much of life, things are relative. Patients will compare postoperative results with preoperative status. Patients who could not see well at near uncorrected will likely be happier by emmetropia than presbyopic myopes who saw well uncorrected before they were made emmetropic. Therefore, myopic presbyopes may be the "sweet spot" for these presbyopic inlays.

C. J. Rapuano, MD

One-year results of simultaneous laser in situ keratomileusis and small-aperture corneal inlay implantation for hyperopic presbyopia: Comparison by age

Tomita M, Waring GO 4th (Shinagawa LASIK Ctr, Tokyo, Japan; Med Univ of South Carolina, Charleston)

J Cataract Refract Surg 41:152-161, 2015

Purpose.—To compare by age the safety, efficacy, and patient satisfaction after simultaneous laser in situ keratomileusis (LASIK) and small-aperture corneal inlay implantation (Kamra) for hyperopic presbyopia.

Setting.—Shinagawa LASIK Center, Tokyo, Japan.

Design.—Retrospective comparative cohort study.

Methods.—Simultaneous LASIK and small-aperture corneal inlay implantation were performed in the nondominant eye of hyperopic presbyopic patients with astigmatism. Patients were divided into groups by age as follows: Group 1 (40 to 49 years), Group 2 (50 to 59 years), and Group 3 (60 to 65 years). The uncorrected (UDVA) and corrected (CDVA) distance visual acuities, uncorrected near visual acuity (UNVA), and patient questionnaire results were compared.

Results.—The study evaluated 277 eyes of 277 patients. All groups achieved a mean UDVA of 20/20, with Group 1, Group 2, and Group 3 gaining 1 line, 2 lines, and 3 lines, respectively. The mean UNVA was J2 with 4 lines gained in Group 1 and J3 with 5 lines gained in Group 2 and Group 3. The mean CDVA and corrected near visual acuity remained the same as at baseline.

Conclusions.—Simultaneous LASIK and small-aperture corneal inlay implantation for hyperopic presbyopia was a safe and effective treatment

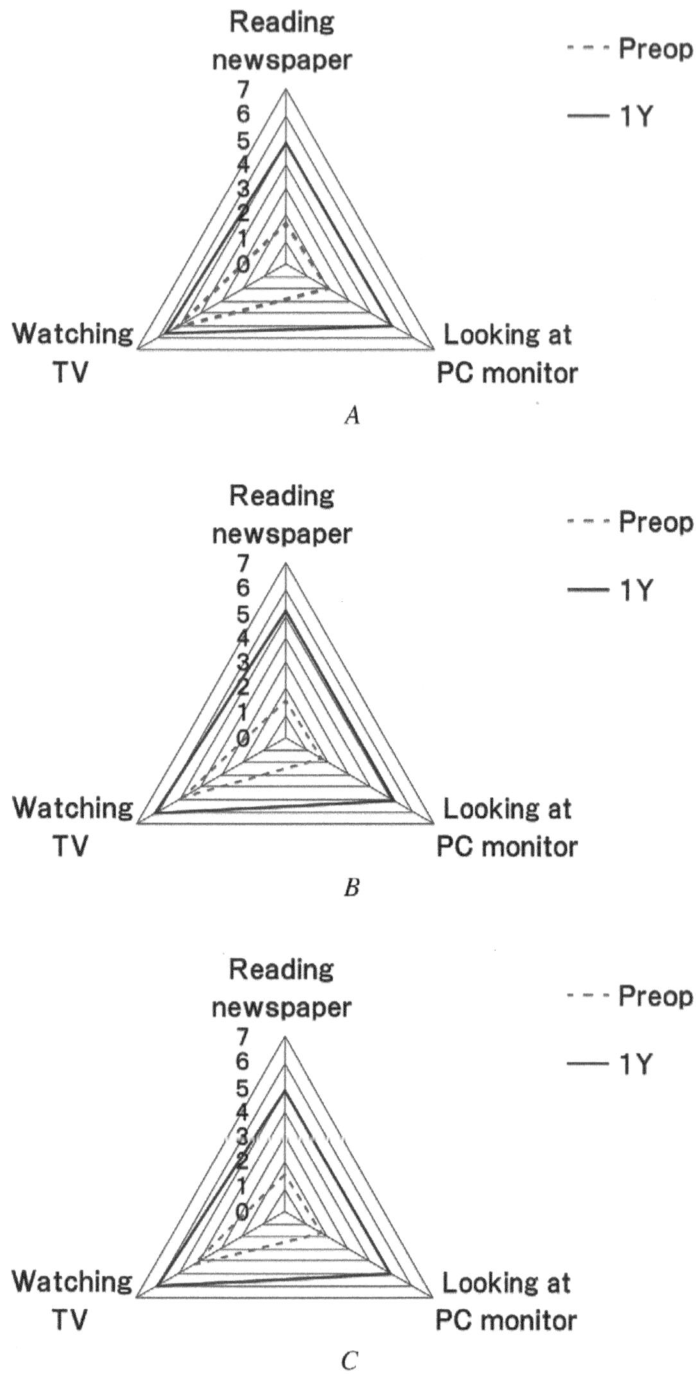

FIGURE 6.—Subjective scores for performing various tasks. *A*: Group 1. *B*: Group 2. C: Group 3 (PC = personal computer; TV = television).(Reprinted from Tomita M, Waring GO 4th. One-year results of simultaneous laser in situ keratomileusis and small-aperture corneal inlay implantation for hyperopic presbyopia: comparison by age. *J Cataract Refract Surg.* 2015;41:152-161, with permission from ASCRS and ESCRS.)

option. Although the outcomes were comparable between groups, Group 3 had the largest gain in UDVA and UNVA and the highest patient satisfaction, despite having the lowest reduction in dependence on reading glasses. Taking age into account might help achieve optimum postoperative outcomes and improved patient satisfaction (Fig 6).

► Hyperopic presbyopes have numerous options for visual correction, including multifocal glasses or contact lenses, monovision in contact lenses, or a variety of standard refractive surgeries. They could also undergo refractive lens exchange or cataract surgery for monovision or with multifocal intraocular lenses. This article reviewed the results of another option, LASIK with a small aperture corneal inlay (Kamra inlay), dividing patients by age group. The results were quite good from an uncorrected distance and near vision perspective and a patient satisfaction standpoint in all 3 age groups (Fig 6).

The Kamra inlay seems to be a reasonable option for patients with minimal to no cataract. But what happens when these patients develop cataracts postoperatively? After all, more than one-third of the patients in this study were 60 to 65 years old. Options for such patients include cataract surgery leaving the inlay in place (case reports indicate cataract surgery can safely be performed in these eyes); removal of the inlay and placing a multifocal IOL or correcting for monovision; or removal of the inlay, performing the cataract surgery, and replacing the inlay immediately after the cataract surgery. Previous reports have demonstrated that pseudophakic eyes can do well with a Kamra inlay. This article adds to the growing body of literature demonstrating this inlay to be effective in a wide variety of patient populations.

C. J. Rapuano, MD

Bifocal refractive corneal inlay implantation to improve near vision in emmetropic presbyopic patients

Malandrini A, Martone G, Menabuoni L, et al (Misericordia e Dolce Hosp, Prato, Italy; Univ of Siena, Italy; et al)

J Cataract Refract Surg 41:1962-1972, 2015

Purpose.—To evaluate the safety and effectiveness of the Flexivue Microlens corneal inlay for the improvement of near vision in emmetropic presbyopic patients.

Setting.—Ophthalmology Department, Misericordia e Dolce Hospital, Prato, Italy.

Design.—Prospective interventional case series.

Methods.—Corneal inlay implantation was performed in nondominant eyes using a 150 kHz femtosecond laser (iFS). Refraction, uncorrected (UNVA) and corrected (CNVA) near visual acuities, uncorrected (UDVA) and corrected (CDVA) distance visual acuities, slitlamp evaluation, wavefront aberrometry, photopic and mesopic contrast sensitivity, anterior segment optical coherence tomography, endothelial cell density,

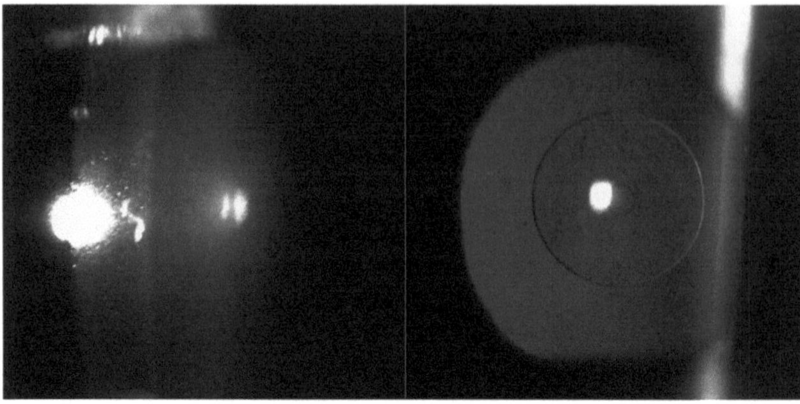

FIGURE 1.—The corneal inlay. (Reprinted from Malandrini A, Martone G, Menabuoni L, et al. Bifocal refractive corneal inlay implantation to improve near vision in emmetropic presbyopic patients. *J Cataract Refract Surg.* 2015;41:1962-1972, with permission from ASCRS and ESCRS.)

and central corneal thickness measurements were assessed preoperatively and at each postoperative visit.

Results.—The study evaluated 81 eyes. In 26 eyes, the mean preoperative UNVA and UDVA were 0.76 logMAR and 0.00 logMAR, respectively, compared with 0.10 logMAR and 0.15 logMAR, respectively, 36 months postoperatively. Sixteen (62%) of 26 treated eyes lost more than 1 line of UDVA, and 5 (19%) lost more than 2 lines of UDVA. Two eyes (8%) lost more than 1 line of CDVA at 36 months. The mean binocular UDVA was 0.00 logMAR preoperatively and 0.02 logMAR at 36 months. The mean spherical aberration increased after surgery. Statistically significant differences in the mean mesopic and photopic contrast sensitivities at higher spatial frequencies were found between treated eyes and nontreated eyes. Explantation was performed in 6 treated eyes because of halos, glare, and a reduced UDVA.

Conclusion.—The corneal inlay might be a safe and effective method of improving UNVA in emmetropic presbyopic patients (Fig 1).

► As of this writing, there are several corneal inlays to treat presbyopia available around the world, only 1 of which is Food and Drug Administration approved for use in the United States: the Kamra inlay, which uses the pinhole effect to increase depth of focus, which results in improved near vision. The Flexiview Microlens used in this study is a 3.2-mm-diameter, transparent, hydrophilic acrylic inlay, placed in the central cornea at a depth of 300 μm. The central zone of the inlay (1.6 mm diameter) has no refractive power, whereas the peripheral zone contains the reading power, which in this series ranged from 1.5 to 3.25 D (Fig 1). The inlay is implanted in the nondominant eye using a femtosecond laser created pocket in patients known to tolerate monovision. Eighty-one eyes were treated in this series, but only 44 (54%) were seen at 12 months and 26 (32%) seen at 36 months.

Putting aside the rather limited follow-up in this series for the moment, the patient's subjective assessment results were pretty good, although certainly not perfect. At 12 months, 37 (84%) said they were very satisfied with their postoperative uncorrected near visual acuity compared to their preoperative uncorrected near visual acuity. Forty (91%) reported using no reading glasses or using reading glasses less than 50% of the time at 12 months, with the same percentage reporting no glare or halo symptoms. However, only 75% of patients reported they would have the surgery again.

Perhaps that is related to 60% of treated eyes losing more than 1 line of uncorrected distance visual acuity and 19% of treated eyes losing more than 2 lines of uncorrected distance visual acuity at 3 years. Eight percent of treated eyes lost more than 1 line of best-corrected distance visual acuity at 3 years. Six eyes (7%) had the inlay removed within the first year, all related to glare and halos and decreased uncorrected distance visual acuity. Fortunately, the inlays were reported to be easily removed, and visual acuity, glare, and halo symptoms returned to baseline within 1 year. Given that the majority of patients were happy, it appears as if the loss of uncorrected distance visual acuity in the treated eye is compensated for by the excellent baseline uncorrected distance visual acuity in the untreated eye. Even so, the 7% explantation rate and 25% of patients saying they would not have the procedure again is a bit concerning to me.

C. J. Rapuano, MD

Avoidance of serious medical errors in refractive surgery using a custom preoperative checklist

Robert M-C, Choi CJ, Shapiro FE, et al (Massachusetts Eye and Ear Infirmary, Boston; Beth Israel Deaconess Med Ctr, Boston, MA; et al)

J Cataract Refract Surg 41:2171-2178, 2015

Purpose.—To implement and measure the effect of a surgical safety checklist on the prevention of serious medical errors (never-events).

Setting.—Boston Eye Group, Boston, Massachusetts, USA.

Design.—Retrospective cohort study.

Methods.—A safety checklist incorporating 28 sources of error was designed and implemented in December 2011 at the Boston Eye Group's refractive surgical center. Consecutive patients who had primary or enhancement laser vision correction (LVC) between July 2009 and February 2014 were included in this study. Before that date, a general checklist fashioned around the World Health Organization time-out procedure was used. The latter subjects were recruited as controls. The perioperative characteristics of both groups were retrospectively compared.

Results.—The study comprised 2951 consecutive patients who had primary or enhancement LVC between July 2009 and February 2014; of these, 1417 patients (2744 eyes) had LVC after the implementation of a presurgical safety checklist. The general checklist fashioned around the World Health Organization time-out procedure was used for 1534

Patient Identification

First name:	**Last name:**	
DOB :	_____/_____/_____	
Surgery:	☐ OD ☐ OS ☐ OU	

Right Eye		**Left Eye**	
Type of procedure	☐LASIK	*Type of procedure*	☐LASIK
	☐PRK		☐PRK
	☐ LASEK		☐ LASEK
Refractive	☐ distance	**Refractive**	☐ distance
aim	☐ intermediate	**aim**	☐ intermediate
	☐ near		☐ near

Target Rx	______	Target Rx	______
Pre-operative refraction (Wavescan, etc)		Pre-operative refraction (Wavescan, etc)	
Sphere	______	Sphere	______
Cylinder	______	Cylinder	______
Axis	______	Axis	______
Laser input		Laser input	
Sphere	______	Sphere	______
Cylinder	______	Cylinder	______
Axis	______	Axis	______
Initials MD:	______	Initials MD:	______
Assistant:	______	Assistant:	______
Optical zone	______	Optical zone	______
Nomogram adjustment	______	Nomogram adjustment	______

Time-out confirmation

Surgeon:
Assistant:

LEGEND: All items above the solid line should be confirmed orally by the patient. He or she should be asked to state their name, date of birth, the procedure(s) being conducted and the refractive aim for each eye being operated.
This checklist can be customized for other refractive surgeries such as Epi-Lasik or corneal inlays by adding selections under the heading Type of procedure.

FIGURE 2.—Paper version of the checklist. As indicated in the legend, items found above the solid line should be confirmed orally by the patient. The checklist is customizable and can be adapted to reflect different surgeons' practices (D.O.B. = date of birth; LASEK = laser-assisted subepithelial keratectomy; LASIK = laser in situ keratomileusis; PRK = photorefractive keratectomy). (Reprinted from Robert MC, Choi CJ, Shapiro FE, et al. Avoidance of serious medical errors in refractive surgery using a custom preoperative checklist. *J Cataract Refract Surg*. 2015;41:2171-2178, with permission from ASCRS and ESCRS.)

patients (2969 eyes). Both groups were comparable in patient age. The most common surgical procedures were laser in situ keratomileusis (78%) and laser-assisted subepithelial keratectomy with mitomycin-C (16%). Although there were 2 (0.07%) serious errors in the prechecklist cohort, none occurred following implementation of the safety checklist protocol ($P = .23$). The medical errors involved wrong refractive aim in 1 patient and wrong person–wrong procedure–wrong aim in another.

Conclusions.—Multiple potential sources of error exist in refractive surgery. The broad-scale implementation of a detailed presurgical safety checklist was helpful in minimizing and preventing serious errors (never-events) during LVC (Fig 2).

▶ An article in 2011 determined ophthalmology had the second highest number and rate of adverse surgical events after neurosurgery.[1] Many, if not most, of these events in ophthalmology are related to intraocular lens (IOL) surgery, due to the large variety and power of IOLs available for implantation. Confusion between right and left eyes is another source of adverse events in ophthalmology. Laser vision correction shares many of the refractive calculation and right eye/left eye types of errors as IOL surgery. In the past several years, numerous groups, including the American Academy of Ophthalmology and hospital safety and accrediting organizations, have developed checklists and timeout procedures to reduce the risk of preventable surgical errors.

These authors looked at their data on more than 5700 laser vision correction surgeries, about half while using a surgeon-verified relatively generic preoperative timeout and the other half using a preoperative safety checklist listing 28 refractive surgery specific sources of error for each eye, verified by both the surgeon and surgical assistant (Fig 2). They reduced their number of "never should happen" errors from 2 to 0 after starting in their new checklist, which is great from my standpoint, although it was not a statistically significant difference, at least partly because of the (fortunate) rarity of these events. Whether we use the checklist in this study or one of our own, some sort of preoperative "pre-flight" checklist involving the patient, surgeon, and surgical assistant should be employed to prevent these "never" events.

I was quite interested in the 2 serious errors reported in this study. One was during a reoperation after hyperopic LASIK to create monovision that mistakenly treated the eye for emmetropia. Instead of a third procedure in that eye, the other (dominant) eye was treated for monovision, fortunately successfully. The second patient was a low myope (who was actually scheduled for laser-assisted in situ keratomileusis [LASIK]) but who was mistakenly treated for moderately high myopia (with laser-assisted subepithelial keratomileusis with mitomycin C), due to a mix up in patients, resulting in moderate hyperopia in both eyes. This patient was treated with hyperopic LASIK 2 months later, achieving 20/20 uncorrected vision in both eyes. The authors point out, and I stress with all our residents and fellows, that the excellent final outcomes in these 2 patients were certainly helped by the fact that the surgeons were honest and forthright about the complications with the patients and their families. Additionally, the surgeons expressed their desire to learn from these mistakes and their willingness to work with the patients to "correct" the problems. In my experience, when untoward surgical events occur, patients and their families are interested in several things from their surgeon: truthfulness, preventing the event from happening again (if possible), and not being abandoned. Explaining what happened without delay, what you are going to do to prevent this from happening to another patient and what you are going to do to "fix" the problem are absolutely invaluable.

C. J. Rapuano, MD

Reference

1. Neilly J, Mills PD, Eldridge N, et al. Incorrect surgical procedures within and outside of the operating room; a follow up report. *Arch Surg*. 2011;146:1235-1239.

Prevalence of laser vision correction in ophthalmologists who perform refractive surgery

Kezirian GM, Parkhurst GD, Brinton JP, et al (Surgivision Consultants, Scottsdale, AZ; Parkhurst Nuvision, San Antonio, TX; Hunter Vision, Orlando, FL; et al)

J Cataract Refract Surg 41:1826-1832, 2015

Purpose.—To determine the prevalence of laser corneal refractive surgery (laser vision correction [LVC]) among ophthalmologists who perform these procedures and to assess the willingness of these ophthalmologists to recommend LVC to immediate family members.

Setting.—Online survey with results analyzed at Surgivision Consultants, Inc., Scottsdale, Arizona, USA.

Design.—Prospective randomized questionnaire study.

Methods.—The 22-question Global Survey on Refractive Surgery in Refractive Surgeons was sent by e-mail to 250 ophthalmologists randomly selected from a database of 2441 ophthalmologists known to have performed LVC at some point in the past decade. Responses were solicited by e-mail, with subsequent telephone reminders to nonresponders.

Results.—Responses were received from 248 (99.2%) of 250 queried individuals, of which 232 (92.8%) met the protocol criteria of currently working as refractive surgeons. Of the 232 subjects, 161 (69.4%) reported that they had refractive errors potentially amenable to treatment with LVC, not including presbyopia. Of the 161 ophthalmologists with treatable refractive errors, 54 (33.5%) reported they were not candidates for LVC for a variety of reasons and 107 (66.5%) reported they were candidates for LVC. Of the LVC candidates, 62.6% reported that they had an LVC procedure in their own eyes. Of the overall 232 subjects, more than 90% recommend LVC for adult members of their immediate family.

Conclusions.—Ophthalmologists who perform LVC were significantly more likely than the general population to have LVC in their own eyes. The prevalence of refractive errors was significantly higher among ophthalmologists performing refractive surgery than in the general population (Fig 2).

▶ Estimates in 2014 suggest that approximately 13% of "appropriate candidates" in the United States have undergone laser vision correction (LVC).

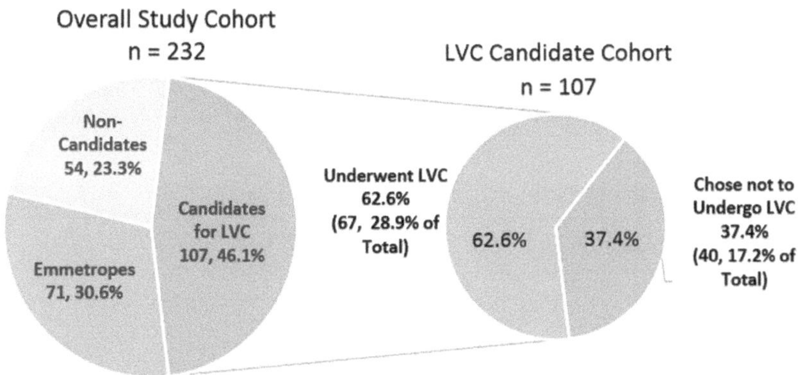

FIGURE 2.—Breakdown of the overall study cohort and LVC cohort. (Reprinted from Kezirian GM, Parkhurst GD, Brinton JP, et al. Prevalence of laser vision correction in ophthalmologists who perform refractive surgery. *J Cataract Refract Surg.* 2015;41:1826-1832, with permission ASCRS and ESCRS.)

The authors report a well-performed survey study investigating the prevalence of LVC in a sample of 250 refractive surgeons. The 99% response rate was excellent. Seventy percent of respondents reported that they had/have refractive errors "potentially amenable to treatment with LVC, not including presbyopia." One-third reported that they were not candidates for LVC, mainly because of refractive error that exceeded Food and Drug Administration (FDA) approvals and dry eye syndrome. Of the LVC candidates, 63% reported that they had undergone LVC, which is over 4 times the rate in the general US population (see Fig 2). Note that 97% of respondents were from the United States.

I found it interesting that the survey did not ask about presbyopia. Given that the mean age of respondents was 52 years old and the mean time since their refractive surgery was 12 years earlier, presbyopia would certainly have been a concern for many of them. Although I started performing refractive surgery in my early 30s (as part of the FDA trials), it was not until I was close to the presbyopic age group that I considered LVC "ready" for me to dive in. But given that I read most of the day and I do not like monovision, I did not undergo LVC. In fact, presbyopia is perhaps the biggest reason my potential refractive surgery patients decide not to proceed with LVC. I think it would have been interesting to know at what age survey respondents actually underwent their LVC.

I also found it intriguing that more than one-third of respondents that had LVC had photorefractive keratectomy, as opposed to laser in situ keratomileusis (LASIK), which is much higher than the general US population. I wonder whether this is because many had LVC before the LASIK era or whether many refractive surgeons feel it is a "safer" procedure than LASIK.

C. J. Rapuano, MD

3 Glaucoma

Risk of Angle-Closure glaucoma With Bupropion and Topiramate

Symes RJ, Etminan M, Mikelberg FS (Univ of British Columbia, Vancouver, Canada)

JAMA Ophthalmol 133:1187-1189, 2015

Importance.—Epidemiologic studies have shown that antidepressants may increase the risk of angle-closure glaucoma. We examined the risk of angle-closure glaucoma with bupropion hydrochloride, a unique, popular antidepressant also marketed as a smoking cessation aid.

Observations.—A nested case-control study was conducted using a large health claims database in the United States from January 1, 2006, to March 31, 2014. The database contained deidentified information pertaining to a cohort of 6 110 723 patients. Cases were defined according to the first coding for angle-closure glaucoma. For each case, 10 control participants were selected and matched to the cases using density-based sampling. Adjusted rate ratios were computed for bupropion, topiramate (positive control group drug), and esomeprazole (negative control group drug). The adjusted rate ratio was 1.09 (95% CI, 0.75-1.59) for bupropion and 2.59 (95% CI, 1.56-4.30) for topiramate. In a prespecified analysis of patients younger than 50 years, the adjusted rate ratio was 1.98 (95% CI, 1.02-3.84) for bupropion and 5.30 (95% CI, 2.54-11.04) for topiramate.

Conclusions and Relevance.—Both bupropion and topiramate are widely prescribed drugs. The risk of angle-closure glaucoma in patients younger than 50 years was twice as high in patients taking bupropion and more than 5 times higher in patients taking topiramate.

▶ In rare cases, topiramate is known to cause bilateral angle closure glaucoma secondary to choroidal effusion. The choroidal effusion typically occurs anteriorly and may be difficult to identify by exam. B-scan ultrasound with attention to the anterior aspect of the posterior segment or ultrasound biomicroscopy may help make the diagnosis. This phenomenon has also been reported with selective serotonin reuptake inhibitors and sulfa medications. Bupropion is a commonly prescribed antidepressant that was also linked to acute angle closure glaucoma via this mechanism in a case report.

This study used health claims data to find patients who took bupropion or topiramate and also experienced angle closure glaucoma. The authors found that patients on bupropion were not generally at a higher risk of developing angle closure glaucoma. However, if only patients younger than 50 years were included in the analysis, bupropion was associated with greater risk of angle closure. Topiramate was associated with a higher risk of angle closure in both analyses, but more dramatically among younger people.

It is important to note that the health claims data did not permit determination of the mechanism of angle closure, so cases may have been unrelated to choroidal effusion. Pharmacologic pupillary dilation is a potential risk of bupropion and could account for angle closure cases. Although most narrow angle is bilateral, a typical case of acute angle closure is unilateral. The attack of angle closure compels the patient to seek care then narrow angle in the fellow eye is identified and both eyes are ultimately treated with laser peripheral iridotomy. Bilateral acute angle closure is more rare and should provoke investigation for a potential inciting factor, including consideration of side effects from systemic medications.

S. J. Fudemberg, MD

Association of Geroprotective Effects of Metformin and Risk of Open-Angle Glaucoma in Persons With Diabetes Mellitus

Lin HC, Stein JD, Nan B, et al (Indiana Univ, Bloomington; Univ of Michigan, Ann Arbor)

JAMA Ophthalmol 133:915-923, 2015

Importance.—Caloric restriction mimetic drugs have geroprotective effects that delay or reduce risks for a variety of age-associated systemic diseases, suggesting that such drugs might also have the potential to reduce risks of blinding ophthalmologic conditions for which age is a major risk factor.

Objective.—To determine whether the caloric restriction mimetic drug metformin hydrochloride is associated with reduced risk of open-angle glaucoma (OAG) in persons with diabetes mellitus.

Design, Setting, and Patients.—Retrospective cohort **study** of **patients** aged 40 years or older with diabetes mellitus and no preexisting record of OAG in a large US managed care network from January 1, 2001, through December 31, 2010.

Exposures.—Quantity of metformin and other prescribed diabetes medications as captured from outpatient pharmacy records.

Main Outcomes and Measures.—Risk of developing OAG.

Results.—Of 150 016 **patients** with diabetes mellitus, 5893 (3.9%) developed OAG. After adjusting for confounding factors, those prescribed the highest quartile of metformin hydrochloride (>1110 g in 2 years) had a 25% reduced OAG risk relative to those who took no metformin (hazard ratio = 0.75; 95% CI, 0.59-0.95; $P = .02$). Every 1-g increase in metformin hydrochloride use was associated with a 0.16% reduction in OAG risk (adjusted hazard ratio = 0.99984; 95% CI, 0.99969-0.99999; $P = .04$), which predicts that taking a standard dose of 2 g of metformin hydrochloride per day for 2 years would result in a 20.8% reduction in risk of OAG. After accounting for potential confounders, including metformin and diabetic medications, the risk of developing OAG was increased by 8%

(hazard ratio = 1.08; 95% CI, 1.03-1.13; $P = .003$) for each unit of increase in glycated hemoglobin level.

Conclusions and Relevance.—Metformin use is associated with reduction in risk of developing OAG, and risk is reduced even when accounting for glycemic control in the form of glycated hemoglobin level. Other diabetes medications did not confer a similar OAG risk reduction. This study suggests that metformin may be affecting OAG risk on multiple levels, some involving improved glycemic control and some involving mechanisms outside glycemic control such as neurogenesis, inflammatory systems, or longevity pathways targeted by caloric restriction mimetic drugs. If confirmed by prospective clinical trials, these findings could lead to novel treatments for this sight-threatening disease.

▶ Caloric restriction and caloric restriction–mimetic drugs such as metformin can reduce risk in a number of age-related diseases, including cardiovascular diseases, diabetes, and a number of cancers. In this retrospective cohort study, the authors evaluate whether the use of metformin in diabetic patients is associated with the incidence of open angle glaucoma (OAG).

Among the 150 016 individuals identified with diabetes, 5893 (3.9%) developed OAG. There was a dose-dependent risk reduction of developing OAG with greater quantities of metformin used. Every 1 g of metformin conferred a 0.16% risk reduction. Therefore, those taking the standard dose of 2 g/day (or 1460 g over 2 years) had a 20.8% OAG risk reduction. This protective effect was present even after controlling for HbA1C levels (Fig 2 in the original article), suggesting a mechanism beyond glycemic levels.

To date, intraocular pressure has been the major therapeutic target in the treatment of glaucoma. Although alternative therapies, such as neuroprotective agents, have experienced major setbacks, investigations are ongoing. Caloric restriction mimetic drugs such as metformin and rapamycin have demonstrated geroprotective (antiaging) effects in other diseases and are potentially a novel target against glaucoma.

D. Lee, MD
S. J. Fudemberg, MD

Measured Changes in Limbal Strain During Simulated Sleep in Face Down Position Using an Instrumented Contact Lens in Healthy Adults and Adults With Glaucoma

Flatau A, Solano F, Idrees S, et al (Univ of Maryland, College Park; The Johns Hopkins Univ School of Medicine, Baltimore, MD; et al)
JAMA Ophthalmol 1-8, 2016

Importance.—Eyes of patients with glaucoma may be damaged during sleep.

Objective.—To measure strains in glaucoma eyes and control eyes produced by mechanical force or deformation of the eye from contact when one side of the face rests against a pillow.

Design, Setting, and Participants.—This study took place in a clinic-based setting among 22 patients with glaucoma and 11 age-matched controls. The research was conducted at Wilmer Eye Institute between February 4, 2014, and December 2, 2014. Data analysis was done from June 3, 2014, to June 30, 2015.

Main Outcomes and Measures.—We used a contact lens sensor (CLS) to measure change in limbal strain associated with placing one side of the face down (FD) on a pillow in simulated sleep. Baseline intraocular pressure (IOP) was measured with a tonometer. The CLS data were collected every 5 minutes during intervals of up to 60 minutes in various positions, including sitting, lateral decubitus, FD (with the CLS-instrumented eye toward the pillow), and supine. Measured changes in limbal strain were related to estimated changes in IOP and to modeled strain produced by changes in IOP.

Results.—Among 22 patients with glaucoma and 11 controls, 17 were female. The mean age for the glaucoma group was 62.6 years, while the mean age for the control group was 61.4 years ($P = .68$). Baseline IOP was also similar for the 2 groups. The mean IOP sitting at the start was 13.7 mm Hg for the glaucoma group and 13.8 mm Hg for the control group ($P = .73$), and the mean IOP lying at the start was 17.5 mm Hg for the glaucoma group and 16.0 mm Hg for the control group ($P = .88$). By multivariable linear regression, FD position was associated with an increase in limbal strain in glaucoma eyes (mean [SE], 44.1 [20.4] mV Eq $P = .03$) but not in control eyes (mean [SE], 13.6 [13.9] mV Eq, $P = .33$). While FD, the increased CLS values in patients with glaucoma did not decrease over time (slope, 0.275 mV Eq/min $P = .53$ by univariable linear regression). Magnitudes of measured changes in limbal strain were greater in glaucoma eyes with past visual field worsening ($P = .006$ by multivariable linear modeling). The mean limbal strain increase among patients with glaucoma in FD position was equivalent to strain expected for a mean (SE) IOP increase of 2.5 (1.1) mm Hg from a baseline IOP of 14.2 mm Hg.

Conclusions and Relevance.—Contact with a pillow in FD position during simulated sleep produced a sustained strain increase in glaucoma eyes, particularly those eyes with past progressive visual field loss. The mean FD change in glaucoma eyes was equivalent to strain increase associated with a mean (SE) sustained IOP elevation of 2.5 (1.1) mm Hg. Further experiments are planned to determine if facial features or a protective eye shield prevents sleep position-induced limbal strains during a mean 8-hour sleep period.

▶ The Triggerfish by SENSIMED is a novel device for 24-hour monitoring of glaucoma patients. It is a contact lens with a strain gauge at the limbus that measures strain associated with changing intraocular pressure (IOP) and mechanical forces applied on the eye. The concept of side preference during sleep and its relationship with asymmetric visual field loss in glaucoma has been previously described. However, direct measurement of IOP during sleep has not been possible. This study utilizes the novel Triggerfish technology to monitor changes in limbal strain and IOP during face-down positioning.

This study demonstrates the changes in limbal strain based on sleep position. Additionally, it shows that increases are sustained in face-down position and more pronounced in glaucoma patients. Limbal strain is an indirect measure of intraocular pressure and the mean limbal strain increase seen in patients with glaucoma is equivalent to 2.5 ± 1.1 mm Hg.

Interestingly, regression analysis found increases in strain were inversely proportional to baseline IOP (Fig 4 in the original article). In other words, patients with lower IOPs tended to have a larger increase in limbal strain in face-down positioning. This seems to be particularly relevant to the so-called normal tension glaucoma population in whom glaucoma damage is apparent despite lower IOPs. This suggests that sleeping patterns might be important in patients with asymmetric glaucoma who are progressing despite good IOP measurements in the office.

D. Lee, MD
S. J. Fudemberg, MD

Failed glaucoma drainage implant: long-term outcomes of a second glaucoma drainage device versus cyclophotocoagulation

Schaefer JL, Levine MA, Martorana G, et al (Univ of Florida, Gainesville; et al)
Br J Ophthalmol 99:1718-1724, 2015

Background/Aims.—To evaluate long-term efficacy of a second glaucoma drainage device (GDD) versus cyclophotocoagulation (CPC) after failure of primary drainage implant.

Methods.—This is a non-randomised, retrospective cohort study. A chart review was conducted of patients who underwent GDD surgery between July 1986 and November 2012 requiring further glaucoma procedures for intraocular pressure (IOP) control. An additional GDD was placed in 15 eyes, while 32 eyes underwent CPC. The main outcome measurement was IOP control and/or time to failure of secondary intervention (IOP >18 mm Hg on two sequential measurements).

Results.—Mean follow-up after the second procedure was 63 ± 65.8 months (range 6–254 months) in the CPC group and 132 ± 91.8 months (range 12–254 months) in the GDD group. Thirty-four percent (11/32 eyes) undergoing CPC later required further treatment at a mean of 13.6 ± 10.7 months with 10/11(91%) of additional interventions occurring within 2 years. Despite an initially high success rate for IOP control in the first 5 years, eventually 60% (9/15 eyes) that underwent a second tube required additional treatment at a mean of 73.4 months with only 2/9(22%) requiring this within the first 2 years. The risk of visual acuity worsening by 2 Snellen lines or more at 12 months was 5/14 for the GDD group (36%) and 4/23(17%) for the CPC group.

Conclusions.—After failure of an initial drainage implant to control IOP, a sequential tube had a high initial rate of success but a relatively high likelihood of long-term failure, generally after 6 years. Eyes that received CPC tended to fail earlier, often within the first year, but had relatively few late failures.

▶ Factors such as variations in surgical technique and varied definitions of success make surgical outcomes analysis challenging in glaucoma. However, it is clear that failure of glaucoma filtration surgery is an obstacle on the path to long-term intraocular pressure (IOP) control. For example, 5-year results from the Tube Versus Trabeculectomy Study revealed the cumulative probability of failure was 29.8% in the tube group and 46.9% in the trabeculectomy group.[1] Importantly, failure in the TVT study was defined as IOP >21 mm Hg or <20% reduction below baseline after 3 months, reoperation, or loss of light perception. The rate of complete success (no glaucoma medications needed) was 25% in the tube group and 29% in the trab group. When the criteria for IOP control were tightened to define failure as IOP >14 mm Hg, the cumulative probability for failure was 52.3% in the tube group and 71.5% in the trab group. These results indicate that patients who undergo glaucoma filtration surgery may subsequently face the prospect of additional glaucoma surgery.

After a failed trabeculectomy despite adjunctive medical management, another trabeculectomy or a tube shunt procedure are typical considerations. In contrast, trabeculectomy is not typically performed after placement of tube shunt. Failed tube shunts are usually followed by an additional tube shunt or cyclodestructive procedure. In general, cyclodestruction has been reserved for refractory glaucoma and believed to have greater risk of hypotony, phthisis, uveitis, and vision loss than tube shunt. Especially as the frequency of tube shunt placement rises, we need to better understand the risks and benefits of subsequent glaucoma surgery.

This article relays the experience of a single center with sequential tube shunt versus laser cyclophotocoagulation (CPC) after a failed tube shunt. The mean follow-up in this series is 11 years, which is extensive compared with other articles on this subject. The authors report failure rate of sequential tube placement was 20% at 4 years, which is in line with previous reports, but ultimately 60% of sequential tubes failed. In the cyclophotocoagulation group, 34% required further intervention and 91% of those interventions occurred within 2 years. Therefore, tubes failed more over time than CPC, but CPC failed earlier. The number of patients with loss of 2 or more lines on Snellen visual acuity testing was greater for the tube group, but the mean follow-up was longer as well.

By virtue of being a retrospective analysis, it is hard to determine why certain patients were treated with CPC versus tube shunt, but this and other factors might affect the study's results. Ideally, a prospective, randomized trial will help determine which surgical intervention should follow failed tube shunts.

S. J. Fudemberg, MD

Reference

1. Gedde SJ, Schiffman JC, Feuer WJ, et al. Treatment outcomes in the Tube Versus Trabeculectomy (TVT) study after five years of follow-up. *Am J Ophthalmol.* 2012;153:789-803.

Optical Coherence Tomography Angiography of the Peripapillary Retina in Glaucoma

Liu L, Jia Y, Takusagawa HL, et al (Oregon Health and Science Univ, Portland; et al)

JAMA Ophthalmol 133:1045-1052, 2015

Importance.—Vascular factors may have important roles in the pathophysiology of glaucoma. A practical method for the clinical evaluation of ocular perfusion is needed to improve glaucoma management.

Objective.—To detect peripapillary retinal perfusion in glaucomatous eyes compared with normal eyes using optical coherence tomography (OCT) angiography.

Design, Setting, and Participants.—Prospective observational study performed from July 24, 2013, to April 17, 2014. Participants were recruited and tested at Casey Eye Institute, Oregon Health & Science University. In total, 12 glaucomatous eyes and 12 age-matched normal eyes were analyzed. The optic disc region was imaged twice using a 3 × 3-mm scan by a 70-kHz, 840-nm-wavelength spectral OCT system. The split-spectrum amplitude-decorrelation angiography algorithm was used. Peripapillary flow index was calculated as the mean decorrelation value in the peripapillary region, defined as a 700-μm-wide elliptical annulus around the disc. Peripapillary vessel density was the percentage area occupied by vessels. The data statistical analysis was performed from October 30, 2013, to May 30, 2014.

Main Outcomes and Measures.—Variability was assessed by the coefficient of variation. The Mann-Whitney test was used to compare the 2 groups of eyes. Correlations between vascular and visual field variables were assessed by linear regression analysis.

Results.—In 12 normal eyes, a dense microvascular network around the disc was visible on OCT angiography. In 12 glaucomatous eyes, this network was visibly attenuated globally and focally. In normal eyes, between-visit reproducibilities of peripapillary flow index and peripapillary vessel density were 4.3% and 2.7% of the coefficient of variation, respectively, while the population variabilities of peripapillary flow index and peripapillary vessel density were 8.2% and 3.0% of the coefficient of variation, respectively. Peripapillary flow index and peripapillary vessel density in glaucomatous eyes were lower than those in normal eyes ($P < .001$ for both). Peripapillary flow index (Pearson $r = -0.808$) and peripapillary vessel density (Pearson $r = -0.835$) were highly correlated with visual field pattern standard deviation in glaucomatous eyes ($P = .001$ for both). The areas under the receiver operating characteristic curve for normal vs glaucomatous eyes were 0.892 for peripapillary flow index and 0.938 for peripapillary vessel density.

Conclusions and Relevance.—Using OCT angiography, reduced peripapillary retinal perfusion in glaucomatous eyes can be visualized as focal defects and quantified as peripapillary flow index and peripapillary vessel density, with high repeatability and reproducibility. Quantitative OCT angiography may have value in future studies to determine its potential usefulness in glaucoma evaluation.

▶ Optical coherence tomography (OCT) angiography is a relatively new tool for evaluating the retina, but it is still a field in its infancy. Using special processing algorithms, comparison of many OCT scans allows a detailed view of circulation in the retina. No exogenous dye is needed for OCT compared with fluorescein angiography, which means it is easier and safer for the patient. OCT angiography provides better resolution of small vascular structures than color Doppler ultrasound, which cannot image small vessels with low flow rate.

OCT angiography is interesting in glaucoma because there is a link, although incompletely understood, between blood flow and glaucomatous damage to the optic nerve. Reduced ocular perfusion of the optic nerve clearly yields optic nerve damage, but the cause of pathologic ocular blood flow changes remains unknown. Perhaps OCT angiography will facilitate the study of blood flow in glaucoma.

In this article, the authors compared OCT angiography of the peripapillary retina between glaucomatous and normal eyes. They found that makers of decreased perfusion could be reproducibly identified. This is a small study, and the authors point out that intraocular pressure–lowering medications might affect blood flow and falsely separate glaucomatous eyes from normals. Nonetheless, their results are encouraging. Ocular blood flow issues are among the leading fields of study in which researchers pursue the etiology of glaucoma. A simple, low-risk, and readily available means of evaluating ocular perfusion in glaucoma could make a big contribution to our field.

S. J. Fudemberg, MD

Fixed-dose combination of AR-13324 and latanoprost: a double-masked, 28-day, randomised, controlled study in patients with open-angle glaucoma or ocular hypertension

Lewis RA, for the PG324-CS201 Study Group (Sacramento Eye Consultants, CA; et al)

Br J Ophthalmol 100:339-344, 2016

Background/Aims.—To evaluate the ocular hypotensive efficacy of fixed-dose combinations of the Rho kinase inhibitor and norepinephrine transport inhibitor AR-13324 (0.01% and 0.02%) and latanoprost (PG324 Ophthalmic Solution) relative to the active components AR-13324 0.02% and latanoprost 0.005%, used bilaterally at night.

Methods.—This was a double-masked, randomised, parallel comparison study in patients with open-angle glaucoma or ocular hypertension. After washout, patients were randomised to one of four treatment arms and treated for 28 days. The primary efficacy variable was mean diurnal intraocular pressure (IOP) at day 29.

Results.—We randomised 298 patients, of whom 292 (98%) completed the study. Mean unmedicated diurnal IOPs (study eye) was 25.1, 25.1, 26.0 and 25.4 in the PG324 0.01%, PG324 0.02%, latanoprost and AR-13324 0.02% groups, respectively. On day 29, mean diurnal IOP decreased to 17.3, 16.5, 18.4 and 19.1 mm Hg, respectively. For the primary efficacy variable of mean diurnal IOP at day 29, PG324 0.02% met the criterion for statistical superiority relative to both latanoprost and AR-13324 0.02% ($p < 0.0001$), providing additional IOP lowering of 1.9 and 2.6 mm Hg, respectively. PG324 0.01% also met the criterion for superiority. The most frequently reported adverse event was conjunctival hyperaemia with an incidence of 41% (30/73), 40% (29/73), 14% (10/73) and 40% (31/78) in the PG324 0.01%, PG324 0.02%, latanoprost and AR-13324 0.02% groups, respectively.

Conclusions.—In this short-term study, the fixed-dose combination of AR-13324 0.02% and latanoprost 0.005% in PG324 Ophthalmic Solution provides clinically and statistically superior ocular hypotensive efficacy relative to its individual active components at the same concentrations. The only safety finding of note was transient asymptomatic conjunctival hyperaemia which was typically of mild severity.

Trial Registration Number.—NCT02207491.

▶ Rho-kinase is an enzyme that affects contractility in the trabecular meshwork (TM). Inhibitors of rho-kinase (RKI) relax contraction of the TM and increases aqueous outflow. RKIs are a potentially new class of IOP-lowering medication. Aerie Pharmaceuticals is developing an RKI for clinical use called Rhopressa, which is undergoing Phase III trials. Additionally, a combination formulation of Rhopressa and latanoprost called Roclatan is also undergoing Phase III clinical trials. This combination medication has the potential to become the first fixed-dose combination including a prostaglandin in the United States if ultimately approved by the Food and Drug Administration (FDA).

This study compared 2 concentrations of Roclatan with Rhopressa and latanoprost. The authors found that Roclatan was more effective than Rhopressa or latanoprost. RKIs are well known to cause conjunctival hyperemia, and the incidence was about 40% for both formulations of Roclatan as well as Rhopressa compared with 14% for latanoprost. Most patients reported the hyperemia as mild for all compounds.

RKIs may become an entirely new class of medications for lowering IOP in glaucoma and are working their way through late stages of the FDA approval process. Further information regarding these medications should be forthcoming in the near future.

S. J. Fudemberg, MD

Estimated trans-lamina cribrosa pressure difference versus intraocular pressure as biomarker for open-angle glaucoma. The Beijing Eye Study 2011

Jonas JB, Wang NL, Wang YX, et al (Capital Med Univ, Beijing, China; et al)

Acta Ophthalmol 93:e7-e13, 2015

Purpose.—To examine whether an estimated trans-lamina cribrosa pressure difference (TLCPD) better than intraocular pressure (IOP) correlated with markers for glaucoma.

Methods.—The population-based Beijing Eye Study 2011 included 3468 individuals. Cerebrospinal fluid pressure (CSFP) was calculated as CSFP [mmHg] = 0.44 × Body Mass Index [kg/m^2] + 0.16 × Diastolic Blood Pressure [mmHg] – 0.18 × Age [Years] – 1.91. TLCPD was IOP–CSFP.

Results.—In the non-glaucomatous population, mean TLCPD was 5.8 ± 4.1 mmHg and mean estimated CSFP was 8.9 ± 3.7 mmHg. IOP was higher ($p = 0.008$), CSFP was lower ($p < 0.001$), and TLCPD was ($p < 0.001$) higher in the glaucoma group than in the non-glaucomatous group. The intergroup difference was highest for TLCPD (2.1 mmHg) followed by CSFP (1.7 mmHg) and IOP (0.4 mmHg). Open-angle glaucoma (OAG) was associated with higher TLCPD [$p < 0.001$; odds ratio (OR): 1.14; 95% confidence intervals (CI): 1.08, 1.19] but not with IOP ($p = 0.22$; OR: 0.96; 95% CI: 0.89, 1.03). In contrast, angle-closure glaucoma (ACG) was associated with higher IOP ($p = 0.03$; *B*: 0.14; OR: 1.15; 95% CI: 1.01, 1.30) but not with TLCPD ($p = 0.98$), after adjustment for age and anterior chamber depth. Retinal nerve fibre layer thickness was associated with lower TLCPD ($p = 0.036$) but not with IOP ($p = 0.96$), after adjusting for gender, age, region of habitation, optic disc area and refractive error. Neuroretinal area and volume were associated with smaller TLCPD ($p = 0.002$, and $p < 0.001$, respectively), after adjusting for gender, optic disc area and refractive error, but not with IOP ($p = 0.43$ and $p = 0.25$, resp.).

Conclusions.—In OAG, but not in ACG, calculated TLCPD versus IOP showed a better association with glaucoma presence and amount of glaucomatous optic neuropathy. It supports the notion of a potential role of low CSFP in the pathogenesis of OAG.

▶ The retinal ganglion cell axons pass through the lamina cribrosa, a sieve-like perforation in the posterior sclera, as they exit the eye. The lamina cribrosa provides the main structural element of the optic nerve head and separates the intraocular space from the retrobulbar space. The pressure gradient between intraocular pressure (IOP) and the orbital cerebrospinal fluid pressure (CSFP), as it surrounds the optic nerve posterior to the lamina, may be a factor in glaucoma. It is possible that imbalance between the IOP and orbital CSFP may cause deformation of the lamina and/or damage to the optic nerve head. Examination of the optic nerve head and lamina cribrosa using optical coherence tomography has shown that posterior deformation of the lamina cribrosa may occur in glaucoma progression, and anterior displacement of the lamina cribrosa may occur with aging.[1] Perhaps patients with glaucomatous optic nerve damage at average IOP, or even low IOP, have a low orbital CSFP.

In this study, CSFP was estimated using a previously derived formula. The translaminar cribrosa counterpressure (TLCPD) is IOP − CSFP. The authors performed this calculation on data from individuals in the Beijing Eye Study 2011. They found that patients with open-angle glaucoma had higher IOP, lower CSFP, and higher TLCPD than patients without glaucoma. In fact, TLCPD was more associated with the presence of glaucoma than IOP in open-angle glaucoma patients. Patients with angle-closure glaucoma also had higher IOP than normals but did not have higher TLCPD.

There are important limitations in the study, including the use of calculated CSFP instead of actual CSFP as measured by lumbar puncture. Nonetheless, the relationship between 2 fluid cavities separated from one another by a relatively thin tissue at the optic nerve head seems intuitively important in glaucoma pathogenesis, especially in light of this and other work.

S. J. Fudemberg, MD

Reference

1. Leung CKS, et al. *Ophthalmology.* 2015;122:1317-1329.

Anterior Segment Imaging Predicts Incident Gonioscopic Angle Closure

Baskaran M, Iyer JV, Narayanaswamy AK, et al (Singapore Natl Eye Centre; et al)

Ophthalmology 122:2380-2384, 2015

Purpose.—To investigate the incidence of gonioscopic angle closure after 4 years in subjects with gonioscopically open angles but varying degrees of angle closure detected on anterior segment optical coherence tomography (AS OCT; Visante; Carl Zeiss Meditec, Dublin, CA) at baseline.

Design.—Prospective, observational study.

Participants.—Three hundred forty-two subjects, mostly Chinese, 50 years of age or older, were recruited, of whom 65 were controls with open angles on gonioscopy and AS OCT at baseline, and 277 were cases with baseline open angles on gonioscopy but closed angles (1–4 quadrants) on AS OCT scans.

Methods.—All subjects underwent gonioscopy and AS OCT at baseline (horizontal and vertical single scans) and after 4 years. The examiner performing gonioscopy was masked to the baseline and AS OCT data. Angle closure in a quadrant was defined as nonvisibility of the posterior trabecular meshwork by gonioscopy and visible iridotrabecular contact beyond the scleral spur in AS OCT scans.

Main Outcome Measures.—Gonioscopic angle closure in 2 or 3 quadrants after 4 years.

Results.—There were no statistically significant differences in age, ethnicity, or gender between cases and controls. None of the control subjects demonstrated gonioscopic angle closure after 4 years. Forty-eight of the 277 subjects (17.3%; 95% confidence interval [CI], 12.8–23; $P < 0.0001$) with at least 1 quadrant of angle closure on AS OCT at baseline demonstrated gonioscopic angle closure in 2 or more quadrants, whereas 28 subjects (10.1%; 95% CI, 6.7–14.6; $P < 0.004$) demonstrated gonioscopic angle closure in 3 or more quadrants after 4 years. Individuals with more quadrants of angle closure on baseline AS OCT scans had a greater likelihood of gonioscopic angle closure developing after 4 years ($P < 0.0001$, chi-square test for trend for both definitions of angle closure).

Conclusions.—Anterior segment OCT imaging at baseline predicts incident gonioscopic angle closure after 4 years among subjects who have gonioscopically open angles and iridotrabecular contact on AS OCT at baseline (Table 3).

► Gonioscopy is the gold standard for visualizing and evaluating angle structures. However, detecting gonioscopic angle closure can be a nuanced technique prone to artifacts. For example, inadvertent compression of the cornea and incident light entering the pupil can contribute to the false perception that the angle is open. Anterior segment ocular coherence tomography (AS-OCT) can potentially circumvent these problems because it requires no external illumination and is a noncontact technique for evaluating the anterior segment and iridocorneal angle. Although AS-OCT has been available for a number of years, it is not routinely used for evaluating the iridocorneal angle among ophthalmologists. Previous reports have reported a high false-positive rate with more eyes having angle closure on AS OCT than gonioscopy.[1] Additionally, defining structures on AS OCT for reference in angle measurement has proven difficult.

This prospective observational study shows that AS-OCT scans suggestive of angle closure despite open angles by gonioscopy can predict future angle closure. In addition, those with more quadrants of angle closure determined by

TABLE 3.—Gonioscopic and Anterior Segment Optical Coherence Tomography Angle Closure After 4 Years (Defined as 2 or More Quadrants Closed)*

No. of Quadrants Closed on Anterior Segment Optical Coherence Tomography at Baseline	No. of Subjects	No. (%) with Gonioscopic Angle Closure After 4 Years†	No. (%) with Anterior Segment Optical Coherence Tomography Angle Closure After 4 Years†
0	65	0 (0)	8/63 (12.7)
1	112	12 (10.7)	50/110 (45.5)
2	112	16 (14.3)	78/109 (78)
3	36	12 (33.3)	31/35 (88.5)
4	17	8 (47.5)	16/16 (100)

*All subjects had no quadrants closed at baseline on gonioscopy.
†$P < 0.0001$, chi-square test for trend.
Reprinted from Baskaran M, Iyer JV, Narayanaswamy AK, et al. Anterior segment imaging predicts incident gonioscopic angle closure. *Ophthalmology.* 2015;122:2380-2384, with permission from American Academy of Ophthalmology.

AS-OCT had a higher chance of developing angle closure on gonioscopy over a 4-year follow-up period (Table 3). The authors suggest that AS-OCT scans showing angle closure should no longer be dismissed as a false positive but should warrant closer follow-up.

The information gleaned from a detailed gonioscopic examination is unparalleled and cannot be replaced by AS-OCT as it stands today. However, this study is yet another example on how modern imaging technology is giving us additional insight into ocular disease processes and may alter treatment and management protocols in the future, as it already has in the evaluation of macular pathology.

D. Lee, MD
S. J. Fudemberg, MD

Reference

1. Lavanya R, Foster PJ, Sakata LM, et al. Screening for narrow angles in the Singapore population: evaluation of new noncontact screening methods. *Ophthalmology.* 2008;115:1720-1727. 1727.e1–2.

Carbonic anhydrase inhibitors as fourth drug in primary glaucomas: Is it worth it?

Juncal VR, Abdo Jorge F, Paranhos A Jr, et al (Federal Univ of São Paulo, Brazil; et al)
Can J Ophthalmol 50:297-301, 2015

Objective.—To evaluate the effectiveness of carbonic anhydrase inhibitors as the fourth drug regarding intraocular pressure (IOP) control in patients with primary glaucomas.

Design.—Single-centre, prospective study.

Participants.—Twenty-five eyes from 25 patients with primary glaucomas treated concomitantly with a topical prostaglandin analogue, a β-blocker, an α-adrenergic agonist, and a carbonic anhydrase inhibitor.

Methods.—Patients followed at the Federal University of São Paulo were enrolled from August to November 2013 and were initially submitted to an ophthalmologic examination where the IOP was measured at 8 AM, 10 AM, and 12 PM. Afterward, patients underwent a 15-day washout of the carbonic anhydrase inhibitor and had their IOP measured again.

Results.—Most patients were female, white, and with a mean age of 66.4 ± 9.7 years. The removal of the fourth drug had a statistically significant effect on the IOP peak (increase of 1.20 mm Hg, $p < 0.01$) and mean (increase of 1.23 mm Hg, $p < 0.01$), but it did not interfere significantly with morning fluctuation of the IOP ($p = 0.83$). After discontinuation of the fourth drug, the IOP increased ≥2 mm Hg in 32% of the patients, and there was a significant increase of the IOP (defined as an IOP change ≥20%) in only 5 patients (20%). Age older than 60 years was associated with 20% of the documented IOP change ($R^2 = 0.19$, $p = 0.03$).

Conclusions.—The removal of a fourth medication does not appear to have a clinically significant impact on IOP control in most patients with glaucoma. However, 32% of the patients experienced an IOP increase ≥2 mm Hg, with age older than 60 years being the only significant predictive factor.

▶ The decision to pursue glaucoma filtration surgery may be a difficult one. Despite more than 40 years of refinement, often-quoted success rates of trabeculectomy are around 80%. For busy glaucoma surgeons, that means every day spent in the operating room will likely yield a surgical failure (as defined by insufficient intraocular pressure [IOP] lowering effect). Much of the total success rate is buoyed by qualified success and the rate of complete success (achieving target IOP without medications) is frustratingly low. Furthermore, there are real and serious risks with filtration surgery. Even when the outcome is successful, patient and surgeon may need to traverse a challenging path of fluctuation and manipulation in the early postop period. It's a very different risk/benefit analysis than cataract surgery, which benefits from better and more predictable outcomes. Nonetheless, filtration surgery has proven to be a potent and essential weapon in the fight against preventable blindness from glaucoma.

This article addresses a practical clinical question regarding the benefit of trying to maximize topical medical therapy when the alternative is usually surgical intervention. Among the 4 major classes of topical IOP lowering agents, prostaglandin analogues, beta-blockers, alpha-adrenergic agonists, and carbonic anhydrase inhibitors (CAIs), the latter is likely the least effective. Furthermore, it is likely that each successive medication added to a patient's regimen functions synergistically, but with diminishing additional benefit. In other words, you get more bang for your buck from the first agent added than the last.

This article evaluated a relatively small sample size but found that the mean and peak IOP rise were statistically significant for a group of patients on all 4 medication classes in whom the topical CAI was withdrawn. Interestingly, the authors found that removal of a topical CAI caused at least a 20% rise in IOP in only 20% of cases. Therefore, although the topical CAI contributed to IOP lowering, the magnitude of change was often small.

The results of this study support the concept that adding a fourth medication may be less effective in the long-term than surgery, but to answer the question fully would require a prospective randomized study to determine the overall impact on outcome of this decision. For some patients, the need for surgery is imminent, whereas others are on the borderline between medical and surgical management. In cases in which there is less urgency, patients may need to come to terms with the prospect of a surgery. Patients who are at peace with the decision to have filtration surgery might be better equipped to deal with the highs and lows of its postoperative course. In clinical practice, sometimes adding a fourth medication is part of a transition period between medical and surgical treatment even though the IOP lowering effect is mild for most patients.

S. J. Fudemberg, MD

The Most Common Barriers to Glaucoma Medication Adherence: A Cross-Sectional Survey

Newman-Casey PA, Robin AL, Blachley T, et al (Univ of Michigan Med School, Ann Arbor; et al)

Ophthalmology 122:1308-1316, 2015

Purpose.—To evaluate the frequency of 11 commonly cited barriers to optimal glaucoma medication adherence among glaucoma patients and to identify barriers contributing to poor adherence.

Design.—Prospective, cross-sectional survey.

Participants.—One hundred ninety adults with glaucoma taking 1 or more glaucoma medication who received care in glaucoma clinics in Ann Arbor, Michigan, and Baltimore, Maryland.

Methods.—Participants completed a survey on demographic and disease characteristics, barriers to optimal glaucoma medication adherence, interest in an eye drop aid, and self-reported adherence (measured by the Morisky Adherence Scale). Descriptive statistics and logistic regression analyses were performed.

Main Outcome Measures.—Frequency and number of barriers to adherence among both adherent and nonadherent patients. Odds ratios (ORs) with 95% confidence intervals (CIs) identifying barriers associated with poor adherence.

Results.—Twenty-seven percent of the sample reported poor adherence. Sixty-one percent of all participants cited multiple barriers and 10% cited a single barrier as impediments to optimal adherence. Twenty-nine percent of subjects cited no barriers, although only 13% of patients who cited no barriers were nonadherent. Among nonadherent patients, 31% or more cited each of the 11 barriers as important. Logistic regression analysis, adjusted for age, revealed that the following barriers were associated with higher odds of nonadherence: decreased self-efficacy (OR, 4.7; 95% CI, 2.2–9.7; $P \leq 0.0001$), difficulty instilling drops (OR, 2.3; 95% CI, 1.1–4.9; $P = 0.03$), forgetfulness (OR, 5.6; 95% CI, 2.6–12.1; $P \leq 0.0001$), and difficulties with the medication schedule (OR, 2.9; 95% CI, 1.4–6.0; $P = 0.006$). For each additional barrier cited as important, there was a 10% increased odds of being nonadherent (OR, 1.1; 95% CI, 1.0–1.2; $P = 0.01$).

Conclusions.—Each of the 11 barriers was important to at least 30% of surveyed patients with poor adherence, with most identifying multiple barriers to adherence. Low self-efficacy, forgetfulness, and difficulty with drop administration and the medication schedule were barriers associated with poor adherence. Interventions to improve medication adherence must address each patient's unique set of barriers.

► Poor adherence to glaucoma therapy is a notoriously large and challenging problem. Intraocular pressure (IOP) control almost always involves the use of topical medication and frequently requires multiple topical medications. The Ocular Hypertension Treatment Study found that, by 5 years, almost 40%

of patients required 2 or more medications to achieve a relatively modest goal of IOP 24 mm Hg or less and reduction from baseline of 20%.[1] Therefore, glaucoma care pits the competing interest of necessary medication use against the inherent difficulty with taking them. This problem is a significant contributor to persistent glaucoma progression rates in the developed world.

This well-organized study evaluated commonly cited barriers to adherence among patients on glaucoma medications to determine whether certain single barriers or groups of barriers stand out as the biggest issues. Interestingly, they found that each of the barriers was important to at least about a third of the surveyed patients, but only 10% of patients thought a single barrier was important. Sixty-one percent cited multiple barriers with 29% citing no barriers as important.

The number 1 barrier was forgetfulness. This would seem an easier barrier than others to overcome in the technological age by using automated reminder systems. However, the authors point out that forgetfulness could be a surrogate response for barriers that seem more confrontational like mistrust of physicians and the health care system. Another interesting finding was that about half of all patients (regardless of adherence status) reported skepticism about their risk of vision loss from glaucoma or skepticism about glaucoma medications mitigating that risk.

With a variety of barriers contributing to nonadherence and varied significance of those barriers to different patients, improving adherence may require tailoring information to individuals. As time for patient-physician interactions in clinic shrinks, it is difficult to address the complex needs of each patient medically and emotionally. Perhaps future advancements like the use of depot medications and surgical interventions with high rates of complete instead of qualified success may reduce the implication of nonadherence. In the absence of major changes in our therapeutic options for glaucoma, research about nonadherence behavior and how to alter it by delivering an appropriate intervention is extremely important.

S. J. Fudemberg, MD

Reference

1. Kass MA, Heuer DK, Higginbotham EJ, et al. The Ocular Hypertension Treatment Study: a randomized trial determines that topical ocular hypotensive medication delays or prevents the onset of primary open-angle glaucoma. *Arch Ophthalmol.* 2002;120:701-713.

A randomised, controlled comparison of latanoprostene bunod and latanoprost 0.005% in the treatment of ocular hypertension and open angle glaucoma: the VOYAGER study

Weinreb RN, for the VOYAGER study group (Shiley Eye Ctr Univ of California, San Diego, La Jolla; et al)

Br J Ophthalmol 99:738-745, 2015

Aim.—To assess the efficacy and safety of latanoprostene bunod (LBN) compared with latanoprost 0.005%, and to determine the optimum drug concentration(s) of LBN in reducing intraocular pressure (IOP) in subjects with open angle glaucoma or ocular hypertension.

Methods.—Randomised, investigator-masked, parallel-group, dose-ranging study. Subjects instilled one drop of study medication in the study eye once daily each evening for 28 days and completed five study visits. The primary efficacy endpoint was the reduction in mean diurnal IOP at Day 28.

Results.—Of the 413 subjects randomised (LBN 0.006%, n = 82; LBN 0.012%, n = 85; LBN 0.024%, n = 83; LBN 0.040%, n = 81; latanoprost, n = 82), 396 subjects completed the study. Efficacy for LBN was dose-dependent reaching a plateau at 0.024%–0.040%. LBN 0.024% led to significantly greater reductions in diurnal IOP compared with latanoprost at the primary endpoint, Day 28 ($p = 0.005$), as well as Days 7 ($p = 0.033$) and 14 ($p = 0.015$). The incidence of adverse events, mostly mild and transient, was numerically higher in the LBN treatment groups compared with the latanoprost group. Hyperaemia was similar across treatments.

Conclusions.—LBN 0.024% dosed once daily was the lower of the two most effective concentrations evaluated, with significantly greater IOP lowering and comparable side effects relative to latanoprost 0.005%. LBN dosed once daily for 28 days was well tolerated.

Clinical Trial Number.—NCT01223378.

▶ The modern age of medical management in glaucoma began with the introduction of timolol in 1978, but most of the medication classes we use today were approved by the Food and Drug Administration (FDA) in the mid-1990s (dorzolamide 1995, brimonidine 1996, latanoprost 1996, dorzolamide-timolol 1998). Combination medications in glaucoma followed (dorzolamide timolol late 1990s, brimonidine-timolol 2007, brinzolamide-brimonidine 2013).[1] If approved by the US FDA, latanoprostene bunod has the potential to introduce a novel mechanism of intraocular pressure (IOP) lowering into clinical care.

In the ocular environment, latanoprostene bunod (LBN) is cleaved into latanoprost acid, a prostaglandin agonist, and butanediol mononitrate, a nitric oxide donating moiety. Nitric oxide synthase was identified in the late 1980s as an endogenous signaling mediator with an important role in the cardiovascular system. Ultimately, this finding led to the development of vasodilating nitrates such as nitroglycerine. Evidence is mounting that nitric oxide may play an important role in glaucoma. The trabecular meshwork (TM) is believed to function like a muscle in that it has contractile properties. If the TM contracts, it restricts flow of aqueous and, conversely, relaxation of the TM improves outflow. Nitric oxide donors have been shown to mediate IOP-lowering effects in both preclinical models and clinical studies, primarily by cell volume and contractility changes in the TM.[2] Given that prostaglandin analogues improve uveoscleral aqueous outflow, the nitric oxide moiety in LBN could provide a synergistic IOP lowering effect through the conventional outflow pathway.

This study is a phase II dose-ranging trial of LBN concentrations compared with latanoprost. The authors found that LBN in certain concentrations was more effective than latanoprost with a similar side effect profile. It is well known that prostaglandin analogues dosed more than once per day are less effective. Treatment effect of LBN 0.006% and latanoprost 0.005%, which deliver the same amount of latanoprost acid, were similar. Interestingly, there was a dose-dependent increase in effect with stronger concentrations of LBN up to a peak, which indicates that the nitric oxide donating moiety may account for the additional treatment effect. Additional study may clarify the significance and mechanism of the additional treatment effect, but the results are encouraging.

The additional IOP lowering effect of the selected concentration of LBN over latanoprost was 1.23 mm Hg. Phase III studies have demonstrated noninferiority to timolol 0.5% dosed twice daily and, at the time of this review's writing, LBN is under review by the FDA with a Prescription Drug User Fee Act date (target for completion of the review) in the third quarter of 2016. The prostaglandin market is a tough one, with generic latanoprost and existing branded prostaglandins. Research into the role of nitric oxide in glaucoma has the potential to provide exciting information in the coming years.

S. J. Fudemberg, MD

References

1. Realini T. A history of glaucoma pharmacology. *Optom Vis Sci.* 2011;88:36-38.
2. Cavet ME, Vittetow JL, Impagnatiello F, Ongini E, Bastia E. Nitric oxide (NO): an emerging target for the treatment of glaucoma. *Invest Ophthalmol Vis Sci.* 2014; 55:5005-5015.

Biomarkers and surrogate endpoints in glaucoma clinical trials

Medeiros FA (Univ of California, San Diego, La Jolla)

Br J Ophthalmol 99:599-603, 2015

Surrogate endpoints are often used as replacements for true clinically relevant endpoints in several areas of medicine, as they enable faster and less expensive clinical trials. However, without proper validation, the use of surrogates may lead to incorrect conclusions about the efficacy and safety of treatments. This article reviews the general requirements for validating surrogate endpoints and provides a critical assessment of the use of intraocular pressure (IOP), visual fields, and structural measurements of the optic nerve as surrogate endpoints in glaucoma clinical trials. A valid surrogate endpoint must be able to predict the clinically relevant endpoint and fully capture the effect of an intervention on that endpoint. Despite its widespread use in clinical trials, no proper validation of IOP as a surrogate endpoint has ever been conducted for any class of IOP-lowering treatments. Evidence has accumulated with regard to the role of imaging measurements of optic nerve damage as surrogate endpoints in glaucoma. These measurements are predictive of functional losses in the disease and may explain, at least in part, treatment effects on clinically relevant endpoints. The use of composite endpoints in glaucoma trials may overcome weaknesses of the use of structural or functional endpoints in isolation. Unless research is dedicated to fully develop and validate suitable endpoints that can be used in glaucoma clinical trials, we run the risk of inappropriate judgments about the value of new therapies.

▶ This article addresses one of the most important problems in glaucoma. The true endpoint in glaucoma is visual disability, meaning vision loss sufficient to affect a patient's quality of life. Typically, glaucoma is slowly progressive and worsens significantly before reaching its true endpoint of visual disability. Therefore, following glaucoma by monitoring its true endpoint is impractical and would miss the significant progression that occurs before damage is sufficient to reach the true endpoint. Surrogate markers are necessary to find progression before irreversible disability occurs. Currently, we use 3 major surrogate endpoints in glaucoma: intraocular pressure, visual fields, and optic nerve imaging. All of them are flawed.

Many clinical trials in glaucoma use alteration in IOP as a primary endpoint. Likewise, treatments in glaucoma are indicated for lowering IOP, not specifically for glaucoma itself. However, patients with a relatively low IOP may experience glaucoma progression, and those with relatively high IOP may never experience glaucoma progression. IOP is the only well-proven modifiable risk factor for glaucoma progression, but its correlation with glaucoma may be indirect. Following only IOP would be a flawed strategy. As well, IOP would be an inappropriate endpoint in trials of potentially neuroprotective agents, which should have a beneficial effect in glaucoma independent of IOP.

Visual field change indicates functional impairment in glaucoma, but lacks a consistent and clear definition. Large clinical trials often use different criteria to judge visual field progression and their methods may be too complex for efficient use in the clinic. Furthermore, correlation between visual field change and quality of life has proven weak at best. Additionally, confirming visual field progression, even with the simplest criteria, may require many visual fields necessitating large, long, and expensive trials to judge the effect of an intervention on visual field progression. Finally, early progression in glaucoma is preperimetric and would be missed on visual field testing.

Optic nerve imaging provides the chance to monitor form and identify progression before it manifests as a functional change. However, current modalities of optic nerve imaging function poorly to judge change with advanced retinal nerve fiber layer loss, when visual impairment and disability may be the most imminent. More fundamentally, there are no clearly determined criteria for judging progression by optic nerve imaging that are tightly correlated to the risk of visual disability from glaucoma.

Research to identify new biomarkers in glaucoma is ongoing. The ripple effect of a new biomarker would be far-reaching. Many risk/benefit decisions in clinical care would be more straightforward if it were easier to determine who is definitely progressing or not. Biomarkers that are less prone to fluctuation than our current surrogates could radically speed the pace of progress in the field by facilitating the capture of good data from smaller studies. Research on new biomarkers is one of the most important endeavors in glaucoma.

S. J. Fudemberg, MD

A Randomized Trial of a Schlemm's Canal Microstent with Phacoemulsification for Reducing Intraocular Pressure in Open-Angle Glaucoma

Pfeiffer N, Garcia-Feijoo J, Martinez-de-la-Casa JM, et al (Johannes Gutenberg-Univ, Mainz, Germany; Hosp Clinico San Carlos, Madrid, Spain; et al)
Ophthalmology 122:1283-1293, 2015

Purpose.—To assess the safety and effectiveness of the Hydrus Microstent (Ivantis, Inc, Irvine, CA) with concurrent cataract surgery (CS) for reducing intraocular pressure (IOP) in open-angle glaucoma (OAG).

Design.—Prospective, multicenter, randomized, single-masked, controlled clinical trial.

Participants.—One hundred eyes from 100 patients 21 to 80 years of age with OAG and cataract with IOP of 24 mm Hg or less with 4 or fewer hypotensive medications and a washed-out diurnal IOP (DIOP) of 21 to 36 mm Hg.

Methods.—On the day of surgery, patients were randomized 1:1 to undergo CS with the microstent or CS alone. Postoperative follow-up was at 1 day, 1 week, and 1, 3, 6, 12, 18, and 24 months. Washout of hypotensive medications was repeated at 12 and 24 months.

Main Outcome Measures.—Response to treatment was defined as a 20% or more decrease in washed out DIOP at 12 and 24 months of follow-up compared with baseline. Mean DIOP at 12 and 24 months, the proportion of subjects requiring medications at follow-up, and the mean number of medications were analyzed. Safety measures included change in visual acuity, slit-lamp observations, and adverse events.

Results.—The proportion of patients with a 20% reduction in washed out DIOP was significantly higher in the Hydrus plus CS group at 24 months compared with the CS group (80% vs. 46%; $P = 0.0008$). Washed out mean DIOP in the Hydrus plus CS group was significantly lower at 24 months compared with the CS group (16.9 ± 3.3 mm Hg vs. 19.2 ± 4.7 mm Hg; $P = 0.0093$), and the proportion of patients using no hypotensive medications was significantly higher at 24 months in the Hydrus plus CS group (73% vs. 38%; $P = 0.0008$). There were no differences in follow-up visual acuity between groups. The only notable device-related adverse event was focal peripheral anterior synechiae (1–2 mm in length). Otherwise, adverse event frequency was similar in the 2 groups.

Conclusions.—Intraocular pressure was clinically and statistically significantly lower at 2 years in the Hydrus plus CS group compared with the CS alone group, with no differences in safety.

► The Hydrus Microstent (Ivantis, Irvine, CA) is a microinvasive glaucoma surgery (MIGS) device that is inserted using an ab interno approach into Schlemm canal. It is intended to function as an intracanalicular scaffold to lower intraocular pressure (IOP). The device is made from nitinol, an alloy of nickel and titanium, which has been used widely in vascular and other medical applications for its properties of shape memory and elasticity. At 8 mm in length, the Hydrus is significantly larger than the 1 mm long iStent (Glaukos). Like the iStent, the Hydrus is an adjunct to cataract surgery and may be placed into the nasal angle through the temporal corneal incision placed during the cataract procedure. It extends about 3 clock hours in Schlemm canal with 1 to 2 mm remaining in the anterior chamber.

This study provides 2-year data of a randomized trial comparing cataract surgery plus the Hydrus to cataract surgery alone. MIGS devices have been characterized by limitations in efficacy, especially when combined with cataract extraction, which is known to lower IOP. The Hydrus data show a statistically significant IOP lowering effect over cataract surgery despite washout of glaucoma medications. This effect largely persisted for the 24-month study period. However, success was defined as a 20% drop in IOP, and washout periods precluded inclusion of patients with advanced disease. Therefore, targets for success were important but still relatively modest.

We are fortunate to be experiencing a period of rapid progress in glaucoma surgery, and information from well-designed studies is critical to assess whether exposing our patients to new technology is doing them a service or a disservice.

S. J. Fudemberg, MD

Trabeculectomy-Related Complications in Olmsted County, Minnesota, 1985 Through 2010

Olayanju JA, Hassan MB, Hodge DO, et al (Mayo Clinic College of Medicine, Rochester, MN; Mayo Clinic, Jacksonville, FL; et al)

JAMA Ophthalmol 133:574-580, 2015

Importance.—Trabeculectomy is the surgical standard of care for patients with medically refractory glaucoma. The use of antimetabolite agents, such as mitomycin, has increased the rate of complications after trabeculectomy.

Objective.—To determine the rate of trabeculectomy-related complications during a 25-year study.

Design, Setting, and Participants.—For this retrospective, population-based study, we enrolled the residents of Olmsted County, Minnesota, who underwent a trabeculectomy from January 1, 1985, through December 31, 2010, at the Mayo Clinic and Olmsted Community Hospital. Data were collected from August 2012 to September 2013 followed by data analysis through January 2014.

Exposures.—After reviewing the patient records, we determined the occurrence of complications, including bleb leak, hypotony, hyphema, choroidal effusion, choroidal hemorrhage, blebitis, and endophthalmitis, as they relate to the mitomycin concentration administered during the operation. We reviewed relevant publications in Ovid, MEDLINE, and PubMed to identify studies representative of the reported trabeculectomy complication rate.

Main Outcomes and Measures.—Cumulative probabilities of short- and long-term complications, determined using the Kaplan-Meier method, and the relation to mitomycin concentration applied during trabeculectomy.

Results.—In 334 patients, 460 eyes underwent trabeculectomy (mean [SD; range] follow-up, 7.7 [5.7; 0-27.7] years). Among them, 159 eyes had complications, with early complications (<3 months) in 100 eyes and late complications (≥3 months) in 59 eyes during the follow-up. Ten eyes had an early and a late complication. The 20-year cumulative chances of early, late, or any complication were 19.7% (95% CI, 16.2%-23.6%), 26.0% (95% CI, 15.0%-36.0%), and 45.0% (95% CI, 38.0%-52.0%), respectively. The cumulative probabilities of vision-threatening complications during 20 years were 2.0% (95% CI, 0%-4.0%) for blebitis and 5.0% (95% CI, 1.0%-9.0%) for endophthalmitis. Association between the rate of trabeculectomy complications and mitomycin dose used was $P = .77$. In total, 98 cases (21.3%) underwent further surgical procedures related directly to the complication.

Conclusions and Relevance.—The rate of trabeculectomy-related complications does not appear to be associated with mitomycin use during a mean follow-up of 7.7 years. The rate of vision-threatening complications appears to be comparable to those of previous studies of shorter duration.

▶ The Rochester Epidemiology Project (REP) was established in 1966 to facilitate study of the natural history of disease. It has maintained a comprehensive medical records linkage system for persons residing in Olmsted County, Minnesota, with Mayo Clinic as the founding and hosting institution.[1] This article evaluated complications of trabeculectomy among patients at Mayo and Olmsted Community Hospital from 1985 through 2010. Previously, the same database was used to evaluate the long-term outcomes of glaucoma filtration surgery from 1965 through 1980.

Surgical outcome analysis is tricky because variations in surgical technique affect results of the analysis and generalizability of the data. For example, among the 8 surgeons who provided primary treatment, all but 1 used a limbus-based conjunctival flap. Fornix-based conjunctival flaps likely have a different rate of bleb leaks than limbus-based flaps. Furthermore, the success rate and complication rate of trabeculectomy are inexorably linked. Pushing for greater success in terms of intraocular pressure (IOP)—lowering effect may predispose to complications such as suprachoroidal hemorrhage or avascular blebs with increased risk of infection. Conversely, protecting against risk of complications with a more conservative approach to IOP lowering predisposes to failure. As well, the study population was homogeneous and does not reflect the multiracial demographic of many glaucoma practices. These are important factors in analyzing complication rates.

Additionally, information reported about complication rates should be balanced by the severity of the complications encountered. The authors found the rate of any complication, early or late, was 45%. However, they also point out that many of the early complications were self-limited. Hyphema or microhyphema accounted for more than half of all early complications and carry a relatively nominal risk to the patient. Even hypotony and choroidal effusion that occur in the early postoperative period may resolve without any sequelae. Therefore, in contrast to the total complication rate of 45%, the chance of vision-threatening complications, such as blebitis and endophthalmitis, during the 20 postoperative years were 2% and 5%, respectively.

Although there are fundamental limitations in generalizing the data from this study, it provides a unique and important perspective about the risk of complications from trabeculectomy with its extensive database and follow-up period.

S. J. Fudemberg, MD

Reference

1. Rocca WA, Yawn BP, St Sauver JL, Grossardt BR, Melton LJ 3rd. History of the Rochester epidemiology project: half a century of medical records linkage in a US population. *Mayo Clin Proc.* 2012;87:1202-1213.

Glaucoma Drainage Devices: Risk of Exposure and Infection

Levinson JD, Giangiacomo AL, Beck AD, et al (Emory Univ, Atlanta, GA)

Am J Ophthalmol 160:516-521, 2015

Purpose.—To identify risk factors for device exposure and intraocular infection following implantation of a glaucoma drainage device.

Design.—Retrospective case series.

Methods.—The medical records of adult patients undergoing glaucoma drainage device implantation at an academic medical center between 2000 and 2010 were reviewed. Main outcome measures included device exposure and intraocular infection.

Results.—Seven hundred and sixty-three cases were identified. These included 702 primary implants (ie, the first drainage device implanted into an eye) and 61 sequential implants. Among 702 primary implants, there were 41 cases of exposure (5.8%). None of the potential risk factors were statistically significant. Implant location was found to be a marginally significant risk factor. The exposure rates for inferior and superior implants were 12.8% (5 of 39) and 5.4% (36 of 663), respectively ($P = .056$). The highest rate of exposure for primary implants occurred in the inferior-nasal quadrant (17.2%, 5 of 29). The rate of exposure for sequential devices was 13.1% (8 of 61), with the highest rate also found in the inferior-nasal quadrant (20%, 5 of 25). Of 49 total exposures, 8 were associated with intraocular infection (16.3%). Exposures over inferior implants were more likely to be associated with infection than exposures over superior implants (41.7% vs 8.1%; $P = .0151$).

Conclusion.—Implant location approached, but did not reach, statistical significance as a risk factor for exposure. Exposures over inferior implants place patients at a higher risk of infection than superior exposures. More studies are needed to identify modifiable risk factors for device exposure.

▶ Theoretically, factors that might affect the health of the conjunctival tissue would seem to increase the risk of erosion. For example, vasculopathic conditions that cause ischemia and lead to neovascular glaucoma, which is a common indication for placement of a glaucoma drainage device, might cause weakness of the conjunctiva and its healing response, leading to erosion. Also, prior surgery, such as trabeculectomy with antimetabolites, might lead to scarring and thinning of the conjunctiva with increased risk of erosion. Failed trabeculectomy is also a common indication for glaucoma drainage devices. Intuitively, mechanical dynamics involving the device position and lid position as well as composition of patch graft material might also affect the risk of erosion. Maybe chronic corticosteroid use in uveitic glaucoma, another common indication for glaucoma drainage devices, thins the conjunctiva. However, research has failed to unequivocally show which factors cause tubes to erode and how to prevent this problem.

This study provides information on a sample size of more than 700 patients from the Emory Eye Center. The rate of intraocular infection among patients with tube erosion was approximately 16%. Inferior shunts eroded more frequently than superior shunts with the highest rate of erosion among inferonasal shunts. Among primary shunts, 93% were implanted superotemporally. This strong predilection for superotemporal placement indicates that primary tubes placed inferonasally may have been placed there secondary to a problem with the superotemporal quadrant, which may have affected their likelihood of erosion. Aside from location of shunt placement, no factors, including type of glaucoma, type of patch, type of shunt, and prior surgery, approached statistical significance.

As the authors point out, to power a study to clearly delineate statistical significance of risk factors, data may need to be pooled from multiple institutions. Identification of modifiable risk factors would provide a real benefit to future recipients of glaucoma drainage devices.

S. J. Fudemberg, MD

Anti-inflammatory Therapy after Selective Laser Trabeculoplasty: A Randomized, Double-Masked, Placebo-Controlled Clinical Trial

Jinapriya D, D'Souza M, Hollands H, et al (Queen's Univ and Hotel Dieu Hosp, Kingston, Ontario, Canada; et al)
Ophthalmology 121:2356-2361, 2014

Purpose.—To investigate the effect of anti-inflammatory therapy on selective laser trabeculoplasty (SLT) outcomes.

Design.—Randomized, double-masked, placebo-controlled trial.

Participants.—Patients with primary open-angle or pseudo-exfoliation glaucoma.

Methods.—Patients undergoing SLT were randomized to receive placebo (artificial tears), prednisolone acetate 1%, or ketorolac tromethamine 0.5% eye drops 4 times per day for 5 days commencing immediately after SLT.

Main Outcome Measures.—Change in intraocular pressure (IOP) from baseline to the 1-month post-SLT visit.

Results.—Mean change in IOP at the 1-month primary outcome time point, as well as all other time points, was not significantly different among groups ($P = 0.99$). Likewise, a repeated-measures, mixed-effects model did not find significant differences in IOP outcome at the 1-month time point ($P = 0.95$). The IOP was reduced in all groups at the 1-month post-SLT time point and all other time points, and no significant differences were found between groups using separate unadjusted cross-sectional analyses of variance ($P > 0.15$ for analyses at all time points). Treatment failure rates were not different among groups ($P = 0.75$), and at 1 year after SLT, the percentage of patients maintaining a 20% IOP reduction ranged from 18% to 22% in the 3 study groups.

Conclusions.—Anti-inflammatory therapy after SLT does not seem to substantially influence the IOP-lowering effect of SLT. In this study of patients with low baseline IOP, SLT showed limited efficacy in achieving a sustained reduction in IOP.

▶ It is unclear exactly how selective laser trabeculoplasty (SLT) actually lowers intraocular pressure (IOP). However, it has been postulated that inflammatory mediators released by the treatment induce extracellular matrix remodeling and improved permeability of Schlemm's canal endothelial cells. It is also unclear which regimen of postoperative antiinflammatory drops, if any, should be standard following SLT. Typically, nonsteroidal antiinflammatory drugs or corticosteroids are given, but these agents may be counterproductive if IOP lowering results from stimulation of the inflammatory cascade.

This study is a prospective, randomized, double-masked, placebo-controlled trial to determine whether antiinflammatory treatment has an effect on SLT outcomes. Its size and clinically relevant definition of success, 20% reduction in IOP from baseline, are strengths. However, it included both initial and adjunctive SLT treatments and the balance between them in different arms of the study is skewed. Adjunctive treatments are less likely than initial treatments to be successful, which may affect comparability of outcomes. Additionally, the steroid arm included more pseudoexfoliation patients than the other arms. It is believed that uptake of laser energy occurs in melanin granules inside trabecular meshwork endothelial cells. Patients with pseudoexfoliation syndrome often have increased pigmentation of the trabecular meshwork and greater uptake of laser energy in SLT, which may affect rates of success and risk of complications such as a spike in IOP. As well, the study treatments were 180 degrees and may not be generalizable to 360-degree treatments.

This study found that anti-inflammatory treatment did not influence the success rate of SLT. Treatment failure rate in all groups was approximately 50% at 1 month and 80% by 1 year, which is disappointing. Perhaps the success rates were affected by the use of 180-degree treatments, baseline pre-SLT IOPs of less than 20 mm Hg, and that 60% to 70% of treatments were adjunctive, although recruitment of patients was typical of clinical practice. If success rates were higher, would there have been more separation between the treatment arms? It seems the ideal regimen or lack thereof remains to be determined. The authors' effort to advance the literature regarding SLT is important and commendable. We need more information about how to best apply SLT including the risk/benefit of repeat treatments, whether to withdraw any glaucoma medications (such as prostaglandin analogues) before SLT, and how to approach post-SLT care.

S. J. Fudemberg, MD

4 Cornea

Multidrug-Resistant *Pseudomonas aeruginosa* Keratitis: Risk Factors, Clinical Characteristics, and Outcomes

Vazirani J, Wurity S, Ali MH (L. V. Prasad Eye Inst, Visakhapatnam, India; L. V. Prasad Eye Inst, Hyderabad, India)

Ophthalmology 122:2110-2114, 2015

Purpose.—To identify risk factors for multidrug-resistant *Pseudomonas aeruginosa* (MDR-PA) keratitis and to report clinical characteristics and outcomes of this infection.

Design.—Retrospective, case-control study.

Participants.—Ninety episodes of *P. aeruginosa* keratitis from a tertiary care eye institution from 2007 through 2014 were identified. Episodes of MDR-PA keratitis were taken as cases. Episodes of drug-sensitive *P. aeruginosa* keratitis during the same period were taken as controls.

Methods.—Chart review of cases and controls. Multidrug resistance was defined as resistance to 3 or more classes of antimicrobial drugs. Logistic regression analysis was used to determine association of baseline characteristics with multidrug resistance. Clinical characteristics and risk factors in each group also were compared.

Main Outcome Measures.—Risk factors for multidrug resistance, including age, gender, eye, duration of symptoms, topical steroid or lubricant ointment use, trauma, prior ocular surgery, presence of a compromised ocular surface, and bandage contact lens use.

Results.—Twenty-three episodes of MDR-PA keratitis (cases) and 67 episodes of drug-sensitive *P. aeruginosa* keratitis (controls) were identified. In the multivariate analysis, lubricant ointment use, presence of a compromised ocular surface, and bandage contact lens use were associated with MDR-PA keratitis. Antimicrobial resistance in the MDR-PA keratitis isolates was least for colistin and imipenem (56.52% each). Corneal perforation was more common in cases (52.17% [12 of 23]) than in controls (11.94% [8 of 67]; $P = 0.0001$). Cyanoacrylate glue application was required in 47.82% of cases (11 of 23), compared with 22.38% of controls (15 of 67; $P = 0.031$). Keratoplasty was more commonly required in cases (47.82% [11 of 23]) than in controls (20.89% [14 of 67]; $P = 0.017$).

Conclusions.—Lubricant ointment use, a compromised ocular surface, and bandage contact lens use are associated with MDR-PA keratitis. Preservative-free lubricant ointment may act as a source or reservoir of infection. Outcomes are worse in MDR-PA keratitis compared with drug-sensitive *P. aeruginosa* keratitis (Table 3).

▶ *Pseudomonas aeruginosa* remains one of our leading sources of bacterial keratitis, especially in contact lens wearers. Fortunately, most cases of *Pseudomonas* are not multidrug resistant in our clinics.

This study suggests a different story in a large tertiary care eye hospital in India. The authors present a retrospective review all culture-proven cases of *Pseudomonas* over a 7-year period. They found 23 episodes of multidrug -resistant *P aeruginosa* (MDR-PA) and 67 drug-sensitive cases, which they used as controls. In the MDR-PA group, 1 eye had 3 distinct episodes of keratitis, while another 1 eye had 2 distinct episodes. There were no episodes of recurrent, distinct infections in the control group.

Based on multivariate analysis, lubricant ointment use, a compromised ocular surface, and bandage contact lens use were associated with multidrug resistance. Because these risk factors may all be present in patients with severe dry eyes or in failed graft, they may be interrelated as the authors discuss. In addition, lubricating ointment was cultured and found to be positive for the same strain of MDR-PA as the patient developed. The authors suggest that lubricating ointment may be a reservoir for the disease and recommend culturing all topical medications used by patients with drug resistance.

TABLE 3.—Antimicrobial Susceptibility Patterns in the Multidrug-Resistant *Pseudomonas aeruginosa* Keratitis Group

Drug	Susceptible Isolates (No.)	Resistant Isolates (No.)	% Resistance
Amikacin	1	22	95.65
Amoxicillin	0	23	100
Amoxyclav	0	23	100
Azithromycin	4	19	82.60
Cefazolin	0	23	100
Cefotaxime	0	23	100
Ceftazidime	3	20	86.95
Ceftriaxone	0	23	100
Chloramphenicol	0	23	100
Ciprofloxacin	0	23	100
Colistin	10	13	56.52
Cotrimoxazole	0	23	100
Gatifloxacin	0	23	100
Gentamicin	0	23	100
Imipenem	10	13	56.52
Moxifloxacin	0	23	100
Ofloxacin	0	23	100
Piperacillin	0	23	100
Piperacillin + tazobactam	0	23	100
Ticarcillin	0	23	100
Tobramycin	0	23	100
Vancomycin	0	23	100

Reprinted from Vazirani J, Wurity S, Ali MH. Multidrug-resistant *Pseudomonas aeruginosa* keratitis: risk factors, clinical characteristics, and outcomes. *Ophthalmology.* 2015;122:2110-2114, with permission from the American Academy of Ophthalmology.

Multidrug resistance was defined as resistance to 3 or more drugs. As displayed in Table 3, colistin and imipenem were the least resistant drugs and therefore, although expensive and potentially difficult to obtain, are the drugs of choice to treat MDR-PA.

Patients with MDR-PA were significantly more likely to develop a perforation and need cyanoacrylate glue and penetrating keratoplasty compared with the control group. Although visual acuity was not a main outcome measure, final visual acuity was worse in the resistant group.

The authors conclude that MDR-PA patients do worse when compared with drug-sensitive cases of *P aeruginosa*. They recommend cultures for all topical medications and found that colistin and imipenem showed least resistance and may be the drugs of choice in this setting.

Although patient demographics were not detailed (eg, contact lens wear, trauma, rural background), given previous reports of bacterial keratitis from India, our patient population in Philadelphia tends to be quite different from rural India. Similarly, our drug-resistance patterns also tend to be different. Nonetheless, we can appreciate the conclusions of this study and consider these issues when concerns regarding drug resistance arise.

P. K. Nagra, MD

Keratoplasty in the United States: A 10-Year Review from 2005 through 2014

Park CY, Lee JK, Gore PK, et al (Montefiore Med Ctr, Bronx, NY; Lions Eye Inst for Transplant and Res, Tampa, FL; et al)
Ophthalmology 122:2432-2442, 2015

Purpose.—To report evolving indications and preferred techniques of corneal transplantation in the United States.

Design.—Retrospective review.

Methods.—Annual reports from the Eye Bank Association of America on corneal graft distribution in the United States from 2005 through 2014 were reviewed.

Main Outcome Measures.—Number and percentage of corneal grafts distributed for various types of keratoplasty and their surgical indications in the United States.

Results.—The total number of corneal transplants increased from 44 277 in 2005 to 46 513 in 2014. In the past decade, penetrating keratoplasty dramatically decreased (from 95% to 42%) and largely has been replaced by various lamellar keratoplasty (LK) techniques (from 5% to 58%). Descemet stripping (automated) endothelial keratoplasty was the most common (50%) type of corneal transplantation performed in the United Stated in 2014. The volume of Descemet membrane endothelial keratoplasty (DMEK) has been doubling every year since 2011 and accounted for 11% of total endothelial keratoplasties in 2014. There was a significant shift in indication for corneal transplantation, with Fuchs' endothelial dystrophy (22%) being the most common, followed

TABLE 1.—Total Number of Domestic Surgery Uses of Corneal Graft Tissue in the United States from 2005 through 2014

Year	Penetrating Keratoplasty	Anterior Lamellar Keratoplasty	Endothelial Keratoplasty: Descemet Stripping Endothelial Keratoplasty/Descemet Stripping Automated Endothelial Keratoplasty	Endothelial Keratoplasty: Descemet Membrane Endothelial Keratoplasty	Keratolimbal Allograft	Keratoprosthesis[†]	Total (No.)
2005	42 063 (94.9)	641 (1.4)	1398 (3.2)*		175 (0.4)	NA	44 277
2006	37 776 (84.4)	806 (1.8)	6027 (13.5)*		138 (0.3)	NA	44 747
2007	34 806 (69.4)	950 (1.9)	14 159 (28.2)*		207 (0.4)	NA	50 122
2008	32 524 (63.5)	1072 (2.1)	17 468 (34.1)*		173 (0.3)	NA	51 237
2009	23 269 (54.9)	774 (1.8)	18 221 (43.0)*		120 (0.3)	222 (0.5)	42 606
2010	21 970 (51.5)	1041 (2.4)	19 159 (44.9)*		130 (0.3)	342 (0.8)	42 642
2011	21 620 (48.6)	932 (2.1)	21 211 (47.7)	344 (0.7)	69 (0.1)	332 (0.7)	44 508
2012	21 422 (46.9)	883 (1.9)	22 301 (48.8)	748 (1.6)	80 (0.2)	236 (0.5)	45 670
2013	20 954 (44.4)	951 (2.0)	23 465 (49.7)	1522 (3.2)	91 (0.2)	223 (0.5)	47 206
2014	19 294 (41.5)	914 (2.0)	23 100 (49.7)	2865 (6.2)	80 (0.2)	260 (0.6)	46 513

Data are no. (%).
NA = not available (United States domestic use only).
*Further classification was not available from 2005 through 2010.
[†]Keratoprosthesis data were available from 2009.
Reprinted from Park CY, Lee JK, Gore PK, et al. Keratoplasty in the United States: a 10-year review from 2005 through 2014. *Ophthalmology.* 2015;122:2432-2442, with permission from the American Academy of Ophthalmology.

by corneal edema occurring after cataract surgery (12%) in 2014. Eye banks supplied precut corneal grafts for 68% of LK techniques in 2014.

Conclusions.—In the United States, there has been a major shift in preferred keratoplasty techniques over the past decade, with a wide adoption of new LK techniques (Table 1).

▶ The past decade has been a time of great enterprise and development in corneal transplantation. Although the results of this study are not surprising, it is a pleasant reminder of the great changes that have occurred in corneal transplantation surgical technique, allowing for more anatomic replacement of corneal tissue.

This review assessed Eye Bank Association of America data from 2005 to 2014, specifically evaluating type of transplantation performed, as well as indication for surgery. As illustrated in Table 1, between 2005 and 2015, the number of full-thickness penetrating keratoplasties decreased by more than half. During these 10 years, however, this decline was balanced by the advent and steady increased in endothelial keratoplasty, predominantly Descemet stripping endothelial keratoplasty, but more recently Descemet membrane endothelial keratoplasty (DMEK) as well. DMEK graft numbers have almost doubled on a yearly basis since first noted in 2011. Overall, the number of corneal grafts used in this country remained relatively stable.

Changes in the most common indications for corneal transplantations were also noted. PBK remained the top surgical indication until 2006, after which a decline was noted, likely due to improvements in phacoemulsification techniques, instrumentation, and intraocular lenses. Fuchs endothelial dystrophy was the most common indication noted for corneal transplantation in this review, accounting for 47.7% of endothelial keratoplasties in 2014, and overall 22% of total grafts over these 10 years.

With the significant increase in lamellar procedures performed, another important finding was that 68% of lamellar procedures used precut tissue. The rapid adoption of lamellar procedures and significant increase in the numbers of these procedures is likely related to this availability of precut tissue through the eye banks.

Overall, this study shows the continued evolution of corneal transplantation that we are experiencing. It will be interesting to see what the next decade brings in the surgical management of corneal pathology.

P. K. Nagra, MD

Terrien Marginal Degeneration: Clinical Characteristics and Outcomes

Chan AT, Ulate R, Goldich Y, et al (Univ of Toronto Med School, Canada; Univ of Toronto, Canada)

Am J Ophthalmol 160:867-872.e1, 2015

Purpose.—To describe outcomes of patients with Terrien marginal degeneration.

Design.—Retrospective case series.

Methods.—Database review of 25 patients (43 eyes) seen over 10 years (2004–2013) at Toronto Western Hospital cornea clinic. Outcome measures included demographics, location of disease, topographic astigmatism, visual acuity, coexisting ocular disease, and surgical management.

Results.—Mean age at presentation was 44 years (range, 20–82 years) and 54% were male. Eighteen patients (72%) had bilateral disease. Mean follow-up was 30.3 months. Mean topographic astigmatism was 4.02 diopters (D) at 5 degrees. Mean change in astigmatism 1 year from baseline was 0.75 D; at 2 years was 1.22 D; and at 3 years was 1.68 D. Mean best spectacle-corrected visual acuity (BSCVA) at presentation was 20/46 and 20/48 at last follow-up. Eyes requiring surgery (23.3%) had mean BSCVA of 20/81 at presentation and 20/106 after surgery. Five eyes perforated: 4 spontaneously, and 1 from trauma. Three eyes (6.9%) presented with pseudopterygium. Two eyes (4.7%) had intracorneal cysts. Fourteen patients (56%) presented with ocular surface inflammation.

Conclusions.—Terrien marginal degeneration is a slow-progressing, bilateral but asymmetric degeneration of the peripheral cornea. Men over 40 are more commonly affected. Stromal thinning, vascularization, lipid deposition, and against-the-rule astigmatism are classic signs. Though typically noninflammatory, a variant form characterized by prominent inflammation exists. Surgery (lamellar graft) can preserve corneal integrity and is indicated when conventional options fail to maintain vision or if perforation is imminent. Perforations are rare but can result in significant vision loss (Table).

▶ Although clinical findings and progression have been well documented in Terrien marginal degeneration, many questions remain such as the underlying etiology, role of inflammation, need for surgical management, and outcome in these patients. The authors of this retrospective review shed some light on these and other issues with Terrien marginal degeneration.

In this review of 43 eyes in 25 patients, a slight male predilection was noted with an average age of 44 years (with a wide range of 20-82). Bilateral disease was noted in 72% of patients. The patients with unilateral disease on initial presentation had a younger mean age of 30, suggesting they may evolve to bilateral disease over time. Superior or superior-nasal involvement was initially noted with against-the-rule astigmatism. A majority of patients (72%) presented initially with loss of vision, and a relatively rapid progression of astigmatism on topography was noted with 1.68 D mean progression by 3 years. These findings contradict the classic understanding that this is a slowly progressive, asymptomatic condition.

Surgical intervention was performed in 23.3% of patients, with a lamellar keratoplasty being the most common treatment (7 of 10 eyes) as illustrated in the Table. Corneal perforation occurred in 5 eyes, 4 eyes spontaneously and 1 due to mild trauma, and these eyes had a worse visual outcome.

Terrien marginal degeneration is traditionally believed to be a noninflammatory condition, although there is some support for an inflammatory variant.

TABLE.—Clinical Characteristics of Patients With Terrien Marginal Degeneration Requiring Surgical Treatment

Case	Patient	Sex	Age	Eye	Ocular Comorbidities	Symptoms: Decreased Vision	Symptoms: Redness/ Soreness	Topographic Astigmatism: Cyl (D)	Topographic Astigmatism: Axis	BSCVA Pre-op	BSCVA Post-op	Other Findings	Perforation	Surgical Treatments
1	1	M	34	OD	Cataract	+		6.67	175	20/100	20/70	Ghost vessels		LK, P&IOL
2	2	M	50	OD	Blepharitis, cataract		+	2.57	41	20/25	20/25	Pseudopterygium		SK, AMG
3	2	M	50	OS	Blepharitis, cataract		+	10.82	32	20/25	20/200	Pseudopterygium	+	LK, P&IOL, AMG
4	3	M	58	OD	Blepharitis, cataract	+	+	5.59	6	20/40	20/200	Rosacea	+	Rupture repair, aphakia + IOL, iridoplasty
5	3	M	58	OS	Blepharitis, cataract	+	+	8.59	148	20/50	20/70	Rosacea		LK
6	4	M	47	OD	Glaucoma	+		N/A	N/A	20/400	20/400		+	PKP, AMG
7	5	F	67	OD	Scleral thinning	+		13.4	8	20/400	20/80			LK
8	6	F	45	OD	Blepharitis	+	+	20.68	93	20/400	20/80			LK, P&IOL
9	7	F	20	OS	Blepharitis	+		8.47	139	20/50	20/200	Intracorneal cyst	+	LK
10	8	M	20	OS				1.67	59	20/25	20/70		+	LK

AMG = amniotic membrane graft; BSCVA = best spectacle-corrected visual acuity; Cyl = cylinder; D = diopters; IOL = intraocular lens; LK = lamellar keratoplasty; N/A = not available; P&IOL = phacoemulsification and intraocular lens; PKP = penetrating keratoplasty; Post-op = postoperative; Pre-op = preoperative; SK = superficial keratectomy.

Reprinted from Chan AT, Ulate R, Goldich Y, et al. Terrien marginal degeneration: clinical characteristics and outcomes. *Am J Ophthalmol.* 2015;160:867-872.e1, with permission from Elsevier Inc.

A majority of patients (14 of 25 patients, 56%) in this study presented with signs of ocular inflammation, raising several questions regarding both the etiology of this condition as well as the role of antiinflammatory medications in its management. The authors found 10 of 25 patients (40%) had concomitant meibomian gland dysfunction and raised additional questions regarding the role of hypersensitivity in the pathogenesis.

The authors recognize that some of their "atypical" findings, such as symptomatic patients with decreased vision, relatively rapid progression on topography, and majority of patients with signs of inflammation may be related to selection bias seen through their referral-based specialty cornea clinic. Nonetheless, it is important to note the spectrum of this condition. In particular, the role of inflammation should be recognized, and certainly further research is warranted to evaluate inflammation as an underlying etiology, how this may affect the progression and management for these patients, as well as distinguishing features from autoimmune-related peripheral ulcerative keratitis.

The authors recommend earlier intervention in cases of impending perforation, as well as patient education on the need for protective eyewear and risk of spontaneous and traumatic perforation. Overall, the authors did a commendable job in furthering our understanding of Terrien marginal degeneration, and we look forward to additional studies.

P. K. Nagra, MD

Bowman Layer Transplantation to Reduce and Stabilize Progressive, Advanced Keratoconus

van Dijk K, Liarakos VS, Parker J, et al (Netherlands Inst for Innovative Ocular Surgery, Rotterdam)

Ophthalmology 122:909-917, 2015

Objective.—To evaluate the clinical outcome of mid-stromal isolated Bowman layer transplantation, a new surgical technique to reduce and stabilize ectasia in eyes with advanced keratoconus, to postpone penetrating keratoplasty or deep anterior lamellar keratoplasty, and to enable continued daily contact lens wear.

Design.—Prospective, nonrandomized cohort study at a tertiary referral center.

Participants.—Twenty-two eyes of 19 patients with progressive, advanced keratoconus not eligible for ultraviolet cross-linking.

Interventions.—The mid-stroma was manually dissected and an isolated donor Bowman layer was positioned within the stromal pocket.

Main Outcome Measures.—Before and up to 36 months after surgery (mean follow-up, 21 ± 7 months), best spectacle-corrected visual acuity (BSCVA), best contact lens–corrected visual acuity (BCLVA), Scheimpflug-based corneal tomography measurements, endothelial cell density, biomicroscopy, refraction, and intraoperative and postoperative complications were recorded.

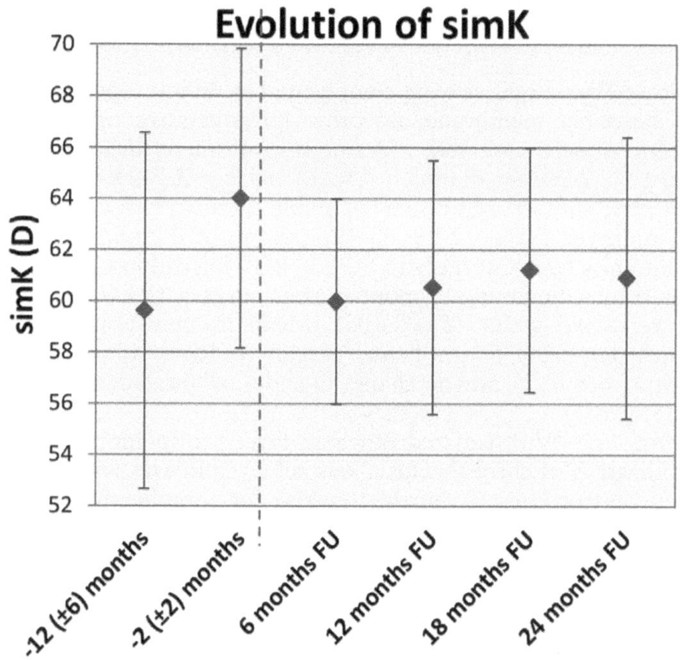

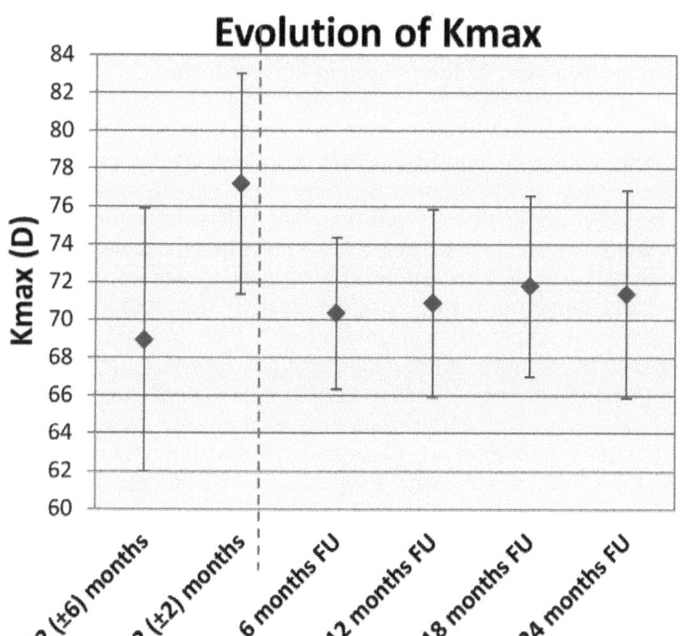

FIGURE 3.—Graphs showing the evolution in mean simulated keratometry (SimK) and maximum keratometry (K_{max}) values. The mean SimK and K_{max} values are displayed. The dashed line indicates the approximate time point of Bowman layer transplantation. Note the preoperative progression, postoperative flattening, and stabilization thereafter. D = diopters; FU = follow-up. (Reprinted from van Dijk K, Liarakos VS, Parker J, et al. Bowman layer transplantation to reduce and stabilize progressive, advanced keratoconus. *Ophthalmology.* 2015;122:909-917, with permission from American Academy of Ophthalmology.)

Results.—Two surgeries were complicated by an intraoperative perforation of Descemet membrane; no other intraoperative or postoperative complications were observed. Maximum keratometry decreased on average from 77.2 ± 6.2 diopters (D) to 69.2 ± 3.7 D ($P < 0.001$) at 1 month after surgery and remained stable thereafter ($P \geq 0.072$). Mean BSCVA improved from 1.27 ± 0.44 logarithm of the minimum angle of resolution units before surgery to 0.90 ± 0.30 logarithm of the minimum angle of resolution units 12 months after surgery ($P < 0.001$), whereas BCLVA remained stable ($P = 0.105$). Mean thinnest-point pachymetry increased from 332 ± 59 μm before surgery to 360 ± 50 μm at the latest follow-up ($P = 0.012$), and no change in endothelial cell density was found ($P = 0.355$).

Conclusions.—With isolated Bowman layer transplantation, reduction and stabilization of corneal ectasia was achieved in eyes with progressive, advanced keratoconus. Given the low risk for complications, the procedure may be performed to postpone penetrating or deep anterior lamellar keratoplasty (Fig 3).

▶ In this prospective study, Melles et al detail their outcomes of midstromal Bowman layer transplantation for the management of progressive, advanced keratoconus. All of the 22 eyes included in this study has documented progression and were ineligible for crosslinking and/or intracorneal ring segments.

Of the 22 eyes, 2 had intraoperative perforation of Descemet membrane, 1 of which did not require additional treatment, the other of which later underwent penetrating keratoplasty. Of the remaining 20 eyes included in the analysis, no additional surgical complications were noted. As illustrated in Fig 3, there was significant initial decrease in mean simK and Kmax readings, followed by stabilization through up to 24 months of follow-up. Significant improvement in best uncorrected vision at 12 months was also noted, although best contact lens–corrected visual acuity showed no change. The flattening of the corneas was associated with a mild hyperopic shift in these myopic patients, as expected.

Although this was a small study, the surgical results of the efficiency of Bowman transplantation in stabilizing progressive keratoconus are promising. Uncorrected vision improved, but unfortunately there was no improvement in best corrected or contact lens–corrected visual acuity. Although the flattening noticed on keratometry readings was significant, the final "flatter" Ks were still steep, and, in association with the corneal scarring and irregular astigmatism noted in the patients preoperatively, would still lead to limited vision.

The real question going forward is where does this procedure fit in our algorithm for treating keratoconus, and in what circumstances should patients undergo this procedure rather than a more definitive penetrating keratoplasty or deep anterior lamellar keratoplasty (DALK)? Larger studies, further evaluating the safety and efficiency of this procedure for advanced, and potentially even moderate, progressive keratoconus, as well as comparing it with penetrating keratoplasty/DALK would provide great insight as to the future role of Bowman layer transplantation.

P. K. Nagra, MD

Long-Term Outcomes of Epithelial Debridement and Diamond Burr Polishing for Corneal Epithelial Irregularity and Recurrent Corneal Erosion

Vo RC, Chen JL, Sanchez PJ, et al (David Geffen School of Medicine at UCLA, Los Angeles, CA)

Cornea 34:1259-1265, 2015

Purpose.—To determine the efficacy of epithelial debridement and diamond burr polishing (ED + DBP) in managing recurrent corneal erosion (RCE) and visually significant epithelial irregularity associated with epithelial basement membrane dystrophy (VS-EBMD).

Methods.—Retrospective, interventional, consecutive case series of all ED + DBP procedures performed between December 1, 2002, and December 1, 2014.

Results.—ED + DBP was performed in 91 eyes (66 patients) for the management of RCE and VS-EBMD. Sixty percent (55/91) of the procedures were performed for RCE, of which 65% (36/55) were associated with EBMD and 22% (12/55) with previous corneal trauma. Forty-six percent (42/91) of the procedures were performed for VS-EBMD, including 6 eyes with RCE. RCE resolved after treatment in 97% of eyes with >3 months of follow-up (mean, 33.2 months; range, 3.5–137.6 months). Corrected distance visual acuity (CDVA) and mean topographic astigmatism improved significantly in the 36 eyes treated for VS-EBMD with >1 month of follow-up. In none of the 22 eyes treated for VS-EBMD with >3 months of follow-up did EBMD recur (mean, 31.7 months; range, 3.2–137.6 months). Surgically induced subepithelial haze was present on last follow-up in 9.4% (8/85) of eyes with >1 month of follow-up, but was not associated with decreased final CDVA in any patient.

Conclusions.—ED + DBP is effective in producing long-term resolution of RCE in 95% of treated eyes and significant improvement in CDVA, decreased topographic astigmatism, and long-term resolution of VS-EBMD in 100% of treated eyes.

▶ As epithelial debridement with diamond burr polishing remains one of the most common in-office procedures, it is important to occasionally review the safety and efficiency of this procedure. The authors presented a retrospective case series of 91 eyes treated for recurrent erosions and visually significant epithelial basement membrane dystrophy (EBMD) with epithelial debridement and diamond burr polishing. In patients treated for visually significant EBMD, the authors found a significant improvement in corrected distance visual acuity. In addition, of the 22 eyes with more than 3 months' follow-up, no recurrence of EBMD was noted. In patients treated for recurrent erosion syndrome, 95% of eyes with at least 3 months' follow-up remained recurrence-free. The main complication the authors noted was haze. Haze was found in the early postoperative period in 21.2% of patients, with 9.4% of eyes with haze at final follow-up. Surgically induced haze was not associated with decreased visual acuity in any patient.

We have also found great success with this procedure. We recently reviewed our results, specifically in the management of recurrent erosion, and found a similar although slightly higher recurrence rate of 14.8% for epithelial debridement with diamond burr. We also found a similar incidence of haze of 22.2% of eyes; haze was deemed visually significant in 12.9% of patients, who were then managed with topical steroids. The haze resolved in all patients and vision improved.[1]

Given the ease of this in-office procedure as well as its safety and efficiency, we wholeheartedly agree with the authors of this study that epithelial debridement with diamond burr polishing is the procedure of choice in the management of visually significant EBMD or recurrent erosion syndrome.

Recurrent corneal erosion (RCE) secondary to epithelial basement membrane dystrophy (EBMD) either acquired as a result of traumatic corneal abrasion or inherited can lead to painful episodes, photophobia, corneal scarring, and, in some cases, infectious corneal ulcer.

Although frequent lubrications with artificial tears/ointments, use of sodium chloride eye drops/ointment, and placement of bandage contact lenses may reduce the severity of the disease and decrease the number of episodes, they do not appear to be therapeutic. Surgical options including anterior stromal micropuncture, epithelial debridement (ED) plus diamond bur polishing (DBP), and ED plus phototherapeutic keratectomy (PTK) offer a more permanent solution.

In this study, medical records of 91 eyes of 66 patients who underwent ED plus DBP were reviewed. In 60% of cases, treatment was performed for RCE, and in 46% it was performed for visually significant epithelial irregularities; furthermore, in 6% of patients, treatment was done for both RCE and visually significant epithelial irregularities. Ninety-five percent of eyes did not have RCE after a mean follow-up time of 33 months. In the group of eyes treated for visually significant EBMD, significant improvement in visual acuities and topographies were observed; this group also had no recurrence of EBMD on the slit-lamp examination.

In my practice, I often offer ED plus DBP to patients with either a visually significant EBMD or RCE secondary to EBMD if conservative treatment with lubricating drops/ointments fails. If there is significant subepithelial and/or anterior stromal scarring, I offer ED plus PTK. Successful outcomes with complete resolution of all symptoms and improvement in visual acuity/quality of vision and topography can be expected in the vast majority of patients with a single treatment.

P. K. Nagra, MD
A. A. Azari, MD

Reference

1. Suri K, Kosker M, Duman F, Rapuano CJ, Nagra PK, Hammersmith KM. Demographic patterns and treatment outcomes of patients with recurrent corneal erosions related to trauma and epithelial and Bowmans layer disorders. *Am J Ophthalmol.* 2013;156:1082-1087.

The Effect of Donor Diabetes History on Graft Failure and Endothelial Cell Density 10 Years after Penetrating Keratoplasty

Lass JH, for the Cornea Donor Study Research Group (Univ Hosps Eye Inst, Cleveland, OH; et al)

Ophthalmology 122:448-456, 2015

Objective.—To examine the long-term effect of donor diabetes history on graft failure and endothelial cell density (ECD) after penetrating keratoplasty (PK) in the Cornea Donor Study.

Design.—Multicenter, prospective, double-masked, controlled clinical trial.

Participants.—One thousand ninety subjects undergoing PK for a moderate risk condition, principally Fuchs' dystrophy or pseudophakic or aphakic corneal edema, were enrolled by 105 surgeons from 80 clinical sites in the United States.

Methods.—Corneas from donors 12 to 75 years of age were assigned by 43 eye banks to participants without respect to recipient factors. Donor and recipient diabetes status was determined from existing medical records. Images of the central endothelium were obtained before surgery (baseline) and at intervals for 10 years after surgery and were analyzed by a central image analysis reading center to determine ECD.

Main Outcome Measures.—Time to graft failure (regraft or cloudy cornea for 3 consecutive months) and ECD.

Results.—There was no statistically significant association of donor diabetes history with 10-year graft failure, baseline ECD, 10-year ECD, or ECD values longitudinally over time in unadjusted analyses, nor after adjusting for donor age and other significant covariates. The 10-year graft failure rate was 23% in the 199 patients receiving a cornea from a donor with diabetes versus 26% in the 891 patients receiving a cornea from a donor without diabetes (95% confidence interval for the difference, −10% to 6%; unadjusted $P = 0.60$). Baseline ECD ($P = 0.71$), 10-year ECD ($P > 0.99$), and changes in ECD over 10 years ($P = 0.86$) were similar comparing donor groups with and without diabetes.

Conclusions.—The study results do not suggest an association between donor diabetes and PK outcome. However, the assessment of donor diabetes was imprecise and based on historical data only. The increasing frequency of diabetes in the aging population in the United States affects the donor pool. Thus, the impact of donor diabetes on long-term endothelial health after PK or endothelial keratoplasty, or both, warrants further study with more precise measures of diabetes and its complications (Fig 1).

▶ Given concerns regarding diabetic corneal endothelial morphology and function, are patients with diabetes acceptable corneal graft donors? This is an especially important question given recent increases in diabetes in the overall population and therefore corneal graft donor pool.

This study reviewed the data from the CDS (Corneal Donor Study) to answer that question. Specifically, the authors evaluated the effect of the donor's

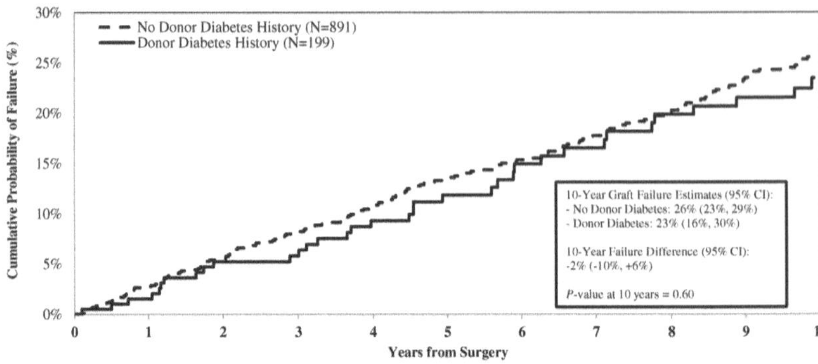

	Years from Surgery										
No Donor Diabetes	**0**	**1**	**2**	**3**	**4**	**5**	**6**	**7**	**8**	**9**	**10**
# at risk at beginning of interval	891	833	771	720	672	601	506	469	432	388	347
# graft failures during interval	24	23	22	19	20	12	14	13	18	10	8
# deaths during interval	23	24	21	19	15	18	17	14	20	2	0
# losses to follow up during interval	4	12	6	9	35	63	5	5	2	2	0
# censored during interval	7	3	2	1	1	2	1	5	4	27	143
Donor Diabetes											
# at risk at beginning of interval	199	191	175	161	153	130	108	102	96	91	75
# graft failures during interval	3	7	1	6	4	4	2	4	2	2	1
# deaths during interval	5	6	9	2	7	4	3	2	3	1	0
# losses to follow up during interval	0	1	4	0	10	14	1	0	0	1	0
# censored during interval	0	2	0	0	2	0	0	0	0	12	36

FIGURE 1.—Graph and table showing graft failure over time according to donor diabetes history. The table beneath the figure presents the number of subjects at risk in the beginning of each year along with the number of graft failures, deaths, losses to follow-up, and censored subjects during the year. CI = confidence interval.(Reprinted from Lass JH, for the Cornea Donor Study Research Group. The effect of donor diabetes history on graft failure and endothelial cell density 10 years after penetrating keratoplasty. *Ophthalmology.* 2015;122:448-456, with permission from American Academy of Ophthalmology.)

diabetes status on corneal graft outcomes and endothelial cell density over 10 years.

Fortunately, the results were encouraging for donors with a history of diabetes. As illustrated in Fig 1, there was no difference in graft failure in patients receiving a graft with and without a donor history of diabetes. In addition, donor diabetes status had no effect on endothelial cell density over the 10 years of the study.

As the authors discussed, there are several limitations to this study. One major issue was determining donor diabetes status. Eye banks are not required to report diabetes as an independent condition contributing to donor death, and therefore diabetes-related diagnoses and/or write-in fields with the diagnoses of diabetes were used to determine diabetic status. In addition, no information regarding the donor's diabetes duration, blood sugar control, and other factors was available.

Nonetheless, this is a reassuring study suggesting donor diabetes status may not influence graft survival. As the authors conclude, as corneal transplantation continues to evolve and with an increase in the donor population with diabetes, additional studies are warranted.

P. K. Nagra, MD

Comparison of ACIOL Retention With IOL Exchange in Patients Undergoing Descemet Stripping Automated Endothelial Keratoplasty

Tannan A, Vo RC, Chen JL, et al (David Geffen School of Medicine at UCLA, Los Angeles, CA)

Cornea 34:1030-1034, 2015

Purpose.—To investigate clinical outcomes in the management of anterior chamber intraocular lenses (ACIOLs) in patients requiring Descemet stripping automated endothelial keratoplasty (DSAEK) for pseudophakic corneal edema.

Methods.—This is a retrospective review of DSAEK procedures performed at a single center between May 1, 2006, and August 1, 2014.

Results.—Forty-three eyes (41 patients) with pseudophakic corneal edema and an ACIOL were identified. In 26 eyes (60.5%), the ACIOL was retained [intraocular lens retention (IOLR) group], and in 17 eyes (39.5%), intraocular lens exchange [(IOLX) group] was concurrent with DSAEK. No significant difference was noted between the IOLR and IOLX groups for the following: the incidence of primary graft failure (7.7% vs. 5.9%; $P = 1.0$); the incidence (3.8% vs. 0.0%; $P = 1.0$) or rate (0.036 per eye-year vs. 0 per eye-year; $P = 0.28$) of secondary graft failure; or the incidence (7.7% vs. 11.8%; $P = 1.0$) or rate (0.056 per eye-year vs. 0.073 per eye-year; $P = 0.69$) of endothelial rejection. However, the incidence (23.1% vs. 58.8%; $P = 0.026$) and rate (0.291 per eye-year vs. 0.475 per eye-year; $P = 0.033$) of increased intraocular pressure were significantly higher in the IOLX group. There were more complications in the IOLX group, although the difference was not significant (7.7% vs. 29.4%; $P = 0.093$).

Conclusions.—There is no significant difference in the incidence of primary graft failure or in the rate of secondary graft failure or endothelial rejection in eyes with ACIOL retention or exchange. However, as IOLX is associated with intraoperative and postoperative complications and an increased rate of postoperative intraocular pressure elevation, we recommend performing DSAEK with retention of well-positioned ACIOLs in these eyes.

► Anterior chamber intraocular lenses (ACIOLs) have traditionally been associated with a higher risk of corneal decompensation and subsequent pseudophakic bullous keratopathy (PBK), especially closed-loop or malpositioned ACIOLs. In the surgical management of PBK in patients with ACIOLs, the decision to perform a lens exchange vs retaining the ACIOL can be difficult. Lens exchange is clearly preferred when the ACIOL is contributing directly to the decompensated cornea or associated with intraocular inflammation (tilted, decentered ACIOL, closed-loop, rigid ACIOL, macular edema, etc). The decision is less clear when dealing with an ACIOL that appears to be well centered and positioned far away from the corneal endothelium.

This retrospective study evaluated this issue by reviewing the surgical management and outcomes of 43 eyes with PBK and ACIOLs. Twenty-six of these eyes had a retained ACIOL with Descemet stripping automated endothelial keratoplasty (DSAEK) alone, and 17 eyes underwent intraocular lens (IOL) exchange with DSAEK. Interestingly, they found no difference in the incidence of graft rejection or failure between the 2 groups. There was a statistically significant higher incidence and rate of elevated intraocular pressure in the IOL exchange group. In addition, more postoperative complications were noted in the IOL exchange group (29.4% compared with 7.7% in the retention group), although this was not statistically significant.

Although this was a small study, it was a well-designed and thoughtful review. The authors specifically evaluated the management of ACIOLs and results of DSAEK in this setting, unlike previous studies, which compared DSAEK with retained ACIOLs to DSAEKs in patients with posterior chamber intraocular lenses (PCIOLs). As the authors point out, DSAEK with a PCIOL is performed in a different anatomic state than is present in patients with ACIOLs and a unicameral chamber, making the comparison difficult. Based on their results, the authors conclude that well-positioned ACIOLs should be retained, given the decreased risk of intraocular pressure issues as well as postoperative complications. Our personal experience has been analogous to that of the authors, in that patients with corneal edema with deep anterior chambers and well-positioned ACIOLs often do well with DSAEK alone.

P. K. Nagra, MD

Graft Failure and Intraocular Pressure Control After Keratoplasty in Iridocorneal Endothelial Syndrome

Quek DT-L, Wong CW, Wong TT, et al (Singapore Natl Eye Centre; Singapore Natl Eye Res Inst; et al)

Am J Ophthalmol 160:422-429.e1, 2015

Purpose.—To describe and compare graft survival and intraocular pressure (IOP) control after penetrating keratoplasty (PK) and Descemet stripping automated endothelial keratoplasty (DSAEK) in eyes with iridocorneal endothelial (ICE) syndrome.

Design.—Retrospective case series.

Methods.—Multicenter study conducted at the Singapore National Eye Centre (SNEC) and Price Vision Group. Twenty-nine consecutive eyes with ICE syndrome that underwent keratoplasty between 1991 and 2011 were identified from the SNEC transplant database and Price Vision Group patient database and the following data extracted: demographics, graft failure, IOP indices, and glaucoma treatment pre- and postkeratoplasty. The main outcome measures were graft failure and need for additional IOP-lowering treatment after keratoplasty.

Results.—The mean follow-up duration was 7.0 ± 4.9 years in the PK group (n = 17) and 4.0 ± 2.6 years in the DSAEK group (n = 12). After a mean of 4.1 ± 3.1 years, 37.9% of grafts (11/29) failed: 7 PK compared to 4 DSAEK (P = .72). The graft failure rate was 50% in eyes with prekeratoplasty glaucoma surgery vs 31.6% in those without (P = .43).

TABLE 2.—Risk Factors for Graft Failure After Keratoplasty in Eyes With Iridocorneal Endothelial Syndrome

Risk Factor	Graft Failures (n = 11)	Non-Graft Failures (n = 18)	*P* Value[a]	Estimated Difference and 95% Confidence Interval of Difference[b]
Age at time of keratoplasty, y	54.7 ± 10.22	55.7 ± 10.40	.776	−9.47<−1.00<7.11
Duration of follow-up, y	7.8 ± 4.4	4.5 ± 3.8	.042	0.1<3.3<6.6
Prekeratoplasty IOP, mm Hg	12.6 ± 3.6	15.8 ± 3.7	.041	−6.2<−3.2<−0.2
Number of quadrants closed on gonioscopy	2.1 ± 0.7	2.0 ± 1.0	.297	−0.6<0.1<0.8
Number of prekeratoplasty glaucoma medications	0.6 ± 1.0	1.0 ± 1.0	.891	−1.2<−0.4<0.4
Mean IOP postkeratoplasty, mm Hg	15.5 ± 3.1	18.7 ± 3.8	.032	−6.1<−3.3<−0.4
Maximum IOP postkeratoplasty, mm Hg	19.9 ± 5.5	24.0 ± 6.8	.113	−9.1<−4.1<0.93
Minimum IOP postkeratoplasty, mm Hg	12.0 ± 3.1	14.6 ± 3.4	.050	−5.2<−2.6<0.04
Number of IOP medications postkeratoplasty	0.6 ± 1.0	1.5 ± 1.1	.029	−1.8<−0.9<−0.1
Ethnicity, n (%)				
Chinese	7 (63.6)	10 (55.6)	.723	
Non-Chinese	4 (36.4)	8 (44.4)		
Female sex (%)	6 (54.5)	11 (61.1)	1.000	
Prekeratoplasty BCVA, n (%)				
6/60 or worse	8 (72.7)	14 (77.8)	1.000	
Better than 6/60	3 (27.3)	4 (22.2)		
Prekeratoplasty glaucoma surgery, n (%)	5 (45.5)	5 (27.8)	.432	
Type of keratoplasty, n (%)				
PK	7 (63.6)	10 (55.6)	.720	
DSAEK	4 (36.4)	8 (44.4)		
Received other procedures during keratoplasty (%)	7 (63.6)	9 (50)	.698	
Received additional glaucoma treatment postkeratoplasty (%)	2 (18.2)	9 (50)	.131	
Received glaucoma operation postkeratoplasty (%)	1 (9.1)	4 (22.2)	.622	

Data presented are proportions or means and standard deviation as appropriate for the variable.

BCVA = best-corrected visual acuity; DSAEK = Descemet stripping automated endothelial keratoplasty; IOP = intraocular pressure; PK = penetrating keratoplasty.

[a]For comparison between individuals with and without graft failure, using χ^2 tests for categorical variables and 2-sample *t* tests for continuous variables.

[b]Estimated difference given by graft failures minus nongraft failures.

Reprinted from Quek DT-L, Wong CW, Wong TT, et al. Graft failure and intraocular pressure control after keratoplasty in iridocorneal endothelial syndrome. *Am J Ophthalmol.* 2015;160:422-429.e1, with permission from Elsevier Inc.

Additional glaucoma treatment was required in 37.9% of eyes (11/29): 41.2% of PK eyes and 50% of DSAEK eyes (*P* =.28) Eyes that had undergone glaucoma surgery before keratoplasty were less likely to require escalation of IOP-lowering therapy postkeratoplasty (9.1% vs 50%, *P* =.03).

Conclusions.—One-third of grafts failed after keratoplasty for ICE syndrome at a mean duration of 4 years and additional IOP-lowering treatment was required in 37.9%. Both PK and DSAEK had similar outcomes with regard to graft failure and IOP control (Table 2).

▶ Corneal decompensation in iridocorneal endothelial (ICE) syndrome can be particularly challenging to manage, given concerns regarding pupillary changes with possible narrowing of the anterior chamber and glaucoma. Endothelial disease is the main etiology of corneal edema, and thus Descemet stripping automated endothelial keratoplasty (DSAEK) would have several benefits over penetrating keratoplasty (PK) for these patients. However, there are few data published on the results of DSAEK compared with PK in the management of ICE syndrome.

This retrospective case series reviewed the surgical management of 29 eyes with ICE syndrome (PK in 17 eyes, DSAEK in 12 eyes). The authors found no difference in graft survival between the PK and DSAEK eyes. However, they did find a higher rate of graft failure in patients with prekeratoplasty glaucoma surgery (50% vs 31.6%), although this was not statistically significant, likely related to the small numbers of eyes. As noted in Table 2, lower mean prekeratoplasty intraocular pressure and fewer postkeratoplasty glaucoma medications were significantly associated with a higher risk of graft failure, likely more commonly found in patients who underwent prekeratoplasty glaucoma surgery. In addition, 37.9% of eyes required additional glaucoma medications postkeratoplasty, underscoring the difficulty in the management intraocular pressure in patients with this condition. Although the authors do not mention postkeratoplasty visual acuity, it would be interesting to evaluate the improvement in vision from prekeratoplasty levels and compare PK vs DSAEK postoperative visual improvement.

Although DSAEK may be more challenging to perform in eyes with ICE syndrome, there are definite benefits of this procedure over PK, including more rapid visual recovery, less induced astigmatism, and improved structural integrity of the cornea. On the basis of the encouraging results of DSAEK compared with PK in this study, specifically looking at graft failure, the authors conclude DSAEK may be the surgical treatment of choice in ICE syndrome.

P. K. Nagra, MD

Relationship between Corneal Guttae and Quality of Vision in Patients with Mild Fuchs' Endothelial Corneal Dystrophy

Watanabe S, Oie Y, Fujimoto H, et al (Osaka Univ Graduate School of Medicine, Suita, Japan)

Ophthalmology 122:2103-2109, 2015

Purpose.—To investigate the effect of the severity of corneal guttae on quality of vision (QOV) in patients with mild Fuchs' endothelial corneal dystrophy (FECD).

Design.—Cross-sectional study.

Participants.—Twenty-three eyes of 14 patients with mild FECD without corneal edema on slit-lamp examination (5 pseudophakic eyes and 18 phakic eyes with mild lens opacity; grade 1.0–2.0 nuclear opalescence, grade 1.0–2.0 nuclear color, grade 1.0 cortical cataract, and grade 1.0 posterior subcapsular cataract on the Lens Opacities Classification System, version III).

Methods.—The area ratio of the corneal guttae (ARCG) in the endothelial cells was measured by multifocal specular microscopy. The QOV parameters, that is, corrected distance visual acuity (CDVA), letter contrast sensitivity (LCS), and intraocular straylight, also were measured. The correlations were assessed between the ARCG and QOV parameters and between the straylight and CDVA and LCS.

Main Outcome Measures.—The ARCG, logarithm of the minimum angle of resolution CDVA, LCS, and straylight.

Results.—Univariate analysis showed that the ARCG was correlated significantly with the CDVA, LCS, and straylight ($R^2 = 0.41$, $P = 0.001$; $R^2 = 0.55$, $P = 0.001$; and $R^2 = 0.39$, $P = 0.002$, respectively). Univariate analysis also showed that straylight was correlated significantly with the CDVA and LCS ($R^2 = 0.47$, $P = 0.001$ and $R^2 = 0.41$, $P = 0.001$, respectively).

Conclusions.—Corneal guttae without edema caused the QOV to deteriorate in eyes with FECD. Patients with higher straylight had worse CDVA or LCS. Intraocular forward light scatter caused by corneal guttae may result in visual disturbances. Quantification of corneal guttae can be useful to evaluate the effect of guttae on the QOV and determine the surgical indications of endothelial keratoplasty for eyes with mild FECD.

▶ Clinically, we have all seen patients with Fuchs endothelial dystrophy without apparent corneal edema who appear more symptomatic than can be explained by their clinical examination. Up to this point, it has been difficult to isolate cornea guttata to evaluate their clinical significance on quality of vision (QOV). This small study, evaluating the effects of guttata in "mild-Fuchs" on quality of vision, attempts to answer the question of what the effect of guttata alone is on QOV.

This unique small study, which included 23 eyes in a mixed group of 18 phakic patients (without visually significant cataracts) and 5 pseudophakic patients, concluded that guttata alone increased forward light scatter and therefore led to visual deterioration. Although this is a plausible explanation, the limitations of this study warrant additional research before this can be definitively accepted.

The several limitations of this study include its small size of 23 patients and lack of control group. There are many other variables in these eyes that may explain the stray-light finding, such as the "mild lens opacities" in the phakic patients and the above-average cornea thicknesses (average of 595 microns in the 23 patients). Matched controls would help eliminate these factors as a source of visual disturbances.

Because of these issues, until further evidence is available, I cannot agree with the conclusion that early endothelial keratoplasty be considered to "remove guttata that affect the QOV parameters." A larger study comparing QOV in well-defined "mild-Fuchs" with a control group, as well as QOV comparison after Descemet stripping automated endothelial keratoplasty/membrane endothelial keratoplasty would help further illustrate whether treating guttata alone is warranted.

Nonetheless, this is an interesting study, taking us a step closer to a better understanding of the visual impact of guttata. As our treatment of Fuchs dystrophy becomes more refined, I look forward to additional studies both demonstrating the effect of guttata and indicating whether surgical management of guttata alone is justified.

P. K. Nagra, MD

Optical Coherence Tomography in the Diagnosis of Scleritis and Episcleritis

Shoughy SS, Jaroudi MO, Kozak I, et al (The Eye Center and the Eye Foundation for Research in Ophthalmology, Riyadh, Saudi Arabia; King Khaled Eye Specialist Hospital, Riyadh, Saudi Arabia; et al)

Am J Ophthalmol 159:1045-1049, 2015

Purpose.—To describe the optical coherence tomography (OCT) findings in eyes with active anterior scleritis and compare the findings to those with episcleritis and normal controls.

Design.—Prospective evaluation of a diagnostic test.

Methods.—We included a total of 30 eyes of 30 patients with unilateral anterior scleral or episcleral inflammation. The contralateral 30 eyes with no active ocular disease served as controls. OCT was performed over the anterior sclera in the inflamed area on all cases. The OCT images were analyzed to determine the thickness of the sclera and the presence or absence of scleral hyporeflective areas representing intrascleral edema.

Results.—There were 17 male and 13 female patients. The mean age was 43 years with an age range of 21–77 years. Eighteen patients had anterior scleritis and 12 patients had episcleritis. The mean transconjunctival scleral thickness was 747 μm (SD ± 68.97) with a range of 616–877 μm in normal eyes, 882 μm (SD ± 87.35) with a range of

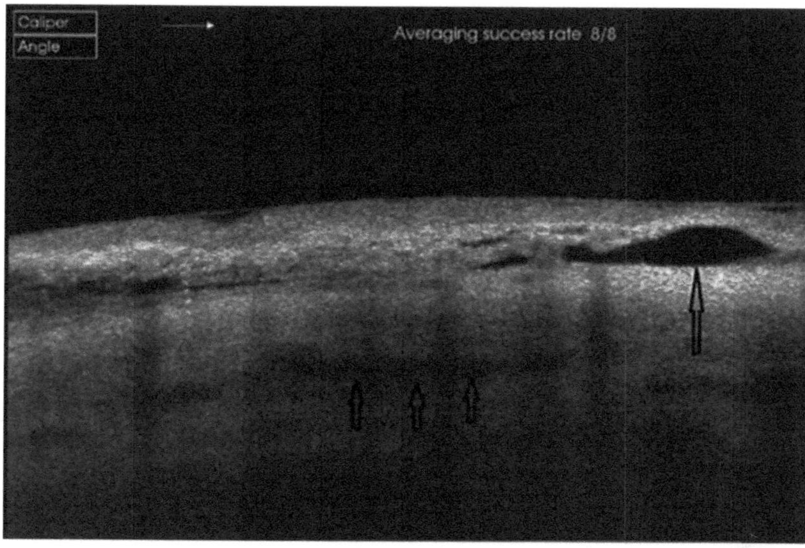

FIGURE 2.—Intrascleral edema in patient with scleritis. Spectral-domain optical coherence tomography section shows hyporeflective pockets in the scleral stroma that represent intrascleral edema in a patient with scleritis (short arrows). Long arrow points to an area representing fluid in the subconjunctival space. (Reprinted from Shoughy SS, Jaroudi MO, Kozak I, et al. Optical coherence tomography in the diagnosis of scleritis and episcleritis. *Am J Ophthalmol.* 2015;159:1045-1049, with permission from Elsevier.)

773–1089 μm in patients with scleritis, and 825 μm (SD ± 85.57) with a range of 718–949 μm in patients with episcleritis.

Conclusions.—Patients with active anterior scleritis showed increased thickness of the sclera and presence of intrascleral hyporeflective areas of edema by OCT compared to patients with episcleritis and normal eyes. OCT adds both qualitative and quantitative information to diagnosis and monitoring of patients with scleritis (Fig 2).

▶ The distinction between scleritis and episcleritis can pose a great clinical challenge in some instances. Diagnosis is often made by a combination of clinical signs and symptoms, but unfortunately, there has been a paucity of objective tests to reliably distinguish the 2 entities. The distinction between episcleritis and scleritis is very important. Scleritis is associated with systemic conditions that may be life threatening in some instances; in addition, treatment of scleritis often requires a prolonged course of systemic medication, such as steroids and/or other immune-modulating agents.

The authors of this study reviewed the structure of the sclera using anterior segment optical coherence tomography (OCT) in 18 patients with diagnosis of scleritis and 12 patients with diagnosis of episcleritis. They used the patient's fellow uninvolved eye as control. The authors found that the sclera in eyes with scleritis were thicker than the sclera in eyes with episcleritis or normal eyes. However, the most interesting OCT feature in eyes with scleritis was the presence of hyporeflective pockets in the scleral stroma. The authors postulated that the hyporeflective areas represent edema secondary to local scleral inflammation (Fig 2). In addition, they observed that upon treatment and resolution of the scleritis, the scleral thickness returned to normal and the intrastromal hyporeflective areas disappeared.

In many instances, distinction between episcleritis and scleritis scan be made based on patient history and clinical examination. However, in some cases, it is difficult to distinguish the 2 entities. In those cases, anterior segment OCT can serve as a great diagnostic tool.

A. A. Azari, MD

Visual Recovery and Endothelial Cell Survival After Descemet Stripping Automated Endothelial Keratoplasty for Failed Penetrating Keratoplasty Grafts—A Cohort Study

Tarantino-Scherrer JN, Kaufmann C, Bochmann F, et al (Cantonal Hosp of Lucerne, Switzerland; et al)

Cornea 34:1024-1029, 2015

Purpose.—To assess visual recovery and donor cell survival after Descemet stripping automated endothelial keratoplasty (DSAEK) for the repair of failed penetrating keratoplasty (PK) grafts.

Methods.—Best spectacle-corrected Snellen visual acuity results after DSAEK were compared with best-ever documented visual acuity (BDVA) results obtained with the previous PK graft in a prospective cohort study. Donor cell survival after DSAEK for PK repair was compared with cell survival after DSAEK for Fuchs endothelial dystrophy and pseudophakic bullous keratopathy. Differences in the logMAR best spectacle-corrected Snellen visual acuity and endothelial cell loss rates were calculated.

Results.—Twenty-eight eyes with DSAEK for PK repair were identified, 21 of which lacked vision-limiting comorbidities. The mean follow-up was 18.4 ± 10.6 months. At 3 months postoperatively, 10/21 eyes (48%) regained their BDVA. By 24 months, only 14% remained with 0.2 logMAR below their BDVA. Endothelial cell counts decreased significantly faster in patients with DSAEK for failed PK ($P = 0.024$) or pseudophakic bullous keratopathy ($P = 0.018$) than in patients with DSAEK for Fuchs endothelial dystrophy.

Conclusions.—DSAEK for the restoration of failed PK grafts promotes rapid visual recovery within the visual limits of the previous PK graft. Increased endothelial cell loss is noted relative to other DSAEK indications, which may result in earlier endothelial graft failure in renovated PK.

▶ Successful outcome of DSAEK in cases of failed penetrating keratoplasty (PK) has been reported in the literature. This method offers a quicker visual recovery and avoids an open sky procedure by only replacing the diseased layer of the failed graft. The authors of this article retrospectively reviewed 28 eyes that underwent DSAEK for failed PK. The authors discovered that there was an improvement in the visual acuity in all eyes in which grafting was performed to improve vision. By 6 months, 45% of patients achieved best corrected visual acuity of their previous PK, and 65% of patients achieved this by 1 year.

Authors of this article also compared the endothelial cell loss in DSAEK for failed PK, DSAEK for PBK, and DSAEK for Fuchs dystrophy. They found significantly greater endothelial cell loss in the group of patients that underwent DSAEK for failed PK and those who underwent DSEK for PBK compared to the group of patients that underwent DSAEK for Fuchs. The cell loss in DSAEK for failed PK was thought not to be surgically induced because the endothelial cell loss at 1 month was not significant.

This study demonstrates that DSAEK under PK is an effective method in recovering patient's preoperative visual acuity but the graft may suffer a significant loss of endothelial cells. As mentioned here, there are inherent advantages to DSAEK, including faster visual recovery, avoidance of an open sky procedure, and elimination of suture-induced astigmatism. However, not every patient is a good candidate for DSAEK under PK; examples of poor candidates include phakic patients, those with AC aqueous shunt devices, presence of anterior chamber intraocular lens, and patients with a high degree of astigmatism related to their PK. These patients may benefit more from a repeat PK.

A. A. Azari, MD

Potency and Sterility of Fortified Tobramycin, Fortified Vancomycin, and Moxifloxacin at 4, 24, and 35°C for 14 Days

Montes JA, Johnson D, Jorgensen J, et al (Univ of Texas Health Science Ctr at San Antonio)

Cornea 35:122-126, 2016

Purpose.—To assess the potency and sterility of ophthalmic antibiotic drops commonly used in the treatment of bacterial keratitis.

Methods.—This was a basic investigation. Three drugs were tested: fortified vancomycin 25 mg/mL, fortified tobramycin 14 mg/mL, and moxifloxacin 5 mg/mL. A bottle of each was stored separately at 4, 24, and 35°C, with the potency determined by microbiological assay at 0, 7, and 14 days. Differences in potency were assessed by 2-way analysis of variance followed by a 1-way repeated-measures analysis of variance with Bonferroni post hoc testing as warranted. Sterility of drugs when handled by patients for varying periods was confirmed by culturing samples on MacConkey and sheep blood agars.

Results.—The concentration of fortified tobramycin and moxifloxacin remained constant over 14 days at the 3 tested temperatures. The concentration of fortified vancomycin remained constant at 4°C, but it declined by 38% ± 1% ($P = 0.001$) at 24°C on day 14 and by 48% ± 1% ($P = 0.001$) and 78% ± 3% ($P = 0.0009$) at 35°C on days 7 and 14, respectively. A total of 49 drops (mean, 7.3 days; range, 1–18 days) were tested for sterility, and all were negative for microbial contamination.

Conclusions.—All 3 drugs remained potent at 4°C for up to 14 days. Fortified tobramycin and moxifloxacin also maintained potency for 14 days at 24 and 35°C. In contrast, fortified vancomycin lost its potency by day 14 at 24°C and by day 7 at 35°C. All in-use antibiotic drops tested were sterile. The results indicate that patients should be cautioned to store vancomycin under refrigerator or at least under cool conditions.

▶ Fortified antibiotics and fourth-generation fluoroquinolones play an important role in treating bacterial keratitis. When fortified antibiotics are dispensed, patients are instructed to keep them on ice at all times in order for them to remain effective. Many patients are unable or forget to carry these drops on ice all the time. Sometimes the drops are kept at room temperature or even left in the car on hot summer days; in these situations, the care provider must make a decision as whether to have the patient continue using the same drops or replace them with new ones.

The authors of this study looked at the potency (defined as stability of concentration as determined by microbiological assay) of 3 commonly used antibiotics for treatment of bacterial keratitis, which included fortified vancomycin, fortified tobramycin, and commercially available moxifloxacin. They found that both fortified tobramycin and commercially available moxifloxacin remained potent at 4°C (temperature if kept on ice), 24°C (room temperature), and 35°C (temperature inside of a car in a relatively hot day) for up to 14 days. However, vancomycin lost its potency significantly at 24°C by day 14, and at 35°C by day 7, but it remained stable at 4°C for up to 14 days. It is interesting to note that although there was a significant drop in concentration of vancomycin at 24°C and 35 °C, the concentration remained well above the minimum inhibitory concentration values for most bacteria.

This study suggests that it is reasonable to continue using topical moxifloxacin and fortified tobramycin for up to 14 days if exposed to higher temperatures, but fortified vancomycin should be replaced under similar conditions. However, the true efficacy and possible toxicity of these drugs (due to possible changes in PH) remain unknown until randomized clinical trials are conducted.

A. A. Azari, MD

Depressive Symptoms in Patients With Dry Eye Disease: A Case–Control Study Using the Beck Depression Inventory

Hallak JA, Tibrewal S, Jain S (Univ of Illinois at Chicago, IL; et al)

Cornea 34:1545-1550, 2015

Purpose.—To measure depressive symptoms in patients with dry eye disease (DED) and controls using the Beck Depression Inventory (BDI) and to determine the association between depressive and DED symptoms.

Methods.—Fifty-three patients with DED and 41 controls were recruited to the study. DED symptoms were assessed using the Symptom Burden Tool and Ocular Surface Disease Index tool. Depressive symptoms were assessed using the BDI. Regression diagnostics were performed to detect outliers. Linear statistical models and polynomial regression were used to determine the relationship between depressive symptoms and DED symptoms. An independent *t* test was performed to determine differences in BDI scores between cases and controls. Scatter plots were generated and linear regression was used to estimate the association between scores. Logistic regression was used for the DED dichotomous outcome and depression status as exposure.

Results.—Regression models revealed that the association is linear more than quadratic or cubic. After adjusting for age, sex, race, and psychiatric medication, the regression coefficient between DED symptoms and depressive symptoms among DED cases was 1.22 (95% confidence interval, 0.27–2.18). DED symptom scores and depression scores were statistically significantly different between DED cases and controls. Adjusted logistic regression revealed an odds ratio of 2.79 (95% confidence interval, 0.96–8.12).

Conclusions.—This study provides further evidence regarding the association between DED and depression and their symptoms. Prospective studies are needed to understand the mechanisms underlying the association between symptoms of depression and symptoms of DED.

▶ It is well known that in patients with dry eye disease, the symptoms do not correlate well with the clinical signs. This discordance presents a great challenge in the treatment and management of this condition. There has been a great interest recently in research investigating the associations among dry eye disease, depression, posttraumatic distress disorder, anxiety, and other psychiatric conditions. Presence of these conditions might cause patients to perceive dry eyes in a different way than most people do, rendering them more symptomatic.

The authors of this article measured the depressive symptoms in patients with dry eye disease and controls. Fifty-three patients with dry eye disease and 41 normal controls were enrolled in this study. The dry eye disease symptoms were assessed by using the Symptom Burden Tool and Ocular Surface Disease Index (OSDI) tool. The depressive symptoms were assessed using the Beck Depression Inventory. The study found that there is a linear relationship between the dry eye disease symptoms and depressive symptoms. The study also found that patients with dry eye disease and depression have higher dry eye disease symptom scores than patients with dry eye disease and no depression.

This study suggests that treating depression may improve the dry eye disease symptoms, allowing it to be managed with less aggressive ocular therapy. However, based on this study, the mechanism of the association between dry eye disease symptoms and depression remains unknown. It is not clear whether the dry eye disease causes depression or vice versa. Also the possibility of antidepressants causing dry eye disease and exacerbating its symptoms must be considered. Future prospective randomized clinical trials are needed to shed more light on the exact relationship between depression and dry eyes.

A. A. Azari, MD

Risk Factors Predicting the Need for Graft Exchange After Descemet Stripping Automated Endothelial Keratoplasty

Nahum Y, Mimouni M, Busin M ("Villa Igea" Hosp, Forlì, Italy; Rambam Health Care Campus, Haifa, Israel; et al)

Cornea 34:876-879, 2015

Purpose.—To identify the risk factors predicting the need for graft exchange after Descemet stripping automated endothelial keratoplasty (DSAEK).

Methods.—This is a retrospective cohort study. The study group included all 117 eyes that underwent or necessitated repeat DSAEK performed between January 2005 and June 2014 at Villa Serena–Villa Igea private hospitals (Forlì, Italy). The control group consisted of 1033 eyes that underwent only primary DSAEK during the same period. Demographic details, indications for primary surgery, ocular preoperative status and comorbidities, donor endothelial cell density (ECD), and postoperative complications were compared between the groups using univariate and multivariate analyses.

Results.—The prevalence of graft failure necessitating graft exchange was 10.2% (117 of 1150 eyes). In univariate analysis, a diagnosis of Fuchs endothelial dystrophy was a protective factor against the risk of repeat DSAEK. Prior trabeculectomy or aqueous shunt implantation, postoperative graft detachment, lower donor ECD, and a rejection episode were all associated with a significantly higher risk of requiring repeat DSAEK. The presence of buphthalmos, anterior chamber intraocular lens, aphakia, or prior penetrating keratoplasty were not risk factors for the failure of DSAEK. Of these variables, multivariate analysis showed that only prior aqueous shunt implantation [odds ratio (OR) = 5.5, 95% confidence interval (CI), 1.4–22.2], lower donor ECD (OR = 0.99, 95% CI, 0.997–0.999), and a documented postoperative rejection episode (OR = 18.2, 95% CI, 7.9–45.0) predicted the need for repeat DSAEK.

Conclusions.—DSAEK grafts have similarly good long-term survival regardless of the indication for surgery, lens status, or ocular comorbidities, with the only exception being the presence of an aqueous shunt.

▶ Descemet's stripping automated endothelial keratoplasty (DSAEK) has become the transplant of choice in cases of endothelial failure. Failure of DSAEK has been reported to be up to 8.2% in the literature. In clinical practice, it is important to identify patients who are at high risk of DSAEK graft failure preoperatively, inform those patients properly about the risk of failure and offer the alternative surgical procedure (penetrating keratoplasty [PK]) in select cases.

This study looked at 1150 eyes that underwent DSAEK in a 9-year period. Authors identified 117 eyes with graft failure (10.2% of all DSAEK cases). Authors of this study found that diagnosis of Fuchs was a protective factor against graft failure, but presence of aqueous shunt device, lower donor endothelial cell count, and a rejection episode were predictors of graft failure.

Interestingly, anterior chamber intraocular lens did not increase risk of failure, which supports previously published works in the literature.

In my practice I have observed a disproportionally higher rate of DSAEK failure in patients with aqueous shunt surgery, which is in line with this study, which found that patients with aqueous shunt surgery are 5 times more likely to have failure of their DSAEK. Although the success of DSAEK graft is still relatively high in those cases, one should consider PK in eyes with aqueous shunt device surgery that had a previously failed DSAEK graft.

A. A. Azari, MD

Anatomic Predictive Factors of Acute Corneal Hydrops in Keratoconus: An Optical Coherence Tomography Study

Fuentes E, Sandali O, El Sanharawi M, et al (Pierre & Marie Curie Univ Paris 6, France)

Ophthalmology 122:1653-1659, 2015

Purpose.—To define the optical coherence tomography (OCT) corneal changes predisposing to acute corneal hydrops among patients with advanced keratoconus.

Design.—Retrospective cohort study.

Participants.—A total of 191 advanced keratoconic eyes from 191 patients with advanced keratoconus cases were studied.

Methods.—Data collected from patients with advanced keratoconus cases were studied during a minimum period of 24 months of follow-up. High-resolution Fourier-domain corneal OCT (5 μm of axial resolution) and corneal topography were performed every 4 months during the follow-up. Several anatomic features at the keratoconus cone were analyzed with OCT, including epithelial and stromal thicknesses, the aspect of Bowman's layer, the presence of Vogt's striae, and stromal opacities. A comparative analysis between anatomic corneal features in eyes that developed corneal hydrops and those that did not develop this complication during the follow-up was performed.

Main Outcome Measures.—Evaluation of anatomic corneal changes at risk of developing a corneal hydrops on the basis of OCT findings.

Results.—Eleven cases of corneal hydrops (5.8%) occurred in our series during a mean follow-up of 30 months (24–36 months). All of these patients were male and younger (23.7 ± 5.9 years) than patients with no acute keratoconus (32.7 ± 11.3 years). Increased epithelial thickening with stromal thinning at the conus and the presence of anterior hyperreflectives at the Bowman's layer level were significantly associated with corneal hydrops, whereas the presence of corneal scarring was a preventive factor. At the healing stage, a pan-stromal scar occurs, with a significant stromal thickening and cornea flattening.

Conclusions.—Increased epithelial thickening, stromal thinning at the keratoconus cone, anterior hyperreflectives at the Bowman's layer level, and the absence of stromal scarring are associated with a high risk of

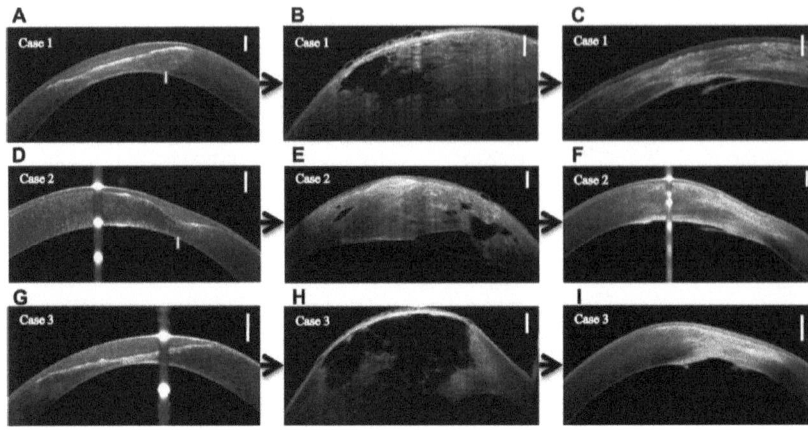

FIGURE 1.—Optical coherence tomography (OCT) scans show the evolution of 3 patients who developed corneal hydrops (before hydrops, acute onset, and healing stage). **A, D, G**, Stage 3a before hydrops; important epithelium thickening, stromal thinning, and anterior hyperreflective anomalies occurring at the Bowman's layer level with clear stroma. *Arrows* indicate Vogt's striae. **B, E, H**, Corneal hydrops (stage 5a); Descemet's membrane rupture with delamination of collagen lamellae, large fluid-filled intrastromal cysts, and epithelial edema formation. **C, F, I**, Healing stage (stage 5b); pan-stromal scarring with a remaining aspect of Descemet's membrane rupture. All scale bars represent 250 μm. (Reprinted from Fuentes E, Sandali O, El Sanharawi M, et al. Anatomic predictive factors of acute corneal hydrops in keratoconus: an optical coherence tomography study. *Ophthalmology.* 2015;122:1653-1659, with permission from American Academy of Ophthalmology.)

developing corneal hydrops. These aspects should be taken into account by the clinician in the evaluation of keratoconus eyes and in the planning of corneal keratoplasty (Fig 1, Table 2).

▶ One of the most dreaded complications of keratoconus is development of acute corneal hydrops, which is characterized by break in the Descemet's membrane and influx of aqueous humor into the corneal stroma, leading to severe pain, corneal edema and scarring, and decreased vision. Furthermore, patients with history of hydrops are poor candidates for the newer surgical technique for this condition, which is deep anterior lamellar keratoplasty, due to difficulty in dissecting the thin and scarred corneal stroma. If a test could identify those patients who are at a higher risk of developing hydrops, early intervention could be implemented, which could potentially, lead to better visual outcome and less patient discomfort and fewer office visits. The authors of this article have addressed this problem by using anterior segment optical coherence tomography (OCT) to identify patients that are at high risk of developing hydrops.

In this article 191 eyes of 191 patients with advanced keratoconus were followed for a mean of 30 months, and the OCT characteristics of patients that developed hydrops (11 patients [5.8%]) were compared with those who did not develop hydrops. The authors classified the OCT findings in patients with advanced keratoconus into 5 stages (Table 2). Patients with stage 3a OCT findings were found to be at the highest risk of developing hydrops, and in fact all the cases of hydrops belonged to this group (11/20). Stage 3a is characterized

TABLE 2.—Optical Coherence Tomography Keratoconus Classification

Stage	Characteristic
1	Thinning of epithelial and stromal layers at the conus. Corneal layers have a normal aspect.
2	Hyperreflective anomalies occurring at the Bowman's layer level and epithelial thickening at the conus: 2a, clear stroma; 2b, stromal opacities.
3	Posterior displacement of the hyperreflective structures occurring at the Bowman's layer level with increased epithelial thickening and stromal thinning: 3a, clear stroma; 3b, stromal opacities.
4	Pan-stromal scar
5	Hydrops stage: 5a, acute onset, characterized by the rupture of Descemet's membrane with delamination of collagen lamellae, large fluid-filled intrastromal cysts, and the formation of epithelial edema; 5b, healing stage, pan-stromal scarring with a remaining aspect of Descemet's membrane rupture.

Reprinted from Fuentes E, Sandali O, El Sanharawi M, et al. Anatomic predictive factors of acute corneal hydrops in keratoconus: an optical coherence tomography study. *Ophthalmology.* 2015;122:1653-1659, with permission from American Academy of Ophthalmology.

by presence of hyperreflective structures at the level of Bowman's membrane, increased epithelial thickening, stromal thinning, and presence of a clear stroma (Fig 1, Table 2). Moreover, presence of Vogt's striae on the OCT of patients with stage 3a was an additional risk factor for developing acute hydrops.

Based on this article, I am more likely to obtain corneal OCT images in patients with advanced keratoconus and offer an early surgical intervention in those that are at higher risk of developing acute hydrops.

A. A. Azari, MD

Effect of Topical Tacrolimus in the Treatment of Thygeson's Superficial Punctate Keratitis

Marquezan MC, Nascimento H, Vieira LA, et al (Federal Univ of São Paulo, Brazil)

Am J Ophthalmol 160:663-668, 2015

Purpose.—To evaluate topical tacrolimus ointment for treating Thygeson's superficial punctate keratitis (Thygeson SPK).

Design.—Retrospective interventional case series.

Methods.—Setting

Institutional practice.

Patient population

Themedical records of 14 patients (9 women; age range, 9–65 years) with Thygeson SPK were reviewed retrospectively. Diagnosis was based on the history and clinical examination.

Intervention

Patients were treated with tacrolimus 0.03% eye ointment instilled into the lower fornix twice daily for the first 2 weeks, followed by nocturnal application. The clinical signs and symptoms were assessed after 1 month of treatment. The drug was tapered with disease improvement.

Main outcome measure(s)

Treatment efficacy and side effects.

Results.—All patients had bilateral disease (average duration, 6 years). All patients, except 2 who used the medication irregularly, had improved visual acuity (VA), symptoms, and signs as long as the medication was applied. Before treatment 28.57% of patients had VA between 20/30 and 20/50, with improvement after treatment to 20/25 or 20/20. Attempts to withdraw the medication resulted in recurrent disease, and, therefore, treatment was not curative during the study period. No significant local medication side effects were reported.

Conclusion.—Tacrolimus eye ointment 0.03% was effective for controlling Thygeson SPK for a long period with good patient tolerance and no noticeable local or systemic side effects. During the average 6-year follow-up, treatment was not curative. Randomized studies are difficult to conduct because of the disease rarity.

▶ Thygeson superficial keratitis is characterized by bilateral raised punctate corneal epithelial lesions leading to foreign body sensation, tearing, ocular irritation, scarring, and decrease in best corrected visual acuity in some cases, prompting the need for treatment. The condition is usually responsive to topical steroids with complete resolution of all signs and symptoms shortly after initiating treatment. Although many cases appear to be cured after initiating topical steroids, some recur and pose a challenge to both the patient and the clinician. Many cases require long-term treatment with topical steroids; however, keeping patients on topical steroids carries the risk of cataract formation and glaucoma. Alternative agents that are particularly helpful in those refractory cases include topical cyclosporine and tacrolimus.

The authors of this study evaluated the efficacy of tacrolimus eye ointment 0.03% in treating patients with chronic Thygeson superficial keratitis (average disease duration of 6 years). They noted complete resolution of all symptoms and improvement in clinical signs in all patients that used the medication regularly. After initial therapy using tacrolimus twice daily for 2 weeks and then daily for 1 month, patients were tapered based on their clinical response. The average treatment period for the drug was 3.2 years in this study, and any attempts to withdraw the drug resulted in recurrence of the disease.

This study establishes the efficacy of topical tacrolimus in treating Thygeson superficial keratitis. Although the drug does not appear to be the cure for this condition, it keeps the disease under good control while it is used. The drug is well tolerated in most patients and does not have the usual side effects of steroids, including cataract formation and elevated intraocular pressure.

In conclusion, topical tacrolimus ointment is a good alternative to topical steroids in cases of chronic Thygeson superficial keratitis refractory to conventional therapy.

A. A. Azari, MD

Re-appraisal of topical 1% voriconazole and 5% natamycin in the treatment of fungal keratitis in a randomised trial

Sharma S, Das S, Virdi A, et al (L V Prasad Eye Inst, Bhubaneswar, Odisha, India; et al)

Br J Ophthalmol 99:1190-1195, 2015

Purpose.—To compare the efficacy of topical 1% voriconazole vs 5% natamycin for the treatment of fungal keratitis.

Methods.—In a prospective, double-masked, randomised, controlled, registered clinical trial, 118 patients with fungal keratitis were treated using identical dosage schedule with either voriconazole (58) or natamycin (60) as inpatients for 7 days and followed up weekly. The outcome measures were percentage of patients with healed or resolving ulcer and final visual acuity at last follow-up (primary) and on day 7 (secondary) in each group.

Results.—More patients ($p = 0.005$) on natamycin (50/56, 89.2%) had healed or resolving ulcer compared with voriconazole (34/51, 66.6%) at last follow-up. The improvement in vision was marginally greater in patients in the natamycin group compared with the voriconazole group at day 7 ($p = 0.04$) and significantly greater at final visit ($p = 0.01$). In univariate analysis, drug, age and mean size of corneal infiltrate and epithelial defect had a significant effect on the final visual outcome. In multivariate analysis, the effect of drug (voriconazole vs natamycin, adjusted coefficient 0.27 (−0.04 to 0.57), $p = 0.09$) was marginal while the effect of age and epithelial defect was significant ($p < 0.001$ for both). In the group treated with natamycin, the final visual acuity was significantly better ($p = 0.005$, Wilcoxon signed-rank test) in patients with Fusarium keratitis but not with Aspergillus keratitis ($p = 0.714$, paired t test).

Conclusions.—When compared with voriconazole, natamycin was more effective in the treatment of fungal keratitis, especially Fusarium keratitis.

▶ Voriconazole has been replacing natamycin for treatment of fungal keratitis in many instances. There is good evidence showing superb diffusion of voriconazole into the aqueous humor and its efficacy in treating fungal keratitis caused by yeast and filamentous fungus. However, some recent clinical trials have contradicted the superiority of voriconazole over natamycin. For example, the Mycotic Ulcer Treatment Trial has shown a benefit of natamycin over voriconazole in treating filamentous fungus specifically *Fusarium* keratitis.[1]

Authors of this study enrolled 118 patients with fungal keratitis and randomized them to either receive topical voriconazole or natamycin using identical dosage schedule. They observed that a higher proportion of patients on natamycin (89.2%) healed their corneal ulcer compared with those on voriconazole (66.6%). Interestingly, of the 18 patients who got worse on voriconazole, 11 were switched to natamycin, and 10 showed improvement. The final visual acuity was better in the group treated with natamycin versus voriconazole; this difference was significant in patients with *Fusarium* keratitis, but it was not significant in patients with *Aspergillus* keratitis. Furthermore, patients who were treated with voriconazole required surgical intervention more often than those who were treated with natamycin.

Based on this study, the presence of filamentous fungus should prompt clinicians to start topical natamycin because it has been shown to be superior to topical voriconazole in several studies including the one cited here. Despite this, voriconazole still remains a potent medication against filamentous fungus, and it should be used in conjunction with natamycin in cases that are poorly responsive to monotherapy with natamycin.

A. A. Azari, MD

Reference

1. Prajna NV, Krishnan T, Mascarenhas J, et al. The Mycotic Ulcer Treatment Trial: a randomized trial comparing natamycin vs voriconazole. *JAMA Opthalmol.* 2013; 131:422-429.

Corneal Fine Needle Diathermy With Adjuvant Bevacizumab to Treat Corneal Neovascularization in Children

Elbaz U, Mireskandari K, Shen C, et al (Univ of Toronto, Ontario, Canada)

Cornea 34:773-777, 2015

Purpose.—To report the outcomes of corneal fine needle diathermy (FND) with adjuvant intrastromal and subconjunctival bevacizumab injection for corneal neovascularization (CN) in children.

Methods.—Medical records of all children who had undergone FND with adjuvant bevacizumab injection were reviewed retrospectively. Treatment efficacy was evaluated by changes in visual acuity, regression of CN, and clearing of lipid deposits with the aid of slit-lamp color images that were taken before surgical intervention and at last follow-up visit. Postoperative complications were recorded and served to assess the safety of the procedure.

Results.—Nine eyes of 9 patients were included in the study. The mean age of the patients was 8.4 ± 4.2 years (4–15 years) and the mean follow-up time was 18.7 ± 12.2 months (5–35 months). Three eyes had a history of herpes simplex keratitis (HSK), 3 eyes had complete corneal anesthesia, 2 eyes had CN following suture tract infection after corneal transplant for HSK scar and limbal dermoid excision, and 1 eye had blepharokeratoconjunctivitis. After treatment, 8 eyes had complete CN resolution, and 1 eye with corneal anesthesia following brain tumor resection had partial regression in vessel distribution and size. Lipid deposition clearance lagged behind CN resolution. Mean duration of CN before treatment was 15.3 ± 14.0 months (1—37 months). Mean corrected distance visual acuity before and after surgery was 0.66 ± 0.31 and 0.50 ± 0.37 logMAR, respectively ($P = 0.02$).

Conclusions.—Corneal FND with adjuvant bevacizumab injection is effective at treating sectorial corneal vessels in children.

▶ Corneal neovascularization in children may be due to several conditions, including bacterial keratitis, herpes simplex virus keratitis, and blepharoconjunctivitis. Corneal neovascularization can lead to corneal edema, lipid deposition, and loss of best corrected visual acuity. Many treatments, including use of laser to coagulate the vessels, intrastromal and subconjunctival bevacizumab, and fine-needle diathermy have been reported in the literature. Most of these methods at best cause a temporary and partial resolution of the corneal neovascularization. Authors of this article reported a very successful outcome with a combination of fine-need diathermy and intrastromal/subconjunctival injection of bevacizumab. The authors performed the procedure by inserting the needle from a 10-0 monofilament nylon suture into the area of corneal neovascularization, then tapping the needle with unipolar cautery achieved blanching of the vessels. This was then followed by intrastromal as well as subconjunctival injection of bevacizumab. Eight of 9 patients who underwent the procedure had complete resolution of the corneal blood vessels after a mean follow-up of 17 months with a single treatment. There was also a significant improvement in the mean visual acuity after the procedure.

Eliminating the corneal neovascularization as described in this article, may lead to decreased corneal edema and resolution of lipid deposits and subsequent improvement in vision, sparing the patients from receiving a corneal transplant. Although this study included pediatric patients, the same results should be expected in adults with corneal neovascularization.

A. A. Azari, MD

5 Retina

Aflibercept, Bevacizumab, or Ranibizumab for Diabetic Macular Edema

The Diabetic Retinopathy Clinical Research Network (Jaeb Ctr for Health Res, Tampa, FL)

N Engl J Med 372:1193-1203, 2015

Background.—The relative efficacy and safety of intravitreous aflibercept, bevacizumab, and ranibizumab in the treatment of diabetic macular edema are unknown.

Methods.—At 89 clinical sites, we randomly assigned 660 adults (mean age, 61 ± 10 years) with diabetic macular edema involving the macular center to receive intravitreous aflibercept at a dose of 2.0 mg (224 participants), bevacizumab at a dose of 1.25 mg (218 participants), or ranibizumab at a dose of 0.3 mg (218 participants). The study drugs were administered as often as every 4 weeks, according to a protocol-specified algorithm. The primary outcome was the mean change in visual acuity at 1 year.

Results.—From baseline to 1 year, the mean visual-acuity letter score (range, 0 to 100, with higher scores indicating better visual acuity; a score of 85 is approximately 20/20) improved by 13.3 with aflibercept, by 9.7 with bevacizumab, and by 11.2 with ranibizumab. Although the improvement was greater with aflibercept than with the other two drugs ($P < 0.001$ for aflibercept vs. bevacizumab and $P = 0.03$ for aflibercept vs. ranibizumab), it was not clinically meaningful, because the difference was driven by the eyes with worse visual acuity at baseline ($P < 0.001$ for interaction). When the initial visual-acuity letter score was 78 to 69 (equivalent to approximately 20/32 to 20/40) (51% of participants), the mean improvement was 8.0 with aflibercept, 7.5 with bevacizumab, and 8.3 with ranibizumab ($P > 0.50$ for each pairwise comparison). When the initial letter score was less than 69 (approximately 20/50 or worse), the mean improvement was 18.9 with aflibercept, 11.8 with bevacizumab, and 14.2 with ranibizumab ($P < 0.001$ for aflibercept vs. bevacizumab, $P = 0.003$ for aflibercept vs. ranibizumab, and $P = 0.21$ for ranibizumab vs. bevacizumab). There were no significant differences among the study groups in the rates of serious adverse events ($P = 0.40$), hospitalization ($P = 0.51$), death ($P = 0.72$), or major cardiovascular events ($P = 0.56$).

Conclusions.—Intravitreous aflibercept, bevacizumab, or ranibizumab improved vision in eyes with center-involved diabetic macular edema, but the relative effect depended on baseline visual acuity. When the initial visual-acuity loss was mild, there were no apparent differences, on average, among study groups. At worse levels of initial visual acuity, aflibercept was more effective at improving vision. (Funded by the National Institutes of Health; ClinicalTrials.gov number, NCT01627249.).

▶ This was a large, randomized, multicenter study conducted by the Diabetic Retinopathy Clinical Research Network that evaluated the safety and efficacy of intravitreal bevacizumab, ranibizumab, and aflibercept for diabetic macular edema. Administration of the anti–vascular endothelial growth factor (VEGF) agent occurred as often as every 4 weeks according to algorithms outlined by the study protocol. The 1-year results demonstrated that there is no significant difference in visual outcomes among these 3 medications when the initial visual acuity was around 20/32 to 20/40. However, in eyes that were 20/50 or worse, the mean improvement in visual acuity was statistically significant in favor of aflibercept over ranibizumab or bevacizumab. There were no significant differences in rates of serious adverse events among these 3 medications.

This is an extremely important trial that reported differences in anti-VEGF agents in the setting of diabetic macular edema. To date, this has not been demonstrated in the setting of neovascular age-related macular degeneration. Obviously, these disease processes are different, especially considering the higher VEGF concentration in diabetic retinopathy compared with macular degeneration. In addition, regardless of the initial visual acuity, the on-label medications, ranibizumab and aflibercept, performed better than bevacizumab. This is also important for treating physicians, health care administrators, and insurance companies to acknowledge.

O. P. Gupta, MD

Darapladib, a Lipoprotein-Associated Phospholipase A_2 Inhibitor, in Diabetic Macular Edema: A 3-Month Placebo-Controlled Study

Staurenghi G, Ye L, Magee MH, et al (Univ of Milan, Italy; GlaxoSmithKline, King of Prussia, PA; et al)
Ophthalmology 122:990-996, 2015

Purpose.—To investigate the potential of lipoprotein-associated phospholipase A_2 inhibition as a novel mechanism to reduce edema and improve vision in center-involved diabetic macular edema (DME).

Design.—Prospective, multicenter, randomized, double-masked, placebo-controlled phase IIa study.

Participants.—Fifty-four center-involved DME patients randomized 2:1 to receive darapladib ($n = 36$) or placebo ($n = 18$).

Methods.—Darapladib 160 mg or placebo monotherapy was administered orally once daily for 3 months, and patients were followed up monthly for 4 months.

Main Outcome Measures.—Mean change from baseline in best-corrected visual acuity (BCVA) and the center subfield and center point of the study eye at month 3 as determined by spectral-domain optical coherence tomography.

Results.—Five patients in the study received intravitreal anti-vascular endothelial growth factor rescue therapy before the day 90 assessment, 2 of 36 (6%) in the darapladib arm and 3 of 18 (17%) in the placebo arm. Administration of 160 mg darapladib for 3 months resulted in statistically significant mean improvements, from baseline to month 3, in BCVA of 4.1 Early Treatment Diabetic Retinopathy Study (ETDRS) letters (95% confidence interval [CI], 2.3–5.8) and of 57 μm in central subfield thickness (95% CI, −84 to −30) in the study eyes. An increase in BCVA of 1.7 ETDRS letters (95% CI, −1.0 to 4.4) and a decrease in center subfield thickness of 34 μm (95% CI, −75 to 6.8) for the placebo group were not significant. No ocular severe adverse events (SAEs) or SAEs considered related to darapladib were reported. One SAE of myocardial infarction, not considered related to darapladib, was reported, and 1 SAE of severe diarrhea was reported in a placebo patient, subsequently withdrawn from the study. Study eye ocular adverse events (AEs) and nonocular AEs were similar between treatment groups.

Conclusions.—Once-daily oral darapladib administered for 3 months demonstrated modest improvements in vision and macular edema that warrant additional investigation of this novel lipoprotein-associated phospholipase A_2 inhibitory mechanism for the treatment of DME.

▶ Anti–vascular endothelial growth factor (VEGF) agents have been primarily explored in the treatment of exudative age-related macular degeneration and diabetic macular edema. Intravitreal injection is the means of administration. This study explores a drug from a new class of medications in the treatment of diabetic macular edema. In addition, this medication is delivered orally. Darapladib is an inhibitor of lipoprotein-associated phospholipase A_2 that was previously used in the treatment of atherosclerosis. The investigators report that the darapladib arm gained more than 4 ETDRS letters and reduced the mean central subfield thickness by more than 50 μm from baseline. This was a 3-month study in which the oral medication was dosed once daily and the results were compared to placebo arm. Intravitreal anti-VEGF agents were administered as rescue therapy. Although the results were modest, the development of alternative therapies to intravitreal anti-VEGF agents is encouraging. These treatments may not surpass the efficacy of intravitreal agents, but they could be used in combination therapy to improve outcomes or reduce the burden of injections.

O. P. Gupta, MD

Anti-Vascular Endothelial Growth Factor Therapy for Proliferative Diabetic Retinopathy: A Systematic Review and Meta-Analysis

Simunovic MP, Maberley DA (Univ of Oxford, United Kingdom; Oxford Univ Hosps NHS Trust, United Kingdom; Moorfields Eye Hosp, London, United Kingdom; Vancouver General Hosp, British Columbia, Canada)

Retina 35:1931-1942, 2015

Purpose.—To systematically review and perform meta-analysis on the available randomized controlled trial data for anti-vascular endothelial growth factor (anti-VEGF) agents in the management of proliferative diabetic retinopathy and its complications.

Methods.—The authors identified randomized controlled trials using anti-VEGF agents, either as stand-alone therapy or combined with other interventions, in the management of proliferative diabetic retinopathy. The primary outcome measures were change in best-corrected visual acuity and (in the context of vitrectomy) duration of surgery and postoperative vitreous hemorrhage. Secondary outcomes were change in central retinal thickness and (in the context of vitrectomy) intraoperative variables suggestive of complex surgery (retinal breaks, intraoperative bleeding, and endodiathermy applications). The quality of evidence for all outcomes was appraised using the GRADE criteria.

Results.—Twenty-two studies involving 1,397 subjects met the criteria for inclusion in this study. One study compared intravitreal ranibizumab with saline, one compared intravitreal pegaptanib to pan-retinal photocoagulation (PRP), one compared intravitreal bevacizumab to PRP, 3 compared combined intravitreal ranibizumab/PRP to PRP, 5 compared combined intravitreal bevacizumab/PRP to PRP alone, and 11 compared combined intravitreal bevacizumab/PPV to PPV alone. When used in conjunction with PRP, there is a high-quality evidence to suggest that intravitreal ranibizumab is associated with superior visual acuity and central retinal thickness outcomes at 3 months to 4 months. In the context of PPV, there is moderate quality evidence to suggest that preoperative intravitreal bevacizumab results in a significant reduction in the duration of surgery, fewer retinal breaks, less intraoperative bleeding, and fewer endodiathermy applications. Although there is evidence to suggest occurrence of early postoperative vitreous hemorrhage is reduced, the quality of evidence in support of this finding is low.

Conclusion.—The use of anti-VEGF agents before PRP results in superior functional and structural outcomes at 3 months to 4 months. The use of anti-VEGF agents before PPV results in decreased duration of surgery, fewer breaks, and less intra-operative bleeding. Although there is evidence for a decreased incidence of early postoperative vitreous hemorrhage, the quality of evidence is low. The available data therefore support the use of anti-VEGF agents as adjuncts to PRP and PPV in patients with complicated proliferative diabetic retinopathy primarily as a means of facilitating, and potentially minimizing the iatrogenic damage resulting from, these procedures.

▶ The medical and surgical management of proliferative diabetic retinopathy is challenging. The gold standard treatment is panretinal photocoagulation (PRP). Pars plana vitrectomy (PPV) is also indicated in more complex cases. However, plenty of patients have suboptimal outcomes even under the best of circumstances. Anti- vascular endothelial growth factor (VEGF) agents are an attractive option in the management of these diseases given that VEGF is one of the main drivers in disease progression. The authors performed a meta-analysis on all randomized, controlled trial data for anti-VEGF agents in the management of proliferative diabetic retinopathy. Twenty-two studies were identified that evaluated the use of anti-VEGF agents in conjunction with PRP and/or PPV. The results of the meta-analysis supported the use of anti-VEGF agents before PRP. At the 3- to 4-month time point, eyes that received anti-VEGF agents before PRP had better functional and structural outcomes compared with PRP alone. In addition, similar findings were reported with the use of anti-VEGF agents before PPV compared with PPV alone. However, the rate of postoperative vitreous hemorrhage following PPV may not be improved with the use of anti-VEGF. Overall, the use of anti-VEGF yielded favorable results in the setting of proliferative diabetic retinopathy. There will be larger, more controlled trials forthcoming that will help outline the role of anti-VEGF agents in this disease process.

O. P. Gupta, MD

Baseline Choroidal Thickness as a Predictor for Response to Anti–Vascular Endothelial Growth Factor Therapy in Diabetic Macular Edema

Rayess N, Rahimy E, Ying G-S, et al (Retina Service of Wills Eye Hosp, Philadelphia, PA; Univ of Pennsylvania, Philadelphia)

Am J Ophthalmol 159:85-91, 2015

Purpose.—To determine the association between baseline subfoveal choroidal thickness and short-term response to intravitreal anti–vascular endothelial growth factor (anti-VEGF) therapy in diabetic macular edema (DME).

Design.—Retrospective, consecutive case series.

Methods.—Fifty-three eyes from 42 patients diagnosed with treatment-naïve DME were treated with 3 monthly intravitreal injections of ranibizumab or bevacizumab. Serial enhanced depth imaging optical coherence tomography scans were used to measure subfoveal choroidal thickness and central macular thickness (CMT). Anatomic response (CMT decrease ≥50 μm) and functional response (best-corrected visual acuity gain ≥1 line) were assessed at 3 months follow-up using univariate and multivariate analyses.

Results.—After 3 monthly anti-VEGF treatments, subfoveal choroidal thickness decreased significantly (225 μm at baseline, 201 μm at 3 months, $P < .0001$). The anatomic responder group (32 eyes) had a greater baseline choroidal thickness (243 ± 15 μm) than the nonresponder group (21 eyes, 198 ± 13 μm, $P = .03$). Similarly, the functional responder group (28 eyes) tended to have a greater baseline subfoveal choroidal thickness (239 ± 12 μm) than the nonresponder group (25 eyes, 211 ± 16 μm, $P = .08$). Multivariate analyses revealed that a greater baseline subfoveal choroidal thickness was associated with a better anatomic (odds ratio = 1.12 for every 10 μm increase, $P = .03$) and functional response (odds ratio = 8.45 for >200 μm vs ≤200 μm, $P = .008$).

Conclusion.—Baseline subfoveal choroidal thickness may help predict which patients with DME will respond more favorably in the short term to intravitreal anti-VEGF pharmacotherapy. In this study, eyes with a thicker baseline subfoveal choroidal thickness had better short-term anatomic and functional responses.

▶ Regardless of the type of macular disease, there is variability in clinical response to anti—vascular endothelial growth factor (anti-VEGF) agents. Identifying pretreatment clinical markers is important for deciding on the treatment and predicting prognosis. This was a retrospective, consecutive series that evaluated the association between baseline subfoveal choroidal thickness and short-term response to anti-VEGF agents for diabetic macular edema. Using univariate and multivariate analysis, the researchers determined that anatomic responders had a greater baseline choroidal thickness (243 ± 15 μm) compared with eyes that did not favorably respond (198 ± 12 μm) to anti-VEGF agents. Anatomic response was defined by optical coherence tomography and vision criteria. Although the theory behind this association remains unclear, similar findings have been corroborated by other investigators. Subfoveal choroidal thickness, macular ischemia, and outer retinal layer function may all be interconnected and contribute to the varied response to anti-VEGF agents in the setting of diabetic macular edema.

O. P. Gupta, MD

Influence of Glycosylated Hemoglobin on the Efficacy of Ranibizumab for Diabetic Macular Edema: A Post Hoc Analysis of the RIDE/RISE Trials

Bansal AS, Khurana RN, Wieland MR, et al (The Northern California Retina Vitreous Associates, Mountain View; et al)

Ophthalmology 122:1573-1579, 2015

Purpose.—To investigate the influence of glycosylated hemoglobin (HbA1c) on treatment outcomes in patients with diabetic macular edema (DME) receiving intravitreal ranibizumab.

Design.—Post hoc analysis of 2 identical phase III clinical trials assessing the efficacy and safety of intravitreal ranibizumab in DME over 36 months (RIDE: NCT00473382/RISE: NCT00473330).

Participants.—A total of 483 adults with vision loss from DME treated with ranibizumab were included in this analysis from RIDE/RISE. Participants received monthly intravitreal ranibizumab (0.3 or 0.5 mg).

Main Outcome Measures.—Differences in visual and anatomic outcomes, and diabetic retinopathy (DR) severity score, between subgroups of patients with baseline HbA1c ≤7% versus HbA1c >7% at 36 months.

Results.—There were 195 patients in RIDE/RISE who were treated with ranibizumab with a baseline HbA1c ≤7% and 288 patients with a baseline HbA1c >7% included in this analysis. The mean improvement in visual acuity (VA) at 36 months was +13 Early Treatment Diabetic Retinopathy Study (ETDRS) letters in patients with baseline HbA1c ≤7% compared with +11 ETDRS letters in the patients with a baseline HbA1c >7% ($P = 0.17$). After adjustment for baseline central foveal thickness (CFT) and duration of diabetes, the mean CFT reduction was −268 μm in patients with a baseline HbA1c ≤7% and −269 μm in patients with a baseline HbA1c >7% ($P = 0.98$; 95% confidence interval, −22.93 to 23.54). The proportion of patients with a ≥2-step improvement in DR severity score was 38% in patients with baseline HbA1c >7% compared with 41% in the patients with a baseline HbA1c >7% ($P = 0.53$). There was no correlation of baseline HbA1c with any visual or anatomic parameter.

Conclusions.—The improvement in VA, anatomic reduction of macular edema, and improvement in DR severity score with ranibizumab treatment seem to be independent of baseline HbA1c.

▶ A variety of studies have linked the severity of diabetic retinopathy with degree of systemic control. In particular, the Diabetes Control and Complications Trial reported an increased risk of complications from diabetic retinopathy in patients with a higher glycosylated hemoglobin (HbA1c). Visual and anatomic outcomes of patients with diabetic retinopathy have also been shown to be superior with lower HbA1c levels. The investigators evaluated the association of HbA1c and outcomes in patients with diabetic macular edema treated in the RISE and RIDE trials. The RISE and RIDE trials were 2 identical, prospective, randomized, phase III clinical trials that reported the use of ranibizumab for diabetic macular edema. The study reported that there was no association between baseline HbA1c and visual or anatomic outcomes. In addition, even in patients that the HbA1c improved or worsened, the visual and anatomic outcomes were independent of this systemic parameter. Future studies could explore whether recalcitrant or recurrent diabetic macular edema is associated with HbA1c control.

O. P. Gupta, MD

Intravitreal conbercept (KH902) for surgical treatment of severe proliferative diabetic retinopathy

Su L, Ren X, Wei H, et al (Tianjin Med Univ Eye Inst, China; Tianjin Children Hosp, China)

Retina 36(5):938-943, 2016

Purpose.—To evaluate the role, safety, and effectiveness of intravitreal conbercept (KH902) injections as an adjunct to vitrectomy in the management of severe proliferative diabetic retinopathy.

Methods.—A randomized controlled trial was performed on 36 eyes of 36 patients affected by vitreous hemorrhage and tractional retinal detachment, which occurred as a consequence of active proliferative diabetic retinopathy. The patients were randomly assigned to two groups. The patients in one of the groups received an intravitreal injection of conbercept in the inferior temporal sector 4 mm from the sclerocorneal limbus with a sterile technique 1 week before vitrectomy.

Results.—In the group without conbercept, intraoperative bleeding occurred in 14 patients (77.8%), and in five of these cases, bleeding was significant. The use of endodiathermy was necessary in 8 patients (44.4%). In 3 patients (16.6%), iatrogenic retinal breaks occurred, and in 1 patient (5.5%), a relaxing retinotomy was performed. Endotamponade with silicone oil was performed in 12 patients (66.6%). In the group treated with conbercept, intraoperative bleeding occurred in 2 cases (11.1%). The use of endodiathermy was necessary in 1 patient (5.5%). No patients experienced iatrogenic breaks or relaxing retinotomy during the surgery. Endotamponade with silicone oil was performed in 2 patients (11.1%).

Conclusion.—Preoperative intravitreal injection of conbercept could reduce the chances of intraoperative bleeding, which are beneficial in the management of proliferative diabetic retinopathy.

▶ Conbercept has been approved in China and is another anti- vascular endothelial growth factor (VEGF) agent for the treatment of exudative macular degeneration. It is a fusion protein similar to aflibercept, and both molecules block VEGF-A, VEGF-B, and placental growth factor. Both ranibizumab and bevacizumab block only VEGF-A isoforms. In addition, conbercept has a higher affinity for VEGF and a longer half-life than aflibercept. Theoretically, this could result in better outcomes with a lower number of injections. In the current study, the investigators evaluated the use of conbercept in the surgical management of severe proliferative diabetic retinopathy. Eyes were injected 1 week before pars plana vitrectomy and compared with eyes that did not receive an injection before surgery. The rate of intraoperative bleeding and use of endodiathermy, iatrogenic breaks, relaxing retinotomy, and silicone oil were less in the conbercept group compared with placebo. The use of anti-VEGF agents in the surgical management of proliferative diabetic retinopathy has already been described. This study confirms that the newest anti-VEGF agent, conbercept, can also be used in a similar fashion with favorable results. Obviously, a highly anticipated study would compare the safety and efficacy of this medication compared with the existing ant-VEGF agents in the setting of exudative age-related macular degeneration and proliferative diabetic retinopathy.

O. P. Gupta, MD

Comparison of Smartphone Ophthalmoscopy With Slit-Lamp Biomicroscopy for Grading Diabetic Retinopathy

Russo A, Morescalchi F, Costagliola C, et al (Univ of Brescia, Italy; Univ of Molise, Campobasso, Italy)

Am J Ophthalmol 159:360-364, 2015

Purpose.—To assess the accuracy and reliability of smartphone ophthalmoscopy, we compared the ability of a smartphone ophthalmoscope with that of a slit-lamp biomicroscope to grade diabetic retinopathy (DR) in patients with diabetes mellitus (DM).

Design.—Clinical-based, prospective, comparative instrument study.

Methods.—This comparative clinical study was performed in 120 outpatients (240 eyes) with type 1 or type 2 DM. After pupil dilation, the patients underwent smartphone ophthalmoscopy with the D-Eye device, followed by dilated retinal slit-lamp examination, to grade DR according to a 5-step scale.

Results.—Overall exact agreement between the 2 methods was observed in 204 of 240 eyes (85%) (simple $\kappa = 0.78$; CI 0.71-0.84) and agreement within 1 step was observed in 232 eyes (96.7%). Compared to biomicroscopy, the sensitivity and specificity of smartphone ophthalmoscopy for the detection of clinically significant macular edema were 81% and 98%, respectively. Smartphone ophthalmoscopy and biomicroscopy could not be used to examine the fundus and grade DR in 9 eyes (3.75%) and 4 eyes (1.7%), respectively, because of cataract and/or small pupil diameter.

Conclusion.—Smartphone ophthalmoscopy showed considerable agreement with dilated retinal biomicroscopy for the grading of DR. The portability, affordability, and connectivity of a smartphone ophthalmoscope make smartphone ophthalmoscopy a promising technique for community screening programs.

▶ Teleophthalmology has improved its accuracy and reliability of detecting and managing retinal diseases. In particular, digital images have been shown to be a sensitive way to detect diabetic retinopathy. In this current study, the investigators compared funduscopic images obtained with a smartphone to slit-lamp biomicroscopy in patients with diabetic retinopathy. All patients underwent smartphone ophthalmoscopy followed by dilated retinal slit-lamp examination. A 5-step grading scale was used to determine the severity of the diabetic retinopathy. There was considerable agreement between the 2 methods. The grade of diabetic retinopathy was exactly the same in 85% of eyes and differed by 1 step in 96.7% of eyes. Moreover, smartphone ophthalmoscopy demonstrated a sensitivity of 81% and specificity of 98% for detecting clinically significant macular edema.

The nonmydriatic camera still remains the most common means to obtain images for retinal screening. Smartphone technology continues to advance and remain a much more accessible means to screen patients that are unable to have a formal examination.

O. P. Gupta, MD

Retinopathy and the Risk of Cardiovascular Disease in Patients With Chronic Kidney Disease (from the Chronic Renal Insufficiency Cohort Study)

Grunwald JE, the CRIC Study Investigators (Univ of Pennsylvania Philadelphia; et al)

Am J Cardiol 116:1527-1533, 2015

Patients with chronic kidney disease (CKD) experience other diseases such as cardiovascular disease (CVD) and retinopathy. The purpose of this study was to assess whether retinopathy predicts future CVD events in a subgroup of the participants of the Chronic Renal Insufficiency Cohort (CRIC) study. In this ancillary investigation, 2,605 participants of the CRIC study were invited to participate, and nonmydriatic fundus photographs were obtained in 1,936 subjects. Using standard protocols, presence and severity of retinopathy (diabetic, hypertensive, or other) and vessel diameter caliber were assessed at a central photograph reading center by trained graders masked to study participant's information. Patients with a self-reported history of cardiovascular disease were excluded. Incident CVD events were adjudicated using medical records. Kidney function measurements, traditional and nontraditional risk factors, for CVD were obtained. Presence and severity of retinopathy were associated with increased risk of development of any CVD in this population of CKD patients, and these associations persisted after adjustment for traditional risk factors for CVD. We also found a direct relation between increased venular diameter and risk of development of CVD; however, the relation was not statistically significant after adjustment for traditional risk factors. In conclusion, the presence of retinopathy was associated with future CVD events, suggesting that retinovascular pathology may be indicative of macrovascular disease even after adjustment for renal dysfunction and traditional CVD risk factors. Assessment of retinal morphology may be valuable in assessing risk of CVD in patients with CKD, both clinically and in research settings.

▶ One of the attractive features of the fundoscopic examination is the direct observation of blood vessels. A variety of systemic diseases manifest characteristic findings in the retina. Most commonly, diabetes, hypertension, inflammatory disorders, infections, and systemic neoplastic processes can be seen in the retina, sometimes before any other systemic findings are seen. Researchers are now looking for clinical indicators in the retina that may serve as a predictive marker for systemic disease. In this study, the prescience of retinopathy (diabetic, hypertensive, or other) and vessel diameter caliber was found to be associated with future cardiovascular events in patients with chronic kidney disease. In particular, the severity of the diabetic retinopathy and larger venular diameter were associated with increased risk of cardiovascular events. These findings add to the growing body of knowledge that retinal findings are associated and may predict systemic disorders. The other interesting application of these findings might be in the setting of teleophthalmology. Patients with an increased risk of systemic medical problems might be readily identified using a nonmydriatic camera.

O. P. Gupta, MD

Treatment outcomes for neovascular age-related macular degeneration patients with initial vision better than 20/40 using a treat-and-extend regimen

Rahimy E, Rayess N, Ho AC, et al (Thomas Jefferson Univ, Philadelphia, PA)
Retina 36(5):875-880, 2016

Purpose.—To determine treatment outcomes in eyes with neovascular age-related macular degeneration having visual acuity better than 20/40 after 1 years to 2 years of ranibizumab or bevacizumab therapy using a treat-and-extend regimen.

Methods.—Retrospective observational case series. Clinical records were reviewed from patients with treatment-naive neovascular age-related macular degeneration and baseline best-corrected Snellen visual acuity >20/40 treated with intravitreal ranibizumab or bevacizumab for a minimum of 1 year using a treat-and-extend regimen. The primary outcome measures were change from initial visual acuity, proportion of eyes losing <3 best-corrected visual acuity lines, proportion of eyes maintaining visual acuity ≥20/40, change from baseline central retinal thickness, and mean number of injections after 1 years and 2 years of follow-up.

Results.—A total of 42 eyes from 40 patients were included. The mean follow-up period was 1.44 years. The mean initial logMAR visual acuity was 0.226, and remained stable at 0.257 and 0.267 after 1 years and 2 years of follow-up, respectively. At baseline, mean central retinal thickness was 305.8 μm, improved to 272.6 μm after 1 year of treatment ($P < 0.001$), and remained stable at 266.2 μm ($P = 0.015$) after 2 years. At 1 year follow-up period, 94.4% of eyes had lost less than 3 Snellen lines, and 94.1% of eyes lost less than 3 Snellen lines after 2 years. The percentage of eyes maintaining visual acuity ≥20/40 was 81% and 75% after each year. Eyes received on average 7.8 injections during the first year of treatment and 6.1 injections over the second year.

Conclusion.—Eyes with neovascular age-related macular degeneration presenting with initial visual acuity better than 20/40 on average maintained vision, lost less than 3 lines of acuity, and achieved anatomical improvements using a treat-and-extend regimen over a 2 year period.

▶ We have been fortunate that anti-vascular endothelial growth factor (VEGF) agents for exudative age-related macular degeneration have resulted in excellent visual acuities despite having poor pretreatment visions. The current study evaluates the treat and extend regimen in patients with vision better than 20/40 at baseline. The minimum follow-up was 1 year and the mean follow-up period was 1.44 years. At 1 year, 81% maintained 20/40 or better vision and at 2 years, it dropped slightly to 75%. An average of 7.8 injections were administered the first year and 6.1 injections in the second year. Overall, the results are favorable. Regardless of the treatment regimen utilized, unfortunately an underlying theme is that there is a component of this disease process that is not met by current anti-VEGF agents. In particular, almost 20% of patients could not maintain 20/40 vision at 1 year and rate increased to 25% at 2 years. Despite being treated with a regimen that minimizes injections and eliminates all signs of exudation as quickly as possible, a proportion of eyes with exudative macular degeneration will lose vision due to an unaddressed need in our current therapy.

O. P. Gupta, MD

Treatment of exudative age-related macular degeneration with ranibizumab combined with ketorolac eyedrops or photodynamic therapy

Semeraro F, Russo A, Delcassi L, et al (Univ of Brescia, Italy; Humanitas Clinical Inst, Milan, Italy; Second Univ of Naples, Italy; Univ of Molise, Campobasso, Italy)

Retina 35:1547-1554, 2015

Purpose.—To evaluate whether ketorolac eyedrops plus intravitreal ranibizumab (IVR) or verteporfin photodynamic therapy plus IVR provides additional benefit over IVR monotherapy for treatment of choroidal neovascularization in age-related macular degeneration.

Methods.—This was a prospective, randomized, pilot study in 75 patients with naive choroidal neovascularization. Patients were randomized 1:1:1 into 3 groups: ranibizumab monotherapy (RM), ranibizumab plus ketorolac, or ranibizumab plus loading-phase reduced-fluence verteporfin photodynamic therapy (RV) groups.

Results.—At 12 months, all groups showed significant improvement in both best-corrected visual acuity and central retinal thickness. The mean best-corrected visual acuity change from baseline to 12 months was −0.14 ± 0.52 logMAR (20/73 ± 20/29), −0.25 ± 0.60 logMAR (20/46 ± 20/27), and −0.10 ± 0.30 (20/97 ± 20/40) logMAR in RM, ranibizumab plus ketorolac, and RV groups, respectively. The mean central retinal thickness change from baseline to 12 months was −125 ± 15 μm, −141 ± 21 μm, and −130 ± 15 μm in RM, ranibizumab plus ketorolac, and RV groups, respectively. Both ranibizumab plus ketorolac and RV groups required fewer IVR treatments than RM.

Conclusion.—Compared with RM and ranibizumab plus verteporfin photodynamic therapy, the combination of 0.45% ketorolac eyedrops 3 times a day and ranibizumab in patients with choroidal neovascularization provided superior best-corrected visual acuity and central retinal thickness outcomes. Both combination regimens required fewer IVR injections than RM during the 12-month follow-up period.

▶ Combination therapy continues to be a valuable option in the effort to limit intravitreal injections or improve outcomes in recalcitrant cases. The investigators compared 0.45% ketorolac eye drops three time daily plus ranibizumab, reduced-fluence photodynamic therapy plus ranibizumab, and ranibizumab monotherapy in patients with exudative age-related macular degeneration.

After 1 year of treatment, the ketorolac plus ranibizumab arm demonstrated superior visual and central retinal thickness outcomes followed by photodynamic therapy plus ranibizumab and then ranibizumab monotherapy. In addition, patients in the ketorolac arm required fewer injections compared with ranibizumab monotherapy. Although many current studies investigate high-ticket new drugs that improve outcomes, this study achieves favorable results by using a generic topical drop. Ketorolac has side effects that need to be monitored, but this study provides a good option that can be applied to your next office day.

O. P. Gupta, MD

Long-Term Outcomes in Eyes Receiving Fixed-Interval Dosing of Anti–Vascular Endothelial Growth Factor Agents for Wet Age-Related Macular Degeneration

Peden MC, Suñer IJ, Hammer ME, et al (Retina Associates of Florida, Tampa)
Ophthalmology 122:803-808, 2015

Purpose.—To report on long-term visual outcomes in patients receiving continuous fixed-interval dosing of anti–vascular endothelial growth factor (VEGF) treatment in neovascular age-related macular degeneration (AMD).

Design.—Single-practice retrospective chart review.

Participants.—One hundred nine eyes with exudative AMD receiving continuous fixed-interval dosing (every 4–8 weeks) of anti-VEGF therapy (ranibizumab, bevacizumab, or aflibercept) for at least 5 years. Eyes were excluded if they averaged fewer than 6.5 injections per year.

Methods.—Snellen visual acuity was recorded at baseline and all subsequent injections. Changes from baseline were calculated at yearly intervals.

Main Outcome Measures.—The primary outcome measure was mean change in letter score at 5, 6, and 7 years; secondary outcomes included the percentage of patients with 20/40 vision or better at 7 years and the mean change in letter score at each yearly time point based on baseline visual grouping (20/40 or better, 20/50–20/100, 20/200 or worse).

Results.—Forty-four, 75, and 109 patients with 7, 6, and 5 years, respectively, of continuous treatment were identified. Mean change in letter score at year 5 was +14.0 letters ($P = 3.9 \times 10^{-9}$), +12.2 letters at 6 years ($P = 1.5 \times 10^{-7}$), and +12.1 letters at 7 years ($P = 3.8 \times 10^{-5}$). Driving vision (20/40 or better) was achieved in 43.2% of treated eyes. Subanalysis revealed that the greatest visual gains at 5 and 7 years were seen in those patients with baseline visual acuity worse than 20/200 (+24.5 and +25.5 letters), followed by those with 20/50 to 20/100 vision (+6.7 and +6.9 letters), and finally those with 20/20 to 20/40 (+3.7 and +3.4 letters). Patients received an average of 10.5 injections per year.

Conclusions.—Continuous fixed-interval dosing of anti-VEGF therapy in patients with exudative AMD results in favorable long-term preservation out to 7 years, with vision stabilizing or improving in 93.2% of eyes. Additionally, 43.2% of patients maintained driving vision in the treatment eye at 7 years compared with 10.1% at baseline. Our data suggest better outcomes with continuous therapy over published results with sporadic, as-needed therapy.

▶ Exudative age-related macular degeneration is still being treated in a variety of ways. Fixed-interval dosing was initially popularized approximately 10 years ago. Since that time, other algorithms have been evaluated, including treat-and-extend and as-needed therapy. In the fixed-interval dosing regimen, the treatment interval is not altered despite varying disease activity. In the treat-and-extend regimen, the treatment interval is altered depending on disease activity. In the as-needed therapy regimen, treatment is only performed if recurrent exudation is noted. The current study, evaluated continuous fixed interval dosing over 5 to 7 years of follow-up.

Patients experienced +14.0 letters, +12.2 letters, and +12.1 letters improvement from baseline at 5, 6, and 7 years of follow-up, respectively. Patients received an average of 10.5 injections per year. More than 40% of patients were seeing 20/40 or better. These results continue to be encouraging regarding the durability of intravitreal injections in the treatment of exudative macular degeneration. On the other hand, the mean visual acuity declined between years 5 to 7. This suggests that assuming the exudation remains under control, there is a component of the disease process that intravitreal injections do not address.

O. P. Gupta, MD

Optical Coherence Tomography Angiography Versus Traditional Multimodal Imaging in Assessing the Activity of Exudative Age-Related Macular Degeneration: A New Diagnostic Challenge

Coscas GJ, Lupidi M, Coscas F, et al (Odeon Ophthalmic Ctr, Paris, France; Centre Hospitalier Intercommunal de Créteil, France; Univ of Perugia, Italy)
Retina 35:2219-2228, 2015

Purpose.—To compare optical coherence tomography angiography (OCTA) with traditional multimodal imaging in patients with exudative age-related macular degeneration in terms of guiding the treatment decision.

Methods.—Prospective case series of 80 eyes of 73 consecutive patients with exudative age-related macular degeneration (39 women, mean age: 79.4 ± 5.3 years) diagnosed with different types of choroidal neovascularization (CNV) (58 Type I, 2 Type II, 6 mixed Type I and II, 3 retinal angiomatous proliferation, and 11 age-related macular degeneration-related polyps). The data obtained from traditional multimodal imaging, based on fluorescein angiography, indocyanine green angiography, and OCT were used to assess the need for treatment, those obtained from OCTA to identify two different patterns of CNV. Traditional multimodal imaging and OCTA findings were then compared with evaluate possible correspondence between treatment decision and CNV aspect on OCTA.

Results.—A CNV lesion was identified as Group A (requiring treatment) in 58 eyes (72.5%) in traditional multimodal imaging. On OCTA in 59 eyes (73.7%), the lesion was defined as Pattern I and the remaining 21 (26.3%) as Pattern II. There was 94.9% correspondence between the Pattern I CNV on OCTA and the cases Group A on conventional multimodal imaging. It was also computed 90.5% correspondence between Pattern II CNV on OCTA and the Group B (not requiring treatment) cases on conventional multimodal imaging. There was high ($P < 0.05$) interobserver agreement both for treatment decision in conventional multimodal and for Patterns (I or II) defining on OCTA imaging analysis.

Conclusion.—This study demonstrates a high level of correspondence, in patients with exudative age-related macular degeneration, between different CNV patterns identified on OCTA and treatment decisions established on conventional multimodal imaging. Although fluorescein angiography remains the gold standard for determining the presence of leakage, and OCT shows fluid accumulation and its variations, OCTA may now offer noninvasive monitoring of the CNV, aiding for each treatment decision during the follow-up.

▶ Optical coherence tomography (OCT) has completely revolutionized our treatment of macular diseases. OCT angiography (OCTA) is also a noninvasive test that generates volumetric angiography images with ability to capture structure and blood flow information. Although the technology is exciting, its application remains unclear. This study compared OCTA imaging to standard imaging modalities in eyes with exudative age-related macular degeneration.

The standard imaging used included fluorescein angiography, indocyanine green angiography, and traditional OCT. The investigators compared the findings in terms of the type of choroidal neovascular membrane as well as those requiring treatment versus those that do not. There was a high level of correspondence between OCTA and conventional imaging in the determination of the type of choroidal neovascular membrane. In addition, very similar treatment decisions were made in these 2 groups. OCTA is an attractive imaging modality to use given that it is noncontact and may soon become more readily available than conventional angiography. However, conventional angiography still provides valuable data regarding the activity of a lesion and resulting leakage.

O. P. Gupta, MD

Association between Antiplatelet or Anticoagulant Drugs and Retinal or Subretinal Hemorrhage in the Comparison of Age-Related Macular Degeneration Treatments Trials

Ying G-S, on behalf of the Comparison of Age-Related Macular Degeneration Treatments Trials Research Group (Univ of Pennsylvania, Philadelphia, et al)

Ophthalmology 123:352-360, 2016

Purpose.—To evaluate the association between use of antiplatelet or anticoagulant drugs and retinal or subretinal hemorrhage in participants with neovascular age-related macular degeneration (AMD) in the Comparison of AMD Treatments Trials (CATT).

Design.—Cohort study within CATT.

Participants.—Participants in CATT with untreated active neovascular AMD (n = 1185).

Methods.—Participants were interviewed for use of antiplatelet or anticoagulant drugs. Trained readers evaluated photographs for the presence and size of retinal or subretinal hemorrhage at baseline and years 1 and 2. Associations between use of antiplatelet or anticoagulant drugs and hemorrhage were evaluated among all participants and by baseline hypertension status using multivariate logistic regression models.

Main Outcome Measures.—Odds ratio for association with antiplatelet or anticoagulant use.

Results.—Among 1165 participants with gradable photographs, 724 (62.1%) had retinal or subretinal hemorrhage at baseline; 84.4% of hemorrhages were 1 disc area (DA) or less, 8.1% were 1 to 2 DA, and 7.5% were more than 2 DA. At baseline, 608 participants (52.2%) used antiplatelet or anticoagulant drugs, including 514 participants (44.1%) using antiplatelets only, 77 (6.6%) using anticoagulants only, and 17 (1.5%) using both. Hemorrhage was present in 64.5% of antiplatelet or anticoagulant users and in 59.6% of nonusers ($P = 0.09$; adjusted odds ratio [OR], 1.18; 95% confidence interval, 0.91–1.51; $P = 0.21$). Neither presence nor size of baseline hemorrhage was associated with the type, dose, or duration of antiplatelet or anticoagulant use. Forty-four of 1078 participants (4.08%) had retinal or subretinal hemorrhage detected on 1- or 2-

year photographs; these hemorrhages were not associated with antiplatelet or anticoagulant use at baseline ($P = 0.28$) or during follow-up ($P = 0.64$). Among participants with hypertension (n = 807), antiplatelet or anticoagulant use was associated with a higher rate of hemorrhage at baseline (66.8% vs. 56.4%; adjusted OR, 1.48; $P = 0.01$), but not size of retinal or subretinal hemorrhage ($P = 0.41$).

Conclusions.—Most retinal or subretinal hemorrhages in eyes enrolled in CATT were less than 1 DA. Among all CATT participants, antiplatelet or anticoagulant use was not associated significantly with hemorrhage, but it was associated significantly with hemorrhage in participants with hypertension.

► The association between antiplatelet or anticoagulation and macular hemorrhage in people with exudative age-related macular degeneration remains unclear. There has been some debate in the literature reporting an increased risk of either retinal or subretinal hemorrhage in patients with macular degeneration that take an antiplatelet or anticoagulant. The Comparison of AMD Treatment Trials (CATT) was a large, randomized, prospective clinical trial comparing the use of bevacizumab to ranibizumab in the setting of exudative macular degeneration. Untreated patients were evaluated at baseline for the use of antiplatelet or anticoagulants and the presence of macular hemorrhage at baseline, year 1, and year 2. Antiplatelet or anticoaglulant use was not significantly associated with retinal or subretinal hemorrhage at baseline, year 1, or year 2. However, it was associated with hypertension at baseline. This is an important trial for ophthalmologists as well as other fields of medicine to understand this relationship.

O. P. Gupta, MD

The Effects of Cataract Surgery on Patients With Wet Macular Degeneration

Saraf SS, Ryu CL, Ober MD (Henry Ford Health Systems, Detroit, MI; Retina Consultants of Michigan, Southfield)

Am J Ophthalmol 160:487-492, 2015

Purpose.—To explore whether cataract surgery contributes to the progression of wet age-related macular degeneration (wet AMD).

Design.—Retrospective cohort study.

Methods.—Retrospective review was performed of consecutive patients with wet AMD who underwent cataract surgery at the midpoint of a 1-year study window. A control arm included wet AMD eyes treated with anti–vascular endothelial growth factor (VEGF) injections that did not undergo cataract surgery for a 1-year period. Best-corrected visual acuity (BCVA), number of anti-VEGF injections, and optical coherence tomography (OCT) features were compared between the 2 arms.

Results.—Forty eyes in the surgical group and 42 in the nonsurgical group were included. BCVA was equivalent in the first half of the study, and became significantly better in the surgical group vs the nonsurgical group (0.23 ± 0.65 vs 0.11 ± 0.59 logMAR improvement, P =.049). There was no change in the number of injections given 6 months before vs after the midpoint in the surgical group (P =.921). The mean OCT central retinal thickness became greater in postsurgical eyes compared to nonsurgical eyes (265.4 ± 98.4 μm vs 216.4 ± 58.3 μm, P =.011). Surgical eyes were more likely to develop new or worse cystoid changes after the study midpoint (13 surgical eyes [54.2%] vs 9 nonsurgical eyes [28.1%], P =.048).

Conclusions.—Cataract surgery leads to vision improvement and does not appear to contribute to worsening of wet AMD. However, anatomic changes based on OCT analysis suggest a subclinical susceptibility to postoperative cystoid macular edema or exacerbation of choroidal neovascularization.

▶ The relationship between cataract surgery and exudative age-related macular degeneration (AMD) remains unclear. In these patients, the visual potential is hard to predict. In addition, the progression of the AMD postoperatively has been debated. The investigators retrospectively evaluated patients with exudative age-related macular degeneration that underwent cataract surgery compared with patients who did not undergo cataract surgery. The visual acuity significantly improved in patients who underwent cataract surgery. In addition, the number of injections was similar preoperatively and postoperatively in the surgical arm. However, eyes in the surgical arm developed new or worsening edema postoperatively compared with the nonsurgical arm. This study adds to the growing body of literature that alleviates concerns of worsening macular degeneration following cataract surgery. Additional work needs to be performed on decreasing postoperative edema. An intravitreal injection timed appropriately before and after cataract surgery may reduce postoperative complications related to the choroidal neovascular membrane.

O. P. Gupta, MD

Noninfectious Vitritis After Intravitreal Injection of Anti-VEGF Agents: Variations in Rates and Presentation by Medication

Williams PD, Chong D, Fuller T, et al (Texas Retina Associates, Dallas, Texas)
Retina 36(5):909-913, 2016

Purpose.—The purpose of this study was to describe and compare the rates and characteristics of noninfectious vitritis after intravitreal injection of bevacizumab (Avastin, Genentech, South San Francisco, CA), ranibizumab (Lucentis, Genentech), and aflibercept (Eylea, Regeneron, Tarrytown, NY).

Methods.—A retrospective case series evaluated intravitreal injections from 2006 to 2013. Cases of inflammatory response were separated into culture-positive endophthalmitis, noninfectious vitritis (not treated with intravitreal antibiotics), and indeterminate. Noninfectious cases were analyzed for rate, presentation, and clinical course.

Results.—A total of 66,356 bevacizumab, 26,161 ranibizumab, and 8071 aflibercept injections were screened. The rates of noninfectious vitritis were 0.10% (67 cases) for bevacizumab, 0.02% (6 cases) for ranibizumab, and 0.16% (13 cases) for aflibercept. The differences were statistically significant based on Chisquare analysis ($P < 0.001$). Mean differences in visual decline were not significant by KruskalWallis analysis ($P = 0.12$), but the percentage of patients with any visual decline did vary by medication according to Fisher exact test ($P < 0.05$). The percentage of patients with complaints of pain, blurred vision, and subjective floaters was not significantly different by medication based on Fisher exact testing ($P = 0.2$, $P = 0.18$, $P = 0.16$, respectively). Bevacizumab and aflibercept cases tended to present in separate chronological clusters.

Conclusion.—The results suggest a difference in rates of noninfectious vitritis for antivascular endothelial growth factor medications. Many cases tended to cluster instead of occurring at a consistent rate each year.

▶ Sterile intraocular inflammation following intravitreal injections has become a well-recognized complication. The investigators reviewed more than 100 000 injections of bevacizumab, ranibizumab, or aflibercept. The rate of noninfectious cases was reported to be 0.1% for bevacizumab, 0.02% for ranibizumab, and 0.16% for aflibercept. The most common complaints on presentation were pain, blurred vision, and worsening floaters without any difference in medication used. Both bevacizumab and aflibercept cases tended to present in clusters rather than a consistent rate throughout the year. Noninfectious vitritis following intravitreal injections is an important distinction from endophthalmitis. This study helps add to the growing body of literature on this topic that is not well understood.

O. Gupta, MD

Association of Compounded Bevacizumab With Postinjection Endophthalmitis

VanderBeek BL, Bonaffini SG, Ma L (Univ of Pennsylvania Perelman School of Medicine, Philadelphia; Erie College of Osteopathic Medicine, Bradenton, FL; et al)

JAMA Ophthalmol 133:1159-1164, 2015

Importance.—Current draft guidelines set forth by the US Food and Drug Administration for compounded or repackaged medications would greatly limit the availability and use of bevacizumab by ophthalmologists across the country. Little evidence beyond highly publicized case reports exists for or against the need for additional regulation of compounded bevacizumab.

Objective.—To determine whether the distribution of bevacizumab through compounding pharmacies increases the risk for endophthalmitis compared with the distribution of single-use vials of ranibizumab from the manufacturer.

Design, Setting, and Participants.—A retrospective cohort study using medical claims data from ambulatory care centers across the United States that were submitted to a large, national US insurer. Cohorts were created using information on 530 382 intravitreal injections administered from January 1, 2005, through December 31, 2012. Any individual from this data set who received an intravitreal injection of bevacizumab or ranibizumab (n = 383 810) and had at least 6 months of data before and 1 month after the injection was eligible. After exclusions (any previous diagnosis of endophthalmitis, multiple injected drugs given on the index day, or intraocular surgery within 15 days of the injection or between the injection and a diagnosis of endophthalmitis), our analysis involved 383 810 intravitreal injections given to 58 612 patients. Data collection and analysis occurred from February 16 through April 7, 2015.

Main Outcomes and Measures.—The odds of developing endophthalmitis after an intravitreal injection of bevacizumab compared with ranibizumab.

Results.—In total, 296 565 injections of bevacizumab were given to 51 116 patients and 87 245 injections of ranibizumab were given to 7496 patients. We found 71 cases of endophthalmitis (49 in the bevacizumab cohort and 22 in the ranibizumab cohort) for an endophthalmitis rate of 0.017% (95% CI, 0.012%-0.021%; 1 case per 6061 injections) for bevacizumab and 0.025% (95% CI, 0.015%-0.036%; 1 case per 3968 injections) for ranibizumab. After controlling for age, race, sex, injection-related diagnosis, and year of injection, we found no significant association with development of endophthalmitis after a bevacizumab injection compared with ranibizumab (odds ratio, 0.66 [95% CI, 0.39-1.09]; $P = .11$).

Conclusions and Relevance.—The results of this study suggest bevacizumab as currently used across the United States does not increase the risk for endophthalmitis; therefore, additional regulations on the use of repackaged bevacizumab may be unnecessary.

▶ The use of compounded drugs has received attention by the scientific and lay press alike. In addition, on-label vs off-label medications in the setting of exudative macular degeneration has been a debated topic. Some have suggested that additional regulations be imposed to ensure the safety of compounded medications. This study sought to determine whether distribution of bevacizumab through compounding pharmacies increases the risk of endophthalmitis compared with single-use vials of ranibizumab from the manufacturer. The researchers used Medicare claims data regarding 53 0382 intravitreal injections of which 383 810 injections met the inclusion and exclusion criteria. The rate of endophthalmitis was 0.017% for the bevacizumab cohort and 0.025% for the ranibizumab cohort. The rate of endophthalmitis was controlled for with multiple variables, and no significant association was found with the development of endophthalmitis with a bevacizumab injection compared with ranibizumab. This study is important given the growing demand for treatment and the increasing cost of care for this disease. Hopefully as we address the concerns of off-label compounded drugs, treating physicians will feel more comfortable with their use.

O. P. Gupta, MD

Benefits of Systemic Anti-inflammatory Therapy versus Fluocinolone Acetonide Intraocular Implant for Intermediate Uveitis, Posterior Uveitis, and Panuveitis: Fifty-four-Month Results of the Multicenter Uveitis Steroid Treatment (MUST) Trial and Follow-up Study

Multicenter Uveitis Steroid Treatment (MUST) Trial Research Group (Univ of Pennsylvania Perelman School of Medicine, Philadelphia)

Ophthalmology 122:1967-1975, 2015

Purpose.—To compare the benefits of fluocinolone acetonide implant therapy versus systemic corticosteroid therapy supplemented (when indicated) with immunosuppression for intermediate uveitis, posterior uveitis, and panuveitis.

Design.—Additional follow-up of a randomized comparative effectiveness trial cohort.

Participants.—Two hundred fifty-five patients with intermediate uveitis, posterior uveitis, or panuveitis randomized to implant or systemic therapy.

Main Outcome Measures.—Best-corrected visual acuity (BCVA), visual field mean deviation (MD), activity of uveitis, and presence of macular edema (per reading center grading) ascertained prospectively.

Methods.—Trial participants were followed-up for 54 months from original randomization.

Results.—The visual function trajectory in uveitic eyes demonstrated a similar ($P = 0.73$) degree of modest (not statistically significant) improvement from baseline to 54 months in both groups (mean improvement in BCVA at 54 months, 2.4 and 3.1 letters in the implant and systemic groups, respectively). Many had excellent initial visual acuity, limiting the potential for improvement. The mean automated perimetry MD score remained similar to baseline throughout 48 months of follow-up in both groups. Overall control of inflammation was superior in the implant group at every time point assessed ($P < 0.016$), although most eyes in the systemic therapy arm also showed substantial improvement, achieving complete control or low levels of inflammation. Although macular edema improved significantly more often with implant treatment within the first 6 months, the systemic group gradually improved over time such that the proportions with macular edema converged in the 2 groups by 36 months and overlapped thereafter ($P = 0.41$ at 48 months).

Conclusions.—Visual outcomes of fluocinolone acetonide implant and systemic treatment for intermediate uveitis, posterior uveitis, and panuveitis were similarly favorable through 54 months. The implant maintained a clear advantage in controlling inflammation through 54 months. Nevertheless, with systemic therapy, most patients also experienced greatly improved inflammatory status. Macular edema improved equally with longer follow-up. Based on cost effectiveness and side-effect considerations, systemic therapy may be indicated as the initial treatment for many bilateral uveitis cases. However, implant therapy is a reasonable alternative, especially for unilateral cases and when systemic therapy is not feasible or is not successful.

▶ Recurrent inflammation can often occur in the setting of intermediate uveitis, posterior uveitis, and panuveitis. In patients who are already on immunomodulatory therapy, the use of local or systemic therapy remains unclear. The MUST trial evaluated the use of fluocinolone acetonide implant (RETISERT) compared with systemic corticosteroid therapy. This was a 54-month study with 255 patients with recurrent inflammation, and patients were randomized to implant or systemic steroids. The overall control of inflammation and macular edema improved more significantly in the implant group compared with systemic steroids. The systemic steroid arm eventually achieved control of inflammation and macular edema, although at a slower rate. This study demonstrates superior performance of local therapy compared with systemic therapy in patients with recurrent inflammation who are already on immunosuppression. Systemic therapy still may be the treatment of choice in patients with bilateral cases or cost considerations, whereas implant therapy might be more appropriate in unilateral cases.

O. P. Gupta, MD

Characteristics and long-term outcome of patients with noninfectious retinal vasculitis

Shulman S, Kramer M, Amer R, et al (Tel Aviv Univ, Israel; Hebrew Univ of Jerusalem, Israel)

Retina 35:2633-2640, 2015

Purpose.—To investigate the characteristics and long-term outcome of patients with noninfectious retinal vasculitis.

Methods.—This was a retrospective multicenter study. Main outcome measures included patients' characteristics, ocular findings, treatment modalities, and best-corrected visual acuity. All patients had at least 12-month follow-up time.

Results.—Eighty-two eyes (45 patients) were included. Median follow-up was 46 months (range, 12-210 months). At presentation, 12 of the 45 patients (26.6%) had a known associated systemic or ocular disease. A diagnosis of a new systemic disease was found in additional 14 of 33 patients (42.5%) and birdshot chorioretinopathy in 3 of 33 patients (9.1%). The most common systemic disease was Behcet disease (17/24 patients 70.8%). Laboratory tests had a low diagnostic value. The most common clinical findings were vitritis (58.5%) and perivascular sheathing (50.5%). Most patients were treated with immunosuppressive medications. Mean best-corrected visual acuity improved significantly during follow-up, patients with Behcet disease and worse visual acuity at baseline were more likely to have visual acuity improvement ($P < 0.001$).

Conclusion.—A new systemic or ocular disease associated with retinal vasculitis was found in more than half of the patients. Behcet disease was the most common newly diagnosed disease. Specific diagnosis leading to proper management is important to maintain favorable long-term visual outcome.

▶ Occasionally retinal vasculitis is observed in the setting of uveitis. Syphilis and tuberculosis are 2 more common infectious causes of vasculitis. The investigators in this study evaluated causes of noninfectious cases. Behcet disease, lupus, and sarcoid were often discovered systemically. Birdshot chorioretinopathy, multiple myeloma, and Crohn disease were also causes. Collectively, approximately 64% of patients in this 45-patient cohort ultimately had an underlying disease. The remaining 36% of cases were defined as idiopathic. In conclusion, in patients who present with retinal vasculitis, a large proportion of patients with have an underlying systemic cause.

O. P. Gupta, MD

Pars Plana Vitrectomy for Symptomatic Epiretinal Membranes in Eyes with 20/50 or Better Preoperative Visual Acuity

Lehpamer BP, Carvounis PE (Baylor College of Medicine, Houston, TX)
Retina 35:1822-1827, 2015

Purpose.—To evaluate pars plana vitrectomy with membrane peel for symptomatic epiretinal membranes in eyes with preoperative best-corrected visual acuity of 20/50 or better.

Methods.—Patients with symptomatic epiretinal membrane and 20/50 or better vision who underwent pars plana vitrectomy with membrane peel by a single surgeon at our institution between January 2007 and January 2014 were identified. The principal outcomes measured were best-corrected visual acuity and central subfield macular thickness at 1, 6, and 12 months of follow-up. Subjective improvement in patient symptoms and complications were also documented.

Results.—Thirty-three eyes of 33 consecutive patients were included in this retrospective case series. Mean preoperative best-corrected visual acuity was 20/40 and improved to 20/28 ($P = 0.00008$) at Month 12. Mean central subfield macular thickness improved from 437 μm preoperatively to 391 μm by Month 1 ($P = 0.00006$) and 388 μm at 12 months ($P = 0.00142$). Seventy-three percent (24 of 33) of patients (95% confidence interval: 55.6-85.1%) reported improvement of visual symptoms during the follow-up period. Of the 13 patients who were phakic preoperatively, 6 patients (46.1%, 95% confidence interval: 23.2-70.9%) underwent phacoemulsification surgery within 1 year of vitrectomy.

Conclusion.—Patients experienced a gradual gain in acuity and improvement of symptoms after pars plana vitrectomy with membrane peel. Cataract progression necessitating cataract surgery is common in phakic patients.

▶ There have been some traditional guidelines for the management of surgical diseases. The threshold to pursue vitrectomy has been lowered due instrument advancement and increased safety. In particular, patients with good visual acuity were previously not operated on regardless of symptoms because the higher rate of complications with vitrectomy. The current study evaluated the outcomes in eyes undergoing pars plana vitrectomy for symptomatic epiretinal membranes that have a preoperative visual acuity of 20/50 or better. This was a retrospective chart review of 33 eyes in which small incision pars plana vitrectomy was performed by a single surgeon. The mean preoperative visual acuity was 20/40 and improved to a mean postoperative visual acuity of 20/28 at 1 year. There was an improvement mean central subfield macular thickness and symptoms. Approximately 46% of patients that were phakic developed a visually significant cataract and underwent surgery. Most of these findings are to be expected. However, this study challenges some of the traditional preoperative guidelines that base surgical intervention on preoperative visual acuity.

O. Gupta, MD

6 Uveitis

Late in-the-bag intraocular lens dislocation in patients with uveitis

Steeples LR, Jones NP (Central Manchester Univ Hosps NHS Foundation Trust, United Kingdom)

Br J Ophthalmol 99;1206-1210, 2015

Background.—Late in-the-bag intraocular lens (IOL) dislocation is an unusual complication of cataract surgery, being strongly associated with pseudoexfoliation, less so with previous vitreoretinal surgery, myopia and uveitis. We present the clinical features, management and outcomes of late spontaneous IOL dislocation in a series of patients with uveitis.

Methods.—A retrospective case series of IOL dislocation affecting patients in the Manchester Uveitis Clinic, UK. The uveitis diagnosis, IOL type, presentation and management are discussed.

Results.—Six patients from out of 1056 undergoing cataract surgery (0.57%) were affected. Uveitis was the only identified risk factor for IOL dislocation, which occurred a mean 10.3 years following uncomplicated cataract surgery by phakoemulsification with endocapsular IOL implantation. The dislocation was in-the-bag in all six cases. Two patients presented with the IOL in the anterior chamber, and required removal of the IOL-bag complex, and are using aphakic refractive correction. Two patients with inferior IOL subluxation have been managed conservatively. Two patients underwent pars plana vitrectomy with sutureless scleral fixation of the existing IOL in one case, and IOL exchange with a scleral sutured IOL in the other.

Conclusions.—IOL dislocation is an uncommon late complication in patients with uveitis. Conservative management is appropriate in patients with tolerable symptoms, or in those with difficult uveitis. Otherwise, fixation of the existing IOL, or removal and implantation of a secondary IOL, may be necessary. Angle-supported, or iris-enclaved IOLs, are not of proven safety in this patient group; scleral-fixated posterior chamber IOLs are the favoured approach in our service.

► It has long been recognized that cataract surgery in patients with uveitis is associated with an increased risk of complications compared to cataract surgery in patients without uveitis.[1] Intraoperative risks include small pupils secondary to posterior synechiae or atrophic pupils, eccentric or improperly sized capsulorhexis, torn anterior capsule, ruptured posterior capsule, asymmetric intraocular lens fixation, lens subluxation or dislocation, corneal edema, and poor wound closure. Postoperatively, there is a higher risk of macular edema, vitreous prolapse, infection, and glaucoma. Nonetheless, improvements in phacoemulsification technology and the use of capsular stains and pupil expanders have improved the outcome in this subset of patients. Less appreciated is the long-term risk of subluxation of the intraocular lens (IOL) within the capsular bag following initially successful surgery.

In this study from Manchester, England, the authors undertook a retrospective analysis of more than 1000 patients with uveitis who underwent uncomplicated cataract extraction with IOL implantation (no zonular dehiscence or intraocular complications reported). Six (0.57%) of the patients suffered dislocated IOLs. No standardized approach to correction of the dislocated IOLs was undertaken. Two lenses dislocated into the anterior chamber and required removal with aphakic correction. Two lenses with only inferior subluxation were managed conservatively, and 2 patients underwent pars plana vitrectomy, with sutureless scleral fixation of the existing IOL in 1 case and IOL exchange with a scleral sutured IOL in the other. The authors noted that in all cases, the capsular bag was fibrotic, and there was capsular phimosis, both of which might contribute to zonular stress. Visual outcomes were generally good, with most patients having significantly improved vision after surgery and most comparable to best-corrected acuity before dislocation.

IOL dislocation is an uncommon but potentially dangerous complication after successful in-the-bag IOL fixation. Various techniques have been described to reposition or replace these dislocated lenses,[2-4] but some of these techniques are not applicable in certain cases (eg, iris fixation of a 1-piece IOL).

The authors point out the many causes of late onset in-the-bag IOL dislocation, including high myopia, trauma, pseudoexfoliation, vitreoretinal surgery, and retinitis pigmentosa. To this list clinicians should certainly add uveitis. However, it is not clear from this study (given the small number of events) what role the type, duration, or severity of uveitis plays. Nonetheless, patients should be reminded that late complications can occur, even after resolution of the uveitis and that they should notify their ophthalmologist promptly if they develop monocular diplopia or other severe vision loss. Given that uveitic cataract surgery is often performed in younger patients, the authors reasonably suggest that late-onset (more than 5 years after surgery) IOL dislocation should be included as part of the patient consent for surgery.

J. P. Dunn, MD

References

1. Mehta S, Linton MM, Kempen JH. Outcomes of cataract surgery in patients with uveitis: a systematic review and meta-analysis. *Am J Ophthalmol.* 2014;158: 676-692.
2. Soiberman U, Pan Q, Daoud Y, et al. Iris suture fixation of subluxated intraocular lenses. *Am J Ophthalmol.* 2015;159:353-359.
3. Gimbel HV, Amritanand A. Suture refixation and recentration of a subluxated capsular tension ring-capsular bag-intraocular lens complex. *J Cataract Refract Surg.* 2013;39:1798-1802.
4. Michaeli A, Soiberman U, Loewenstein A. Outcome of iris fixation of subluxated intraocular lenses. *Graefes Arch Clin Exp Ophthalmol.* 2012;250:1327-1332.

Persistence of Ebola Virus in Ocular Fluid during Convalescence

Varkey JB, Shantha JG, Crozier I, et al (Emory Univ School of Medicine, Atlanta, GA; Infectious Diseases Inst, Kampala, Uganda; et al)

N Engl J Med 372;2423-2427, 2015

Among the survivors of Ebola virus disease (EVD), complications that include uveitis can develop during convalescence, although the incidence and pathogenesis of EVD-associated uveitis are unknown. We describe a patient who recovered from EVD and was subsequently found to have severe unilateral uveitis during convalescence. Viable *Zaire ebolavirus* (EBOV) was detected in aqueous humor 14 weeks after the onset of EVD and 9 weeks after the clearance of viremia.

▶ Rarely if ever has a case report of a patient with uveitis attracted as much attention in both the lay and medical press as this harrowing description of an ebola virus survivor who developed blinding unilateral uveitis after recovery. The patient, who was treated at Emory University Hospital in Atlanta, developed ocular burning, foreign-body sensation, and photophobia. He progressively developed bilateral chorioretinal scars, followed by scleritis, panuveitis, glaucoma, heterochromia, and vision loss to the 20/400 level in his left eye. Testing of aqueous humor obtained by paracentesis was positive for ebola virus by reverse transcriptase polymerase chain reaction (RT-PCR). Treatment with topical, periocular, and oral corticosteroids, and the oral antiviral drug favipiravir. The uveitis resolved and visual acuity recovered to 20/15.

Of particular note was that peripheral blood tested negative for ebola virus RNA by quantitative RT-PCR testing, as did tear-film tests obtained before and 24 hours after the paracentesis. Comparison of the ocular fluid and the blood obtained during the patient's prior ebola virus disease showed a single nonsynonymous mutation, as well as 2 silent mutations and 2 mutations in noncoding regions. The significance of these mutations was not clear but was in contrast to another case report in which viral consensus sequences acquired over several days from a single patient showed no changes.[1]

As with all case reports, there are perhaps more questions than answers. The pathogenesis of the uveitis is not clear. The high viral load at the time the uveitis was rapidly worsening could reflect either a lytic viral infection or an immunologic reaction to the ebola virus. The authors suggest their patient's uveitis was a direct cytopathic effect of active replication of ebola virus persisting in an immune-privileged site. Nor is it clear that the antiviral therapy used was a factor in the patient's improvement. Further studies of drugs active against ebola virus are urgently needed; to date, the results have been disappointing. The incidence of post-ebola uveitis is uncertain,[2] although there are ongoing studies, such as the Partnership for Research on Ebola Virus in Liberia, that will assess the efficacy of several trial vaccines against ebola, new drugs to treat ebola virus disease, and the natural history of the disease. Finally, the community health risks posed by patients with post—ebola virus disease uveitis require further investigation. Fortunately, the authors point out that the risk of spread of ebola virus during the uveitic phase is likely low, given the negative RT-PCR results from conjunctival and tear specimens.

The authors point out the similarities between this case of ebola virus uveitis and herpetic uveitis, with acute onset, unilateral involvement, and high intraocular pressure, which in the latter case has been attributed to a direct consequence of active viral replication.[3] One fortuitous outcome of this horrific epidemic may be a renewed interest in the pathogenesis of different viruses in uveitis.

J. P. Dunn, MD

References

1. Trenchard T. Survivors cope with new ebola after-effects. Al-Jazeera. 2014. http://www.aljazeera.com/news/africa/2014/12/survivors-cope-with-new-ebola-after-effects-20141215735215613 84.html.
2. http://www.nih.gov/news-events/news-releases/study-ebola-survivors-opens-liberia. Accessed January 21, 2016.
3. Amano S, Oshika T, Kaji Y, et al. Herpes simplex virus in the trabeculum of an eye with corneal endotheliitis. *Am J Ophthalmol.* 1999;127:721-722.

Autologous antibodies to outer retina in acute zonal occult outer retinopathy

Tagami M, Matsumiya W, Imai H, et al (Kobe Kaisei Hosp, Nada-Ku, Japan; Kobe Univ Graduate School of Medicine, Japan)
Jpn J Ophthalmol 58:462-472, 2014

Purpose.—Our aim was to use molecular biological methods to study evidence of autoimmune disease in five patients with acute zonal occult outer retinopathy (AZOOR).

Methods.—Ophthalmologic data and sera were collected from all patients, who underwent visual field (VF) examination, optical coherence tomography (OCT), and multifocal electroretinogram (mfERG) recording. Serum was prepared from each patient's blood and analyzed for anti-retinal antibody activity using immunohistochemistry and Western blot analysis on mouse and human retinas. We also searched for antigen proteins using mass spectrometry.

Results.—Symptoms were blurred vision in three patients and VF defects in two; all had enlargement of the Mariotte blind spot by VF testing. OCT findings in areas corresponding to the scotoma revealed disruptions of junction borders between inner and outer segment lines. mfERGs amplitudes were reduced in each corresponding scotoma area. Immunohistochemical serum staining revealed the target antigen was present in all photoreceptors of the mouse sensory retina. Western blot analysis using patient serum samples revealed some possible candidate antigens. Mass spectrometry could not determine the causative antigen; however, a list of candidates was discovered.

Conclusion.—We determined that AZOOR could be an autoimmune disease. All AZOOR patients tested using molecular biological methods had antiretinal antigens.

▶ One of the areas in which uveitis remains a science in relative infancy is the understanding of disease pathogenesis. With the exception of ocular infectious disease, the pathophysiology of most uveitides remains uncertain. Thus, although we use the term "idiopathic" for those conditions in which no associated disease (eg, seronegative spondyloarthropathy) or laboratory test (eg, HLA A29) is identified, the vast majority of uveitis remains idiopathic (or more accurately, "undifferentiated"[1]). Without a better understanding of pathogenesis, treatment regimens are likely to be less effective and more toxic. So it is with acute zonal occult outer retinopathy (AZOOR), a rare and frequently blinding disease first described by Gass in 1992 and characterized by zonal dysfunction of photoreceptors emanating outward from the optic nerve with sharp visual field defects.[2] Gass himself theorized an infectious etiology,[3] whereas Jampol and Becker[4] suggested an autoimmune mechanism, comparable to carcinoma-associated retinopathy.[5]

In this article from Japan, Tagami et al provide evidence that AZOOR is an autoimmune retinal disease mediated by an autoantibody. Patients meeting the criteria for AZOOR (sudden onset, nearly normal fundus examination, disruption of the inner and outer segments line (ellipsoid) on spatial domain optical coherence tomography (SD-OCT), and reduced multifocal electroretinogram amplitude corresponding to blind spot enlargement seen on visual field testing) had serum drawn for immunohistochemistry and Western blot analysis. Mouse and human retinas (obtained from patients undergoing retinectomy for rhegmatogenous retinal detachment) were used for immunohistochemistry as lysates in Western blot and mass spectrometry analyses. Immunohistochemistry testing demonstrated that the target antigen was present in the photoreceptors of the mouse sensory retina, sometimes in the outer nuclear layer and sometimes in the outer segments. Western blot analysis and mass spectrometry suggested several possible antigens, including 31-, 45-, and 60-kDa bands. The authors were able to overcome some of the logistical problems associated with immunohistochemistry, such as rapid tissue degradation after death, by performing all protein sampling within 30 minutes and using perfusion fixation techniques in the mice.

The advent of new imaging modalities such as SD-OCT to more precisely evaluate the different layers of the retina, combined with electrophysiologic testing, has helped identify the location of various posterior uveitides. The addition of the immunohistochemistry studies of Tagami et al have strongly identified a humoral mechanism in the pathophysiology of AZOOR. The next step will be the development of more precise drugs that target the autoimmune process and encourage research into other diseases with a humoral basis, such as neoplastic and non-neoplastic autoimmune retinopathies.

Caution is indicated when interpreting these results. First, the target autoantigen in the photoreceptors is not the only one involved in AZOOR. Second, although the authors demonstrated that an autoimmune mechanism is present in the development of AZOOR, their assertion that "steroid therapy ... might potentially be an effective treatment for some AZOOR patients" has not generally been borne clinically. The search for more effective (and safer) immunomodulatory therapies goes on.

J. P. Dunn, MD

References

1. Jabs DA, Busingye J. Approach to the diagnosis of the uveitides. *Am J Ophthalmol.* 2013;156:228-236.
2. Gass JD. Acute zonal occult outer retinopathy. Donders Lecture: The Netherlands Ophthalmological Society, Maastricht, Holland, June 19, 1992. *J Clin Neuroophthalmol.* 1993;13:79-97.
3. Gass JD. Are acute zonal occult outer retinopathy and the white spot syndromes (AZOOR complex) specific autoimmune disease? *Am J Ophthalmol.* 2003;135:380-381.
4. Jampol LM, Becker KG. White spot syndromes of the retina: a hypothesis based on the common genetic hypothesis of autoimmune/inflammatory disease. *Am J Ophthalmol.* 2003;135:376-379.
5. Thirkill CE, FitzGerald P, Sergott RC, et al. Cancer-associated retinopathy (CAR syndrome) with antibodies reacting with retinal, optic nerve, and cancer cells. *N Engl J Med.* 1989;321:1589-1594.

Uveitis Reactivation in Children Treated With Tumor Necrosis Factor Alpha Inhibitors

Lerman MA, Lewen MD, Kempen JH, et al (The Children's Hosp of Philadelphia (CHOP), PA; Tufts Medical Ctr, Boston, MA; Univ of Pennsylvania, Philadelphia; et al)

Am J Ophthalmol 160:193-200.e1, 2015

Purpose.—To evaluate reactivation of pediatric uveitis during/following treatment with tumor necrosis factor alpha inhibition (anti-TNFα).

Design.—Retrospective cohort study.

Methods.—We assessed the incidence of uveitis reactivation in children ≤18 years who had achieved uveitis quiescence under anti-TNFα. Survival analysis was used to calculate reactivation rates while still on (primary outcome), and following discontinuation of (secondary outcome), anti-TNFα. Potential predictive factors were assessed.

Results.—Among 50 children observed to develop quiescence of uveitis under anti-TNFα, 39 met criteria to be "at risk" of the primary (19 for the secondary) outcome. 60% were female, ~half had juvenile idiopathic arthritis, and most were treated with infliximab. Overall, the estimated proportion relapsing within 12 months was 27.8% (95% confidence interval [CI]: 15.9%–45.8%); the estimated probability of reactivation was higher following (63.8% [95% CI: 38.9%–87.7%]) vs before (21.6% [95% CI: 10.8%–40.2%]) anti-TNFα discontinuation. Among those who discontinued anti-TNFα, the likelihood of reactivation was higher for those treated with adalimumab vs infliximab (hazard ratio [HR]

13.4, $P = .01$, 95% CI: 2.2–82.5) and those with older age at uveitis onset (HR 1.3, $P = .09$, 95% CI: 1.0–1.7). The duration of suppression, on medication, did not significantly affect the likelihood of reactivation when quiescence was maintained for ≥1.5 years.

Conclusions.—Approximately 75% of children remaining on anti-TNFα following achievement of uveitis quiescence remain quiescent at 1 year. However, most reactivate following anti-TNFα discontinuation. These results suggest that infliximab more often is followed by remission, off medication, than adalimumab. The data do not suggest that maintenance of suppression for more than 1.5 years decreases the reactivation risk.

▶ Tumor necrosis factor (TNF) inhibitors have become an important second- or third-line drug in the treatment of noninfectious uveitis in both children and adults. In children in particular, steroid-sparing immunosuppression is often needed to control uveitis safely to reduce the risk of glaucoma and cataract as well as the growth and adrenal suppression that is more common in children than adults treated with oral corticosteroids. Adalimumab and infliximab are the most commonly used TNF-inhibitors for patients with uveitis. Previous studies have confirmed that these drugs can induce quiescence of disease in 75% of children within 1 year of treatment and that children with juvenile idiopathic arthritis (JIA)-associated uveitis were most likely to respond.[1] Typically, patients are treated with immunosuppressive therapy for up to 2 years after the medication has proven well tolerated and effective, followed by tapering and discontinuation over 3 to 12 more months while the patient is followed closely for evidence of recurrence.[2] The effectiveness of this approach (as opposed to a shorter regimen) is unproven.

In this retrospective cohort study, the authors sought to determine whether a longer duration of initial therapy decreases the likelihood of reactivation of uveitis in children. Reactivation was defined as observation of active uveitis after achievement of quiescence. Quiescence was defined as achieving either "slightly active" or "inactive" uveitis while on < 2 drops per day of topical corticosteroids and no oral corticosteroids sustained for > 2 visits spanning > 28 days.

The authors found a 28% risk of reactivation of uveitis by 12 months in patients after initial quiescence while still on anti-TNF therapy. Even more disappointing was the high rate of reactivation (64% within 12 months) after discontinuing therapy. A longer duration of suppression before discontinuation of therapy was not associated with a greater likelihood of remission. The risk of reactivation was lower in patients treated with infliximab than adalimumab. However, the study was retrospective, nor was it designed to assess differences between the 2 drugs. Confounding variables included a higher percentage of adalimumab-treated patients with JIA-associated uveitis, which is a chronic disease and therefore perhaps more likely to recur after cessation of therapy. In addition, patients younger than 8 years of age were more likely, but the older patients in the study may have been more likely to have received prior non-TNF inhibitor immunosuppressive therapy (eg, methotrexate), and the study did not control for this possibility. Finally, duration of disease prior to treatment was not controlled for.

In summary, the authors concluded that maintaining control of uveitis for more than 1.5 years before discontinuation of anti-TNF therapy dose not appear to affect the risk of reactivation. If their findings are borne out in controlled studies, they will have significant consequences on the overall cost of uveitis therapy and the follow-up regimen. It remains unproven whether children initially responsive to anti-TNF therapy remain comparably responsive to the same drug regimen if there is reactivation of uveitis.

J. P. Dunn, MD

References

1. Lerman MA, Burnham JM, Chang PY, et al. Response of pediatric uveitis to tumor necrosis factor-a inhibitors. *J Rheumatol.* 2013;40:1394-1403.
2. Jabs DA, Rosenbaum JT, Foster CS, et al. Guidelines for the use of immunosuppressive drugs in patients with ocular inflammatory disorders: recommendations of an expert panel. *Am J Ophthalmol.* 2000;130:492-513.

Cost-effectiveness of alternative strategies for interferon-γ release assays and tuberculin skin test in tuberculous uveitis

Ang M, Nguyen HV, Kiew SY, et al (Singapore Natl Eye Centre; Duke-NUS Graduate Med School, Singapore)
Br J Ophthalmol 99;984-989, 2015

Background.—Although tuberculous uveitis remains a major cause of ocular morbidity in the developing world, there is no consensus on which diagnostic test or testing strategy is the most cost effective. In this study we carried out a cost-effectiveness analysis to determine the most cost-effective diagnostic test strategy.

Methods.—In this prospective study, we recruited 102 patients from Singapore National Eye Centre with signs suggestive of tuberculous uveitis. Using prospective data from this cohort and from published meta-analyses, we modelled the incremental cost effectiveness of the following strategies: tuberculin skin test (TST) only; interferon-γ release assay (IGRA) only; IGRA following a positive TST result; and dual-test strategy, conducting TST and IGRA at presentation. Incremental cost-effectiveness ratios (ICERs) were calculated for each strategy and analysed using a willingness-to-pay threshold of $50 000 per quality-adjusted life year (QALY) gained.

Results.—In our population, the least cost effective was the IGRA-only strategy. The dual-test strategy was the most cost effective, with an improvement of 0.017 QALY at an incremental cost of $190 relative to the TST-only strategy (ICER $11 500); while the TST-only strategy was more cost effective than the third strategy, using IGRA following a positive TST result (ICER $3610). This remained consistent while varying the costs of IGRA and TST, the incidence of tuberculosis and tuberculous uveitis, as well as the diagnostic accuracy of IGRA and TST found in previous studies in various populations.

Conclusions.—The dual-test strategy (performing TST and IGRA at presentation) was the most cost effective strategy for the diagnosis of tuberculous uveitis in our population.

▶ Tuberculous uveitis can be a difficult diagnosis to confirm. The clinical manifestations are protean, and the majority of patients have no clinical or radiologic pulmonary abnormalities.[1] Even uveitis experts disagree on the importance of known risk factors for tuberculosis (TB) and the morphology of the disease when making the diagnosis, as well as the optimal duration of anti-TB therapy and the time after which anti-TB medication can be safely discontinued in patients who have not responded to therapy.[2] There is a low sensitivity to tests used to confirm the presence of an infectious cause in many types of uveitis, such as acid-fast bacillus stains and polymerase chain reaction testing. Consequently, the diagnosis of tuberculous uveitis is often based on findings compatible with ocular TB (chronic granulomatous with broad-based posterior synechiae, serpiginous choroiditis, choroidal tubercles, or retinal vasculitis)[3] in combination with a positive tuberculin skin test (TST) or interferon-gamma releasing assay (IGRA). However, the sensitivity and specificity of these tests remain unclear.[4] The authors point out that recommendations for diagnostic testing differ between the Centers for Disease Control and Prevention in the United States and National Institute of Health and Care Excellence in the United Kingdom.

In this article from Singapore, the authors performed a cost-effective analysis of the use of TST, IGRA (QuantiFERON-Gold in-tube, Cellestis Inc, Australia), both, or IGRA only after a positive TST in the diagnosis of tubercular uveitis. One hundred and two patients were studied, of whom 52 tested positive by TST and 50 by IGRA. Twenty-four of these patients underwent TB therapy; 22 patients completed therapy, of whom 20 had no active uveitis at the conclusion and 2 had recurrent/persistent inflammation requiring long-term treatment with systemic immunosuppression (9.1% recurrence rate). Two patients started treatment but discontinued because of side effects, 1 of whom had persistent inflammation. Among the 78 patients not receiving anti-TB therapy, 13 (16.7%) had recurrent or persistent inflammation despite anti-inflammatory treatment alone.

The results suggested that the simultaneous testing of TST and IGRA for patients with suspected tuberculous uveitis would be the most cost-effective strategy for decision makers willing to pay $11 500 or more per quality adjusted life year (QALY) gained (well below the accepted threshold of $50 000 per QALY commonly cited).[5] The recommendation for a dual-test strategy was based on the findings of a higher positive predictive value (thus reducing the cost of false-positive results) and a decreased likelihood of recurrence of uveitis (thus reducing ocular morbidity). In addition, some patients who tested positive for either TST or IGRA alone declined to receive treatment, and these patients were also more likely to have recurrent uveitis. However, if the willingness-to-pay (WTP) threshold were below $11 500, then the "TST only" strategy would be recommended as the cheapest alternative for our population.

A variety of caveats are necessary for the clinician. The number of patients studied was small. There was no gold standard for the diagnosis of TB, such as a positive sputum culture or smear. Given the absence of cough or an abnormal chest x-ray in the majority of patients with tuberculous uveitis, however, such limitations are inherent. The authors did not describe what constituted a positive TST. The failure of 2 patients to respond to anti-TB therapy alone may not indicate an incorrect diagnosis of tuberculous uveitis; it is not uncommon that supplemental corticosteroids (or immunosuppressive drugs) are necessary to completely control the inflammation.[3]

Finally, any quality-of-life analysis makes assumptions regarding the number of QALY; the authors used a utility obtained from the literature for consistency. They also used a conventional WTP threshold of $50 000 per QALY. Treatment costs were based on which treatment course was followed. Diagnostic, medical, and drug costs vary between countries (and between states), and factors such as the use of directly observed therapy influence the outcome of therapy. Therefore, the results of this study may not be applicable in different health care environments.

J. P. Dunn, MD

References

1. Patel SS, Saraiya NV, Tessler HH, Goldstein DA. Mycobacterial ocular inflammation: delay in diagnosis and other factors impacting morbidity. *JAMA Ophthalmol.* 2013;131:752-758.
2. Lou SM, Larkin KL, Winthrop K, Rosenbaum JT. Uveitis Specialists Study Group. Lack of consensus in the diagnosis and treatment for ocular tuberculosis among uveitis specialists. *Ocul Immunol Inflamm.* 2015;23:25-31.
3. Ang M, Hedayatfar A, Zhang R, et al. Clinical signs of uveitis associated with latent tuberculosis. *Clin Experiment Ophthalmol.* 2012;40:689-696.
4. Ang M, Kiew SY, Wong WL, et al. Discordance of two interferon-gamma release assays and tuberculin skin test in patients with uveitis. *Br J Ophthalmol.* 2014;98: 1649-1653.
5. Grosse SD. Assessing cost-effectiveness in healthcare: history of the $50,000 per QALY threshold. *Expert Rev Pharmacoecon Outcomes Res.* 2008;8: 165-178.

Association of Systemic Lupus Erythematosus With Uveitis

Gallagher K, Viswanathan A, Okhravi N (Moorfields Eye Hosp Natl Health Society Foundation Trust, London, England; et al)
JAMA Ophthalmol 133;1190-1193, 2015

Importance.—Systemic lupus erythematosus (SLE) can be associated with uveitis. The reported prevalence of SLE in patients with uveitis varies from 0.1% to 4.8%. Accordingly, the positive predictive value of antinuclear antibody testing in diagnosing SLE in a patient with uveitis varies enormously. An accurate estimate of SLE prevalence in uveitis is needed to establish the value of routine antinuclear antibody testing in patients with uveitis.

Observations.—A literature review using the Medline database was performed to find studies reporting data on uveitis etiology from January 1, 1984, to March 20, 2015. Studies were included where there were sufficient data to draw conclusions on the prevalence of SLE as an etiological factor in uveitis. Data for 53 315 patients were reviewed and 63 studies from 30 countries were included. The prevalence of SLE as a cause of uveitis was estimated to be 0.47% (95% CI, 0.41%-0.53%). The positive predictive value of routine antinuclear antibody testing was 2.9% (95% CI, 2.65%-3.19%).

Conclusions and Relevance.—Systemic lupus erythematosus is a rare cause of uveitis. Routine antinuclear antibody testing has a low positive predictive value for SLE. These data suggest such testing should be reserved for patients where there is a higher pretest probability of SLE.

▶ It has been well recognized for decades that systemic lupus erythematosus (SLE) is only rarely associated with uveitis.[1] Furthermore, residents have been encouraged to rule out SLE in the workup of patients with uveitis by obtaining antinuclear antibody (ANA) testing despite clear evidence that such testing is far more likely to yield a false-positive than a true-positive result,[1] thus generating additional and unnecessary tests and/or consultation with a rheumatologist, consuming valuable health care dollars, and causing anxiety for patients. In this Brief Report from the United Kingdom, Gallagher et al undertook a large, multinational literature review to determine the prevalence of SLE as a cause of uveitis (0.47%) and calculated the positive and negative predictive results.

Of more than 50 000 cases reviewed, uveitis associated with lupus occurred in just 0.47% of patients: 72 cases of anterior uveitis, 3 cases of intermediate uveitis, 26 cases of posterior uveitis, and 4 cases of panuveitis. For a sensitivity and specificity of diagnosing SLE of 70%, the positive predictive value of routine antinuclear antibody testing was 2.9%. The authors note that even with sensitivity and specificity of 92% and 98%, respectively (as has been reported in other studies), the positive predictive value was still only 5.47% and the negative predictive value 99.99%. In other words, there were 19 false-positive test results for every true-positive result even with the most favorable assumptions of ANA test reliability.

Their results confirm the importance to the clinician of (1) obtaining a proper history before ordering diagnostic ANA tests and (2) restricting the use of ANA tests to patients with a higher pretest probability of SLE. Signs more suggestive of SLE might be either ocular (choroidopathy, optic neuropathy, retinal arteritis, scleritis) or systemic (pleuritis, systemic vasculitis, dermatitis, renal disease, etc).

Although this article is limited to the utility of ANA testing in patients with uveitis, clinicians should follow a similar diagnostic approach with other laboratory tests (eg, human leukocyte antigen testing, serum angiotensin converting enzyme, infectious disease tests). The workup should be parsimonious and use a Bayesian analysis that takes into account not only the sensitivity and specificity of a test but the positive and negative predictive value.[2] The old adage that you should never order a test if you don't know what to do with the result remains valid.

J. P. Dunn, MD

References

1. Rosenbaum JT, Wernick R. The utility of routine screening of patients with uveitis for systemic lupus erythematosus or tuberculosis: a Bayesian analysis. *Arch Ophthalmol.* 1990;108:1291-1293.
2. Jabs DA, Busingye J. Approach to the diagnosis of the uveitides. *Am J Ophthalmol.* 2013;156:228-236.

Quantitative Analysis of Peripheral Vasculitis, Ischemia, and Vascular Leakage in Uveitis Using Ultra-Widefield Fluorescein Angiography

Karampelas M, Sim DA, Chu C, et al (Moorfields Eye Hosp Natl Health Service Foundation Trust, London, United Kingdom; et al)

Am J Ophthalmol 159:1161-1168.e1, 2015

Purpose.—To investigate the relationships between peripheral vasculitis, ischemia, and vascular leakage in uveitis using ultra-widefield fluorescein angiography (FA).

Design.—Cross-sectional, consecutive case series.

Methods.—Consecutive ultra-widefield FA images were collected from 82 uveitis patients (82 eyes) in a single center. The extent of peripheral vasculitis, capillary nonperfusion, and vessel leakage were quantified. Parameters included: (1) foveal avascular zone area and macular leakage, (2) peripheral diffuse capillary leakage and ischemia, (3) peripheral vasculitis, and (4) leakage from neovascularization. Central macular thickness measurements were derived with optical coherence tomography. Main outcome measures were correlations between central and peripheral fluorangiographic changes as well as associations between visual function, ultra-widefield FA–derived metrics, and central macular thickness.

Results.—Although central leakage was associated with peripheral leakage ($r = 0.553$, $P = .001$), there was no association between foveal avascular zone size and peripheral ischemia ($r = 0.114$, $P = .324$), regardless of the underlying uveitic diagnosis. Peripheral ischemia was, however, correlated to neovascularization-related leakage ($r = 0.462$, $P = .001$) and focal vasculitis ($r = 0.441$, $P = .001$). Stepwise multiple regression analysis revealed that a poor visual acuity was independently associated with foveal avascular zone size and central macular thickness (R^2-adjusted $= 0.45$, $P = .001$).

Conclusions.—We present a large cohort of patients with uveitis imaged with ultra-widefield FA and further describe novel methods for quantification of peripheral vascular pathology, in an attempt to identify visually significant parameters. Although we observed that relationships exist between peripheral vessel leakage, vasculitis, and ischemia, it was only macular ischemia and increased macular thickness that were independently associated with a reduced visual acuity.

▶ The use of ultra wide-field fluorescein angiography (FA), which provides a 150-degree image (as opposed to the maximum 60-degree field obtained with conventional FA), is becoming more common in the diagnosis and management of uveitis.[1,2]

This study, from Moorfields Eye Hospital in London, is the largest published case series of ultra wide-field FA images in patients with uveitis and the first quantitative analysis of parameters such as areas of capillary nonperfusion, vessel leakage, and active vasculitis. The authors note the advantages of wide-field imaging: fewer images are required to cover the retina, the intensity of light used is more tolerable for patients, and the optics of the system permit improved imaging through small pupils. Peripheral assessment of vasculitis and ischemia is arguably the greatest benefit, permitting the documentation of peripheral retinal changes not previously possible with conventional FA. Indeed many types of uveitis appear to develop early or isolated peripheral vasculitis, a finding reinforced by experimental animal models where the peripheral retina is an initial site of cellular infiltration.

The authors quantified macular ischemia and leakage as well as peripheral ischemia, leakage, focal vasculitis, and neovascularization-related leakage. A peripheral ischemic index was than calculated by measuring in pixels the area of capillary nonperfusion expressed as a percentage of the total image area. They were able to correlate peripheral retinal ischemia with neovascularization-related leakage, confirming the observation that the risk of retinal neovascularization in patients with uveitis is proportional to the degree of retinal ischemia. Peripheral ischemia was correlated with focal peripheral retinal vasculitis but not diffuse capillary leakage. There was also a significant correlation between diffuse peripheral vascular leakage and macular edema. The authors theorized that the association could be explained by incomplete suppression of inflammation and persistent cellular infiltrate in the periphery. If this were the case, then cases of chronic inflammatory macular edema despite adequate immunosuppression—as defined by lack of vasculitis on conventional fluorescein angiography—may actually respond to increased therapy.

As a cross-sectional study, the article does not shed light on the utility of wide-field imaging in the ongoing management of patients with uveitis. Transient changes of little significance might be overemphasized. No effort was made to control for type, severity or duration of uveitis, treatment, or visual acuity. In addition, there are optical limitations to ultra wide-field angiography. The inferior and superior retinal areas are not seen as well as the nasal and temporal areas, and the size of peripheral areas of pathology may be overestimated. Nonetheless, further supportive studies of wide-field angiography may define an important role for its use in the management of uveitis and the prevention of long-term complications.

J. P. Dunn, MD

References

1. Campbell JP, Leder HA, Sepah YJ, et al. Wide-field retinal imaging in the management of noninfectious posterior uveitis. *Am J Ophthalmol*. 2012;154:908-911.
2. Leder HA, Campbell JP, Sepah YJ, et al. Ultra-wide-field retinal imaging in the management of non-infectious retinal vasculitis. *J Ophthalmic Inflamm Infect*. 2013;3:30.

Epidemiology of uveitis in a Western urban multiethnic population. The challenge of globalization

Llorenç V, Mesquida M, Sainz de la Maza M, et al (Hosp Clinic of Barcelona, Spain; et al)

Acta Ophthalmol 93:561-567, 2015

Purpose.—To report the anatomical pattern and etiological spectrum of uveitis in an urban multi-ethnic population from Barcelona, Spain. General and specific epidemiological data for the most prevalent aetiologies are also calculated.

Methods.—A cross-sectional study of consecutive uveitis cases was performed between 1 January 2009 and 31 December 2012. Exogenous endophthalmitis, surgery-related, post-traumatic and toxic uveitis along with masquerade syndromes were excluded. Anatomical (Standard Uveitis Nomenclature criteria) and aetiological patterns (by tailored tests), age, sex, geographical origin and laterality were analysed. Mean incidence and prevalence were calculated for a mid-period reference population.

Results.—From 1022 patients included, 52% were anterior uveitis (AU), 23% posterior, 15% panuveitis and 9% intermediate uveitis. Aetiologically, 26% were unclassifiable, 29% infectious, 25% associated with systemic immune diseases, and 20% corresponded to ocular-specific syndromes. Among classified causes, herpesvirus (12%), toxoplasma (7%), Behçet's disease (BD) (5%), HLA-B27-isolated AU (5%), ankylosing spondylitis (5%), tuberculosis-related uveitis (TRU) (5%), birdshot chorioretinopathy (3%) and sarcoidosis (3%) were the most frequent. Non-Spanish origin was recorded in 22%, with 47% of Vogt-Koyanagi-Harada and 36% of toxoplasma cases coming from South America, 10% of BD and 11% of TRU from Africa and 24% of TRU cases from Asia. A mean annual incidence of 51.91 cases/100 000 inhabitants was found for the referral population.

Conclusion.—In our referral area, 74% of the uveitis cases can be correctly classified. A large myriad of uveitis aetiologies with a strong geographical origin burden are found in Western urban multi-ethnic populations.

▶ Epidemiologic surveys of uveitis typically reflect the era and geography from which they are drawn. Infectious diseases such as acute retinal necrosis and AIDS-related cytomegalovirus retinitis were unknown before the 1970s. White dot syndromes such as birdshot retinochoroidopathy are much more frequently recognized today. Geographic factors account for regional differences in the prevalence of uveitides such as Behçet disease (BD; more common in Turkey, the Middle East, or Japan, but also more common in Hawaii and the West Coast of the United States compared with the central United States because of the higher concentration of Japanese Americans on the West Coast), Vogt-Koyanagi-Harada disease (more common in the Middle East and South America), and sarcoidosis (more common in the southern United States and northern Europe).

In recent years, globalization has resulted in large migrations of populations due to poverty, civil war, and economic opportunity. Barcelona, Spain, is one such area where population demographics have shifted. Llorenc et al undertook a cross-sectional study of consecutive uveitis cases, excluding exogenous endophthalmitis, surgery-related, posttraumatic, toxic uveitis, and masquerade syndromes. Their findings suggested that geographic origin is an increasingly important risk factor for uveitis in large Western urban centers with multiethnic populations.

The mean annual incidence of uveitis was 52 cases per 100 000 population, which is comparable to some uveitis epidemiology studies[1] but higher than others.[2,3] Non-Spanish origin was found in 22% of patients. The anatomic breakdown of uveitis (roughly one-half anterior uveitis, one-quarter posterior uveitis, 15% panuveitis, and 9% intermediate uveitis) was comparable to uveitis surveys of comparable urban areas. There were roughly equal percentages of unclassifiable, infectious, ocular-specific, and systemic immune disease-associated etiology. What was most interesting was the breakdown from location of origin. Tuberculosis-related uveitis occurred in 5% of the patients, but a disproportionately large percentage of these patients were from Africa and especially Asia. Nearly half the cases of Vogt-Koyanagi-Harada disease and more than a third of cases of toxoplasmosis occurred in patients from South America.

Geography, genetics, and the environment are intertwined in the cause of some forms of uveitis. BD, for example, is most common in the Far East and the Mediterranean Basin in the latitudes corresponding to the old Silk Route. The disease is relatively common in Hawaii, which has a large Japanese American population. There are conflicting studies regarding the extent to which the risk of developing BD is modified by moving to a country with a historically low prevalence of the disease. For infectious diseases such as toxoplasmosis and TB, it is also unclear to what extent migration affects the risk of developing disease, because both diseases commonly result from reactivation of infection that occurred early in life.

For clinicians, the take-home point of this study is that a simple demographic history is important in patients with uveitis. Genetics and place of origin may be valuable predictors of disease risk.

J. P. Dunn, MD

References

1. Gritz DC, Wong IG. Incidence and prevalence of uveitis in Northern California; the Northern California Epidemiology of Uveitis Study. *Ophthalmology.* 2004; 111:491-500.
2. Acharya NR, Tham VM, Esterberg E, et al. Incidence and prevalence of uveitis: results from the Pacific Ocular Inflammation Study. *JAMA Ophthalmol.* 2013; 131:1405-1412.
3. Suhler EB, Lloyd MJ, Choi D, Rosenbaum JT, Austin DF. Incidence and prevalence of uveitis in Veterans Affairs Medical Centers of the Pacific Northwest. *Am J Ophthalmol.* 2008;146:890-896.

Outcome of Treatment of Uveitic Macular Edema: The Multicenter Uveitis Steroid Treatment Trial 2-Year Results

Tomkins-Nezer O, for the Multicenter Uveitis Steroid Treatment Trial Research Group (Univ College London, United Kingdom; et al)

Ophthalmology 122:2351-2359, 2015

Purpose.—To evaluate the 2-year outcomes of uveitic macular edema.

Design.—Longitudinal follow-up of a randomized cohort.

Participants.—At baseline, 148 eyes of 117 patients enrolled in the Multicenter Uveitis Steroid Treatment (MUST) Trial had macular edema, and 134 eyes of 108 patients completed 2-year follow-up.

Methods.—Patients enrolled in the study were randomized to either systemic immunosuppression or intravitreal fluocinolone acetonide implant therapy. Macular edema was defined as thickening of the retina (center point thickness ≥240 μm) on time-domain optical coherence tomography (OCT) of macula.

Main Outcome Measures.—Improvement in macular edema (≥20% reduction in central point thickness on OCT), resolution of macular edema (normalization of thickness on OCT), and best-corrected visual acuity (BCVA).

Results.—Between randomization and 2-years' follow-up, 62% and 25% of eyes in the systemic and implant groups, respectively, received at least 1 supplemental regional corticosteroid injection. By 2-years' follow-up, macular edema improved in 71% of eyes and resolved in 60%. There were no differences between treatment groups in the proportion of eyes with macular edema improving (systemic therapy vs. implant, 65% vs. 77%; $P = 0.20$) and resolving (52% vs. 68%; $P = 0.28$), but eyes randomized to implant had more improvement in macular thickness (median decrease of 180 vs. 109 μm in the systemic therapy group; $P = 0.04$). Eyes with baseline fluorescein angiographic leakage were more likely to improve than those without (76% vs. 58%; $P = 0.03$). Overall, there was a mean 5-letter (1 line) improvement in BCVA at 2 years. Mean changes in BCVA from baseline at 2 years by macular edema response status were: resolution, +10 letters; improvement without resolution, +10 letters ($P = 0.92$); little to no change, 6 letters ($P = 0.19$); and worsening, −16 letters (worsening acuity; $P = 0.0003$).

Conclusions.—About two thirds of eyes with uveitic macular edema were observed to experience improvement in the edema and visual acuity with implant or systemic treatment. Fluocinolone acetonide implant therapy was associated with a greater quantitative improvement in thickness. Fluorescein angiography leakage was associated with a greater likelihood of improvement in macular edema.

▶ The Multicenter Uveitis Steroid Treatment (MUST) Trial is a multicenter study of patients with active or recently noninfectious intermediate, posterior, and panuveitis who are randomized to either systemic therapy or the fluocinolone acetonide 0.59 mg intravitreal implant (Retisert, Bausch & Lomb, Rochester, NY). Systemic therapy included oral corticosteroids and/or immunomodulatory therapy at the discretion of the clinician, with standardized treatment and monitoring regimens.[1] Macular edema was assessed both by optical coherence tomography (OCT; for retinal thickness) and fluorescein angiography (for vascular leakage), with standard protocols used to assess the severity. Macular edema was further characterized as cystoid or diffuse.

In this 2-year analysis of patients enrolled in the MUST Trial, there was improvement in 71% and resolution in 60% of eyes with uveitic macular edema. Although the fluocinolone acetonide implant-treated eyes showed a greater overall improvement in retinal thickness, the differences were not significant between the 2 groups in the proportion of patients with reduction in macular thickness or in visual acuity improvement (about 10 letters on ETDRS testing). The authors concluded that either approach is reasonable and usually effective for treatment of uveitic macular edema.

Several additional points are noteworthy for clinicians. First, eyes with macular edema in patients treated with systemic therapy more frequently required supplemental adjunctive periocular or intravitreal corticosteroid injections, although usually just 1 or 2 over the course of the study. Second, eyes with angiographic leakage at presentation showed 2.3-fold higher odds of improvement in macular edema in retinal thickness, perhaps indicating a more severe pathology to the uveitis. It has been shown that retinal thickness (measured by OCT) correlates better with visual acuity than fluorescein angiography.[2] However, macular leakage cannot be rule out in the absence of retinal thickening, or vice versa.[3] Thus, despite its inconvenience and potential risks, there remains a role for fluorescein angiography in the evaluation of patients with uveitis. However, even in eyes without angiographic leakage at presentation, 58% showed reduction in macular edema with treatment. Finally, the study did not show any significant correlation between visual improvement and the type of macular edema (cystoid or diffuse) or the presence or absence of an epiretinal membrane (ERM).

Several limitations to the study exist. Time-domain OCT (TD-OCT) rather than spectral-domain OCT (SD-OCT) was used to assess retinal thickness. TD-OCT is probably comparable to SD-OCT for evaluation of retinal thickness but is inferior for evaluating severity of ERM, so the lack of association of ERM and reduction in macular edema may not be accurate. In addition, the implant-treated eyes received a fluocinolone acetonide implant rather than the dexamethasone 0.7-mg intravitreal implant (Oxurdex, Allergan, Irvine, CA) that is used more commonly nowadays because of convenience (although it has a much shorter duration of drug delivery). It is unclear whether different forms of regional corticosteroid injection regimens or the use of nonsteroid injections (eg, intravitreal methotrexate or anti-VEGF agents) would provide different outcomes. The POINT and MERIT studies will assess these options.[4] Finally, the limited numbers of patients with specific types of uveitis in randomization resulted in limited power in some subgroup analysis.

J. P. Dunn, MD

References

1. Multicenter Uveitis Steroid Treatment Trial Research Group, Kempen JH, Altaweel MM, Holbrook JT, Jabs DA, Sugar EA. The multicenter uveitis steroid treatment trial: rationale, design, and baseline characteristics. *Am J Ophthalmol.* 2010;149:550-561.
2. Nussenblatt RB, Kaufman SC, Palestine AG, Davis MD, Ferris FL 3rd. Macular thickening and visual acuity. Measurement in patients with cystoid macular edema. *Ophthalmology.* 1987;94:1134-1139.
3. Kempen JH, Sugar EA, Jaffe GJ, et al. Multicenter Uveitis Steroid Treatment (MUST) Trial Research Group. Fluorescein angiography versus optical coherence tomography for diagnosis of uveitic macular edema. *Ophthalmology.* 2013;120: 1852-1859.
4. https://americanuveitissociety.wildapricot.org/Resources/Documents/MUST%20Memo.pdf. Accessed January 10, 2016.

Efficacy and Safety of Intravenous Secukinumab in Noninfectious Uveitis Requiring Steroid-Sparing Immunosuppressive Therapy

Letko E, for the AIN457A2208 Study Group (Corneal Consultants of Colorado, Littleton; et al)
Ophthalmology 122:939-948, 2015

Purpose.—Secukinumab, a fully human anti–interleukin-17A monoclonal antibody, exhibited promising activity in a proof-of-concept study when administered in intravenous (IV) doses to patients with active, chronic, noninfectious uveitis. This study compared the efficacy and safety of different IV and subcutaneous (SC) doses of secukinumab in patients with noninfectious uveitis.

Design.—Multicenter, randomized, double-masked, dose-ranging, phase 2 clinical trial.

Participants.—Thirty-seven patients with active noninfectious intermediate uveitis, posterior uveitis, or panuveitis who required corticosteroid-sparing immunosuppressive therapy.

Methods.—Patients were randomized to secukinumab 300 mg SC every 2 weeks for 4 doses, secukinumab 10 mg/kg IV every 2 weeks for 4 doses, or secukinumab 30 mg/kg IV every 4 weeks for 2 doses. Intravenous or SC saline was administered to maintain masking. Efficacy was assessed on day 57 (2–4 weeks after last dose).

Main Outcome Measures.—Percentage of patients with treatment response, defined as (1) at least a 2-grade reduction in vitreous haze score or trace or absent vitreous haze in the study eye without an increase in corticosteroid dose and without uveitis worsening or (2) reduction in corticosteroid dosages to prespecified levels without uveitis worsening. Percentage of patients with remission, defined as anterior chamber cell and vitreous haze scores of 0 or 0.5+ in both eyes without corticosteroid therapy or uveitis worsening.

Results.—Secukinumab 30 mg/kg IV and 10 mg/kg IV, compared with the 300 mg SC dose, produced higher responder rates (72.7% and 61.5% vs. 33.3%, respectively) and remission rates (27.3% and 38.5% vs. 16.7%, respectively). Statistical and clinical superiority for the 30 mg/kg IV dose compared with the 300 mg SC dose was established in a Bayesian probability model. Other measures, including time to response onset, change in visual acuity, and change in vitreous haze score, showed numeric trends favoring IV dosing. Secukinumab, administered in IV or SC formulations, appeared safe and was well tolerated.

Conclusions.—Intravenous secukinumab was effective and well tolerated in noninfectious uveitis requiring systemic corticosteroid-sparing immunosuppressive therapy. Greater activity with IV dosing suggests that patients may not receive sufficient drug with SC administration. High-dose IV secukinumab may be necessary to deliver secukinumab in therapeutic concentrations.

► Multiple cytokines have been implicated in the pathogenesis of noninfectious uveitis, including tumor necrosis factor-alpha, interferon-gamma, and multiple interleukins such as IL-1, IL2, and IL6. IL-17A is produced in experimental models of T cell–mediated uveitis and has been implicated in the uveitides such as Behçet disease.[1] IL-17A–blocking drugs have been shown to reduce ocular inflammation in animal models.[2] One trend in uveitis therapy has been to identify specific inflammatory pathways that can be targeted with biologic drugs. In this study from the Massachusetts Eye Research Study Institute, the authors performed a double-masked, dose-ranging study of secukinumab, a fully humanized monoclonal antibody that binds to and neutralizes human IL-17A, in the treatment of noninfectious intermediate, posterior, or panuveitis. Because a prior study of patients with non-Behçet uveitis had not demonstrated efficacy of the drug using either of 2 subcutaneous doses of secukinumab,[3] the authors chose to evaluate both intravenous and subcutaneous regimens of the drug in patients with noninfectious uveitis requiring systemic steroid-sparing immunosuppressive therapy. Tapering of concurrent prednisone therapy was performed by standardized protocol. Improvement in vitreous haze and reduction of corticosteroid dosages to a specified level served as the primary end points.

The authors found that intravenous secukinumab (30 mg/kg every 4 weeks for 2 doses or 10 mg/kg every 2 weeks for 4 doses) was more effective than subcutaneous secukinumab 300 mg every 2 weeks for 4 doses. Pharmacokinetic analysis showed that the intravenous formulations produced serum concentrations 5 to 10 times higher than those achieved with the subcutaneous regimen. All 3 regimens were well tolerated, with the most common adverse effects including headache, fatigue, and nasopharyngitis. Only 1 patient had to discontinue therapy (because of a flare-up of uveitis).

The authors found a more rapid time to uveitis control with the intravenous formulations and suggested that initial control of noninfectious uveitis might be obtained with intravenous secukinumab, followed by maintenance therapy with a more patient-friendly subcutaneous regimen, but the study was not designed to evaluate this hypothesis.

As with other studies of biologic agents for the treatment of uveitis, caution is warranted. The study population was small, and no subgroup analyses for specific uveitides was possible. Practically speaking, the role of any drug in the treatment of uveitis is dependent not only on its efficacy but also its availability to the clinician. It will be some time and require more studies before patients and their treating doctors will know whether secukinumab is effective, approved for use by the Food and Drug Administration, or available to patients at an affordable cost due to increasingly onerous insurance plans. Nonetheless, the results of this study offer hope for a promising new way to treat noninfectious uveitis after earlier trials using a different delivery provided disappointing results.

J. P. Dunn, MD

References

1. Sugita S, Kawazoe Y, Imai A, Yamada Y, Horie S, Mochizuki M. Inhibition of Th17 differentiation by anti-TNF-alpha therapy in uveitis patients with Behçet's disease. *Arthritis Res Ther.* 2012;14:R99.
2. Zhang R, Qian J, Guo J, Yuan YF, Xue K. Suppression of experimental autoimmune uveoretinitis by anti-IL-17 antibody. *Curr Eye Res.* 2009;34:297-303.
3. Dick AD, Tugal-Tutkun I, Foster S, et al. Secukinumab in the treatment of noninfectious uveitis: results of three randomized, controlled clinical trials. *Ophthalmology.* 2013;120:777-787.

7 Oculoplastic Surgery

Predicting the Development of Orbitopathy in Graves Thyroidopathy Patients: The Potential Role of TSI Testing

Takakura A, Kirkeby K, Earle K, et al (California Pacific Med Ctr, San Francisco)

Ophthal Plast Reconstr Surg 31:369-372, 2015

Objective.—To determine whether thyroid-stimulating immunoglobulin (TSI) testing can predict the risk of development of Graves orbitopathy in newly diagnosed Graves thyroidopathy patients.

Design.—Retrospective cohort, from 2008 to 2013.

Setting.—The Thyroid Referral Center at California Pacific Medical Center.

Participants.—A retrospective cohort of newly diagnosed Graves thyroidopathy patients from the California Pacific Medical Center Thyroid Referral Center. Patients were included if they had TSIs drawn at or near the time of diagnosis of Graves thyroidopathy. Patients were excluded from the study if they had a long-standing diagnosis of Graves thyroidopathy, orbitopathy at time of diagnosis, no TSIs drawn, or follow up of less than 6 months.

Main Outcome Measures.—Patients were followed for the development of orbitopathy as determined by their endocrinologists. Results were adjusted for family history, smoking status, age, radioiodine ablation treatment, and race.

Results.—Thirty-three patients met inclusion criteria out of a screened population of 506 patients. Eight out of 33 patients (24%) developed orbitopathy. The mean time from diagnosis of Graves' thyroidopathy to development of orbitopathy was 11.6 months (median: 7.5 months, range: 1 to 20 months). The mean initial TSI value was 421.3 in those that developed orbitopathy compared to 245.9 in those who had at least 6 months of documented follow-up and did not develop orbitopathy ($p = 0.04$). Those in the top tercile of initial TSI values were 14 times as likely to develop orbitopathy (relative risk (RR) = 14.0, $p = 0.02$; multivariate adjusted RR = 13.08, $p = 0.03$). Family history, smoking status, age, radioiodine ablation, thyroidstimulating hormone, and race were not statistically significant predictors.

Conclusions.—TSI level greater than 400 at time of presentation of Graves thyroidopathy may be a useful predictor of risk for development of orbitopathy. This information will help to identify patients likely to benefit from early referral to an ophthalmologist for possible preemptive therapy to prevent the development of orbitopathy. Prospective cohort

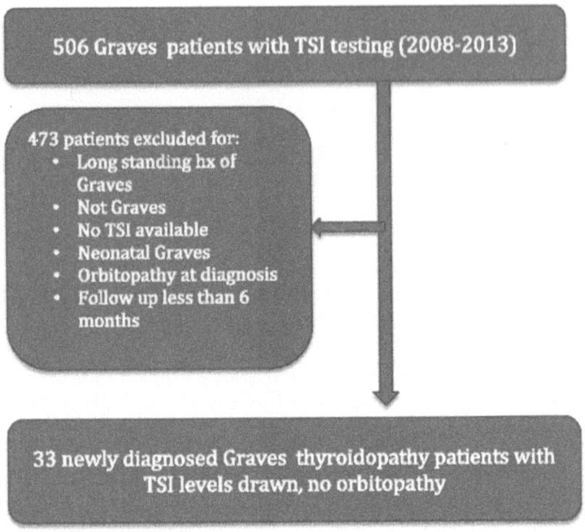

FIGURE 1.—Patient selection flow chart with the various reasons for which patients were excluded from the study. Five hundred and six patient charts reviewed from the EPIC database with a diagnosis code of Graves disease/autoimmune thyroidopathy and TSI testing from 2008–2013. Patients were excluded if they had a long standing history of Graves disease, a diagnosis other than Graves, no initial TSIs available at time of diagnosis, neonatal Graves, orbitopathy at diagnosis, or follow up less than 6 months. Of these, 33 patients met the inclusion criteria. (Reprinted from Takakura A, Kirkeby K, Earle K, et al. Predicting the development of orbitopathy in graves thyroidopathy patients: the potential role of TSI testing. *Ophthal Plast Reconstr Surg.* 2015;31:369-372, with permission from The American Society of Ophthalmic Plastic and Reconstructive Surgery, Inc.)

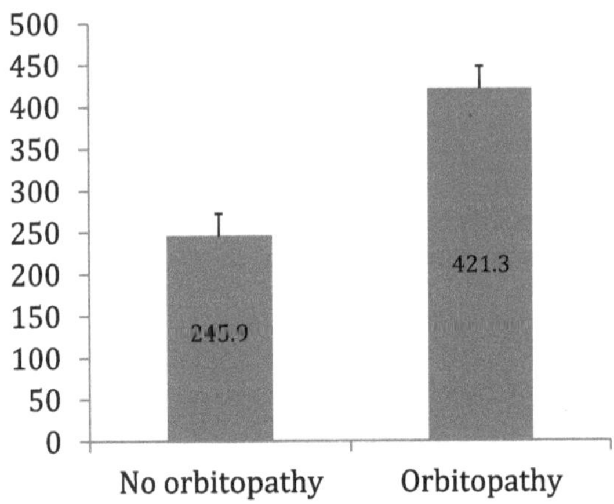

FIGURE 2.—Mean TSI of patients with versus without orbitopathy. Compared with those Graves patients without orbitopathy, patients who developed orbitopathy had a significantly higher average initial TSI level at time of diagnosis of Graves disease. (Reprinted from Takakura A, Kirkeby K, Earle K, et al. Predicting the development of orbitopathy in graves thyroidopathy patients: the potential role of TSI testing. *Ophthal Plast Reconstr Surg.* 2015;31:369-372, with permission from The American Society of Ophthalmic Plastic and Reconstructive Surgery, Inc.)

TABLE 1.—Patient Characteristics and Time to Development of Orbitopathy

Patient	Age	Gender	Race (1 = White, 2 = African-American, 3 = Asian, 4 = Hispanic, 5 = Other)	Family Hx	Smoking Status	Initial TSI	Developed Orbitopathy	Time to Development of Orbitopathy (months)
1	24	F	1		Former	697	Yes	22
2	53	M	3		Never	111		
3	29	F	2	Yes	Former	125		
4	60	F	1		Never	325		
5	21	F	1	Yes	Never	97		
6	74	F	1	Yes	Never	230		
7	34	F	3		Former	258		
8	32	F	1	Yes	Never	117	Yes	3
9	38	F	1		Never	336		
10	26	F	2	Yes	Never	447	Yes	14
11	56	F	1		Current	190		
12	54	M	1	Yes	Never	404	Yes	1
13	39	F	1		Never	265		
14	34	F	3		Former	258		
15	59	F	3	Yes	Never	330	Yes	10
16	54	F	3	Yes	Never	519		
17	28	F	1	Yes	Never	207		
18	39	F	3	Yes	Never	265		
19	32	F	1	Yes	Never	543	Yes	17
20	45	M	1		Current	297		
21	43	F	1	Yes	Never	308		
22	78	F	4		Never	259		
23	37	F	4	Yes	Former	457	Yes	14
24	14	F	3		Never	653		
25	48	F	2		Never	289		
26	45	F	1		Never	330		
27	50	F	3	Yes	Never	93		
28	42	F	3	Yes	Never	375	Yes	12
29	55	F	1		Never	240		
30	32	M	3		Current	105		
31	45	M	3		Current	140		
32	45	F	5		Never	155		
33	61	F	1		Former	93		

Thirty-three patients met inclusion criteria. The mean age at initial presentation was 43 years old. The majority of the patients were white and female. Nearly half reported a family history of thyroid eye disease. Ten patients (30.3%) were current/former smokers. Of the 8 patients (24%) that developed orbitopathy, the mean time from diagnosis of thyroidopathy to orbitopathy was 11.6 months.

Reprinted from Takakura A, Kirkeby K, Earle K, et al. Predicting the development of orbitopathy in graves thyroidopathy patients: the potential role of TSI testing. *Ophthal Plast Reconstr Surg.* 2015;31:369-372, with permission from The American Society of Ophthalmic Plastic and Reconstructive Surgery, Inc.

studies are needed to definitively establish the metrics for TSI as a predictor of orbitopathy (Figs 1 and 2, Table 1).

▶ This is a simple study that looked at the initial thyroid-stimulating immunoglobulin (TSI) levels in Graves thyroidopathy patients and compared patients who did and did not develop Graves orbitopathy (GO). Of the 506 Graves thyroidopathy patients, 473 were excluded (Fig 1). When looking at the remaining 33 patients with Graves thyroidopathy, those developing orbitopathy had an average TSI of 421 versus those who did not develop GO had an average TSI of 245.9 (Fig 2, Table 1).

There is a lot we still do not understand about the relationship of TSI levels and GO. This study suggests 1 very useful relationship. Any patient who presents with a TSI greater than 400 needs to be followed more closely for the development of GO. This study is especially useful for endocrinologists and primary care physicians who may not be as familiar with early ocular signs of GO. These patients should be watched more closely, possibly referred to an ophthalmologist for evaluation, and then the possibility and signs and symptoms of GO need to be discussed with the patient.

R. B. Penne, MD

Efficacy of Vismodegib (Erivedge) for Basal Cell Carcinoma Involving the Orbit and Periocular Area

Demirci H, Worden F, Nelson CC, et al (Univ of Michigan, Ann Arbor)
Ophthal Plast Reconstr Surg 31:463-466, 2015

Purpose.—Evaluate the effectiveness of vismodegib in the management of basal cell carcinoma with orbital extension and/ or extensive periocular involvement.

Methods.—Retrospective chart review of 6 consecutive patients with biopsy-proven orbital basal cell carcinoma and 2 additional patients with extensive periocular basal cell carcinoma who were treated with oral vismodegib (150 mg/day) was performed.

Results.—Basal cell carcinoma extended in the orbit in 6 of 8 patients (involving orbital bones in 1 patient), and 2 of 8 patients had extensive periocular involvement (1 with basal cell nevus syndrome). Vismodegib therapy was the only treatment in 6 patients, off-label neoadjuvant in 1 patient, and adjuvant treatment in 1 patient. Orbital tumors in all 4 patients who received vismodegib as sole treatment showed partial response with a mean 83% shrinkage in tumor size after a median of 7 months of therapy. In the 2 patients receiving vismodegib as neoadjuvant or adjuvant therapies, there was complete response after a median of 7 months of therapy and no evidence of clinical recurrence after discontin uing therapy for a median of 15 months. The 2 patients with extensive periocular involvement experienced complete clinical response after a median 14 months of treatment. During treatment, the most common side effects were muscle spasm (75%) followed by alopecia (50%), dysgeusia (25%), dysosmia, and episodes of diarrhea and constipation (13%).

Conclusions.—Basal cell carcinoma with orbital extension and extensive periocular involvement responds to vismodegib therapy. The long-term prognosis remains unknown, and additional prospective studies are indicated (Table).

▶ Vismodegib was approved by the Food and Drug Administration a few years ago as a treatment option for locally aggressive and metastatic basal cell

TABLE.—Patient Characteristics

Case	Age/Sex/ Race	Duration of Basal Cell Carcinoma History (years)	Involved Side	Location of Basal Cell Carcinoma	Orbit Involvement	TNM Classification	Systemic Disease	Type of Therapy	Duration of Therapy (months)	Follow up* (months)	Response	Complications
1	60/M/W	20	Left	Orbit, zygomatic, frontal and sphenoid bones	Yes (diffuse)	T4N0M0	None	Medical	5	5	Partial	Mild alopecia
2	79/M/W	7	Left	Nasal upper and lower eyelids, medial canthal area and orbit	Yes (medial)	T3bN0M0	None	Medical	13	13	Partial	None
3	63/F/W	7	Left	Nasal left lower and upper eyelids, medial canthus, and orbit	Yes (anteromedial)	T3bN0MO	None	Medical	7	7	Partial	Mild dysgeusia, muscle spasms
4	86/M/W	7	Right	Medial canthus, and orbit	Yes (medial)	T3bN0M0	None	Medical	7	7	Partial	Mild muscle spasms
5	79/M/W	10	Left	Lower eyelid, cheek, medial canthus, and orbit	Yes (medial)	T3bN0M0	None	Neoadjuvant to decrease the tumor size before surgery	5	21	Complete	Severe muscle spasms, episodes of diarrhea, and constipation
6	60/M/W	11	Right	Nasal upper eyelid, medial canthal area, and orbit	Yes (superonasal)	T3bN0M0	None	Adjuvant for postsurgical positive margins	8	19	Complete	Severe muscle spasms, alopecia, dysosmia
7	73/M/W	30	Left	Lower eyelid, cheek, and upper lip	No	T3aN0M0	None	Medical	9	12	Complete	Mild dysgeusia and dysosmia, muscle spasms, and alopecia
8	65/F/W	50	Bilateral	Forehead, eyebrow, and bilateral lower eyelids	No	T3aN0M0	Basal cell nevus syndrome	Medical	18	18	Complete	Mild muscle spasms, alopecia, tinnitus, and rhinorrhea

TNM, Tumor/Node/Metastasis (TNM) Classification.
*Since the beginning of treatment.
Reprinted from Demirci H, Worden F, Nelson CC, et al. Efficacy of vismodegib (erivedge) for basal call carcinoma involving the orbit and periocular area. *Ophthal Plast Reconstr Surg*. 2015;31:463-466, with permission from The American Society of Ophthalmic Plastic and Reconstructive Surgery, Inc.

carcinoma. This article reports on the success of treatment on 8 patients (Table). Six had orbital involvement, and 2 had extensive periocular involvement. The patients with orbital tumors all had partial response to treatment and those with skin and eyelid involvement had complete response. There were significant side effects, which can limit the use of this medication, including muscle spasm, alopecia, dysgeusia, and dysosmia.

Vismodegib has use in advanced basal cell carcinoma primarily when surgery is not an option. All ophthalmologists should at least be familiar with this medication, and its potential use. The optimal time to use this and what the risk is for recurrence after it has been stopped remain factors that need to be studied. I hope that as this medication is used more commonly, it will become easier to get insurance approval and the parameters of optimal use and duration will become clear.

R. B. Penne, MD

The Effect of Eyelid Cooling on Pain, Edema, Erythema, and Hematoma after Upper Blepharoplasty: A Randomized, Controlled, Observer-Blinded Evaluation Study

Pool SMW, van Exsel DCE, Melenhorst WBWH, et al (Univ Med Ctr Groningen, The Netherlands; Isala Clinics Zwolle, The Netherlands; Bergman Clinics Heerenveen and Zwolle, The Netherlands)

Plast Reconstr Surg 135: 277e-281e, 2015

Background.—The purpose of this study was to investigate the efficacy of eyelid cooling to reduce postoperative pain, edema, erythema, and hematoma after upper blepharoplasty.

Methods.—After bilateral upper blepharoplasty in 38 consecutive patients, one eyelid per patient was randomized for cooling with an ice pack, and the other eyelid was left uncooled. Pain was scored by the patients using a visual analogue scale (0 to 10) 1 hour and 1 day after surgery. Degree of edema, erythema, and hematoma were scored by the patients on a four-point rating scale (no, minimal, moderate, or severe) 1 hour, 1 day, 1 week, and 2 months after surgery. Light photography was obtained 1 week after surgery for scoring the degree of bruising on a four-point rating scale by a blinded observer.

Results.—Pain did not differ between cooled and uncooled eyelids on the day of surgery. However, pain in cooled eyelids was significantly lower 1 day after surgery ($p = 0.046$), yet absolute pain scores were low (median, 0 and 0.5, on a scale of 10). Edema, erythema, or hematoma did not differ between cooled and uncooled eyelids on any of the time points studied.

Conclusions.—Cooling of eyelids after upper blepharoplasty does not reduce edema, erythema, or hematoma of the eyelids, but reduces pain 1 day after surgery. However, because the degree of pain seems clinically irrelevant and because the majority of patients indicate that they have no preference for cooling over noncooling, eyelid cooling after upper blepharoplasty as a rule of thumb can be abandoned.

Clinical Question/Level of Evidence.—Therapeutic, II.

▶ The use of ice postoperatively for blepharoplasty is considered routine. This simple randomized, controlled, observer-blinded study looks at the effectiveness of this traditional postoperative regimen.

This was a small study of 38 patients post-blepharoplasty in which 1 eyelid received an icepack and the other did not. The ice was applied immediately postoperatively, the night of surgery, and 3 times the next day. Pain, edema, erythema, and hematoma were graded by the patient 1 hour, 1 day, 1 week, and 2 months after surgery. A photo was taken 1 week after surgery and graded by a blinded observer. The results with all these points was no difference between the cooled and noncooled eyelid with the exception of pain being less at 1 day postoperatively in the cooled eyelid. However, the amount of pain noted in both eyes was low. Finally, when asked whether they preferred the cooled or noncooling treatment, 28.8% preferred cooling, 39.5% preferred noncooling, and 31.6% had no preference.

This article certainly questions the effectiveness of ice postoperatively after upper lid blepharoplasty, which for most surgeons is routine. I do not think this will make me stop using ice postoperatively in my patients undergoing eyelid surgery, but it does make me think about its real effectiveness.

R. B. Penne, MD

Contrast Sensitivity Testing in Functional Ptosis and Dermatochalasis Surgery

Fowler BT, Pegram TA, Cutler-Peck C, et al (Univ of Tennessee Health Science Ctr, Memphis; et al)

Ophthal Plast Reconstr Surg 31:272-274, 2015

Purpose.—To assess whether taped versus untaped contrast sensitivity testing reliably predicts improvement following eyelid-lifting surgery in patients with ptosis and/or dermatochalasis.

Methods.—This prospective study compared pre- and postoperative near contrast sensitivity in patients presenting to 2 ophthalmic plastic surgery practices with functional dermatochalasis and/or ptosis as determined by Humphrey visual field testing. Contrast sensitivity was measured using Mars near cards, held at 40 cm under standard lighting conditions. Logarithmic contrast sensitivity scoring cards were used for analysis. Marginal reflex distance was also collected. Pairwise comparison was used to assess the preoperative and postoperative contrast sensitivity scores. This study was conducted under the approval of the institutional review board.

Results.—Seventy-eight eyes of 41 patients with ptosis +/ dermatochalasis underwent eyelid-lifting surgery. The mean preoperative untaped contrast sensitivity was 1.30. The mean preoperative taped and postoperative log contrast sensitivities were 1.52 (11.85% increase) and 1.51 (11.44% increase), respectively. The difference between the 2 groups was not statistically significant ($p = 0.864$). The marginal reflex distance improved by a mean of 2.0 ($p < 0.0005$).

Conclusions.—Contrast sensitivity improves significantly following blepharoplasty and ptosis surgery. The degree of improvement in contrast sensitivity can accurately be predicted by preoperative taped/untaped testing. Contrast sensitivity testing may provide an additional screening modality for functional dermatochalasis and ptosis. In the future, contrast sensitivity may provide an additional preoperative assessment tool in patients who do not meet traditional visual field screening standards or who are unable to perform classic visual field testing.

▶ The necessity to justify ptosis surgery is likely to increase in the future as payers more closely scrutinize procedures being performed. This is a simple article that looks at contract sensitivity and patients with ptosis. The results were recorded with the lids in their ptotic position, with lids taped up, and after ptosis repair. The results showed a statistically significant improvement in contrast sensitivity in both the taped eyelids and postoperative when compared with the preoperative ptotic eyelids.

Everyone who does ptosis surgery has had many patients say how much brighter things seem after surgery, even with a mild lift of the eyelids. This study scientifically measures that improvement that our patients note. Although the standard test to determine whether ptosis surgery is justified is a visual field, contrast sensitivity really demonstrates the improved vision a patient achieves after ptosis surgery.

It is possible that testing like this may help to justify ptosis surgery and the visual improvement it provides in the future. Contrast sensitivity is a simple test that can be done anywhere. The cards are around $400, but that is a lot less than a visual field machine. The downside is that the testing is unlikely to be reimbursable with the diagnosis of ptosis.

R. B. Penne, MD

Multinational Comparison of Prophylactic Antibiotic Use for Eyelid Surgery

Fay A, Nallasamy N, Bernardini F, et al (Harvard Med School, Boston, MA; Duke Univ Eye Ctr, Durham, NC; Oculoplastica Bernardini, Genova, Italy; et al)
JAMA Ophthalmol 133:778-784, 2015

Importance.—Antibiotic stewardship is important in controlling resistance, adverse reactions, and cost. The literature regarding antibiotic use for eyelid surgery is lacking.

Objectives.—To determine standard care and assess factors influencing antibiotic prescribing practices for eyelid surgery.

Design, Setting, and Participants.—A survey study was conducted from February 2, 2014, to March 24, 2014. The survey was distributed to 2397 oculoplastic surgeons in private and academic oculoplastic surgery practices in 43 countries. All surgeons were members of ophthalmic plastic and reconstructive surgery societies. Data were analyzed by geographic location. Linear regression was performed to quantify contributions to rates of prescribing postoperative antibiotics for routine eyelid surgical procedures.

Main Outcomes and Measures.—Rates of prescribing prophylactic intravenous, oral, and topical antibiotics as well as factors that influence surgeons' prescribing practices.

Results.—A total of 782 responses were received from 2397 surgeons (average response rate, 36.7%; 2.5% margin of error) from 43 countries. Topical antibiotic use was common in all regions (85.2%). Perioperative intravenous antibiotic use was uncommon in all regions (13.5%). Geographic location was the greatest predictor of antibiotic prescribing practices (range, 2.9% in the United Kingdom to 86.7% in India; mean, 24%). Within Europe, Italy had the highest rate of antibiotic prescriptions for eyelid surgery (41.7%) and the United Kingdom had the lowest rate (2.9%.) In South America, Venezuela had the highest rate of antibiotic prescriptions for eyelid surgery (83.3%) and Chile had the lowest rate (0%). The practice locations that were associated with routinely prescribing postoperative oral antibiotics were India (odds ratio [OR], 15.83; 95% CI, 4.85-51.68; $P < .001$), Venezuela (OR, 13.47; 95% CI, 1.43-127.19; $P = .02$), and Southeast Asia (OR, 2.80; 95% CI, 1.15-6.84; $P = .02$). Conversely, practice location in the United Kingdom (OR, 0.048; 95% CI, 0.0063-0.37; $P = .004$), Australia and New Zealand (OR, 0.15; 95% CI, 0.033-0.67; $P = .01$), and the United States and Canada (OR, 0.41; 95% CI, 0.23-0.72; $P = .002$) were associated with decreased rates of postoperative oral antibiotic use. Surgeons' concern for allergic reactions was associated with decreased rates of prescribing antibiotics (OR, 0.34; 95% CI, 0.23-0.49; $P < .001$), while surgeons' concern for infection was associated with increased rates of prescribing antibiotics (OR 1.80; 95% CI, 1.45-2.23; $P < .001$).

Conclusions and Relevance.—These results from members of ophthalmic plastic and reconstructive surgery societies confirm that antibiotic prescribing practices for routine eyelid surgical procedures vary widely throughout the world. No standard of care has been established that would require the routine use of postoperative prophylactic antibiotics following eyelid surgery (Box).

► This article looks at the rate of use of prophylactic antibiotics in eyelid surgery worldwide. This was done through a survey (Box) of oculoplastic surgeons in 43 counties and looked at rate of intravenous (IV), oral and topical antibiotics. Worldwide IV antibiotics were used by 13.5% of respondents, oral antibiotics by 23.6% of respondents, and topical antibiotics by 87.9% of respondents when performing eyelid surgery (Fig in the original article).

Box: Primary Survey Questions[a]

Where did you complete your oculoplastic training?
Where do you currently practice?
How long ago did you finish your oculoplastics training?
In which type of setting did your fellowship primarily take place (university vs private practice)?
In which type of setting do you primarily practice currently (university vs private practice)?
In which type of setting do you primarily practice currently (urban vs rural)?
Do you routinely give your patients intravenous antibiotics prophylactically (ie, within 60 minutes of surgery) for routine, elective eyelid surgery?
Do you typically give your patients oral antibiotics after routine, elective eyelid surgery?
Do you typically apply topical antibiotics immediately after routine, elective eyelid surgery?
Do you typically prescribe topical antibiotics for postoperative (home) care after routine, elective eyelid surgery?
Please indicate the reason(s) you follow your individual antibiotic regimen:
Have you changed your antibiotic regimen practices since you completed your training?
To the best of your knowledge and experience, what would you estimate is the rate of wound infection following routine eyelid surgery when prophylactic or perioperative oral or intravenous antibiotics were not used?
Upon return examination after prescribing oral antibiotics, do you routinely question your patients about adverse effects of antibiotics?
To the best of your knowledge, please estimate the percentage of patients who develop allergic reactions with the use of oral antibiotics:
To the best of your knowledge, please estimate the percentage of patients who develop gastrointestinal upset or diarrhea with a 1-week course of oral antibiotics:
In which of the following cases would you routinely administer intravenous, perioperative antibiotics?

[a] Secondary questions not shown.

Reprinted from Fay A, Nallasamy N, Bernardini F, et al. Multinational comparison of prophylactic antibiotic use for eyelid surgery. *JAMA Ophthalmol.* 2015;133:778-784, with permission from American Medical Association.

The factors that determined the use of antibiotics were training, where the surgeon practiced and perception of the risk of infection postoperatively. India and Venezuela has the highest rate of prophylactic oral antibiotics use, whereas the United Kingdom, Australia/New Zealand, and the United States had the lowest rate (Table in the original article).

There is no support in the medical literature for the use of prophylactic systemic antibiotics in routine eyelid surgery. There are a number of reasons not to use systemic antibiotics unless necessary; these include both reactions the patient may have as well the overall risk of increasing antibiotic resistance worldwide.

I fully agree that prophylactic systemic antibiotics in eyelid surgery are not indicated. This article illustrates the wide variation in antibiotic use worldwide. There is even a question on whether routine antibiotic ointment is needed for postoperative wounds after eyelid surgery. I still use antibiotic ointment in my practice but am not sure there really is a medically proven reason for its use. I never use systemic antibiotics for routine eyelid surgery.

R. B. Penne, MD

Prevalence of canaliculitis after smartplug insertion during long-term follow-up

Klein-Theyer A, Boldin I, Rabensteiner DF, et al (Med Univ of Graz, Austria)
Br J Ophthalmol 99:1134-1136, 2015

Purpose.—To evaluate the long-term prevalence of canaliculitis associated with the use of SmartPlugs.

Methods.—This retrospective study included 42 eyes of 25 dry eye patients at our institution who received a SmartPlug insertion between 2004 and 2008. Irrigation of the lacrimal system was performed in all patients prior to SmartPlug insertion to ensure the patency of the system. The median follow-up time was 7.9 (5.6—10.5) years after plug insertion.

Results.—Six patients (seven eyes) of 25 patients (42 eyes) developed canaliculitis. The prevalence of canaliculitis per patient was 24%, and the prevalence of canaliculitis per SmartPlug was 16.6%. The median time from SmartPlug insertion to the onset of canaliculitis was 4.7 (1.4—6.0) years. The median age of the affected patients was 61.5 (36—74) years. Five of these patients were women and one was man. The pathogens were identified as *Actinomyces* in four eyes and as *Staphylococcus aureus* in three eyes. In five patients (six eyes), the canaliculitis was resolved by the application of topical antibiotics and repeated lacrimal irrigations with antibiotics and povidone-iodine. In one patient, a canaliculotomy was necessary to cure the condition.

Conclusions.—The late onset of complications after SmartPlug insertion requires long-term observation to identify the majority of complications associated with SmartPlugs. In our patients with a follow-up of up to 10.5 years, the use of SmartPlugs was associated with the highest prevalence of canaliculitis published thus far.

▶ The concerning result from this study is that the higher rate of canaliculitis (16.6%) is attributed to a longer follow-up (median 7.9 years). Because there is often no way to know whether an intracanalicular plug is still present, the rate may be even higher with additional follow-up. The positive in this study was that 5 of 6 patients were successfully treated with topical antibiotics and repeated irrigation with antibiotics and povidone-iodine. How long these patients were followed after irrigation is not noted, but it appears that irrigation was successful in pushing the plug out because it was not present on ultrasound evaluation.

There are 2 conclusions from this study. First do not use Smartplugs unless absolutely necessary. This is not a new conclusion. The successful treatment with repeated irrigation with antibiotics and povidone-iodine is something not previously advocated. In my experience, this can be very painful, which may limit its use, but it should be considered for treatment.

R. B. Penne, MD

Canalicular laceration repair using a viscoelastic injection to locate and dilate the proximal torn edge

Örge FH, Dar SA (Case Western Reserve Med Ctr Univ Hosp, Cleveland, OH)
J AAPOS 19:217-219, 2015

Background.—Canalicular lacerations are common complications of eyelid trauma in the pediatric population. Irrigating air, water, and colored or viscous agents through the intact canaliculus have been suggested to identify the torn proximal edge. We report our experience in repairing canalicular lacerations using a novel viscoelastic injection technique with a Monoka monocanalicular stent.

Methods.—The medical records of patients <18 years of age who underwent repair of a canalicular laceration with a monocanalicular stent using superficial viscoelastic deployment to locate the torn canaliculus were retrospectively reviewed. Demographics, cause of eyelid injury, surgical management using our novel viscoelastic injection technique, and outcome were analyzed.

Results.—A total of 38 children with lid lacerations were identified, of whom the 17 with canalicular involvement were included (mean age, 6.27 years). Canalicular injury in these 17 was due to dog bite (9 patients) and shearing trauma (8 patients). In 11 patients, the injury was located in the lower lid; in 4, the upper lid; and in 2, combined upper and lower lids. All patients had good anatomic repair and on follow-up had negative dye disappearance tests and were free of tearing.

Conclusions.—Deploying viscoelastic superficially near, and injecting into the injured canaliculus can improve visualization of the operative field by retracting the surrounding tissue and tamponading any bleeding, which aids in location and dilation of the torn canaliculus initially and in subsequent steps, eases intubation into the lubricated torn canaliculus

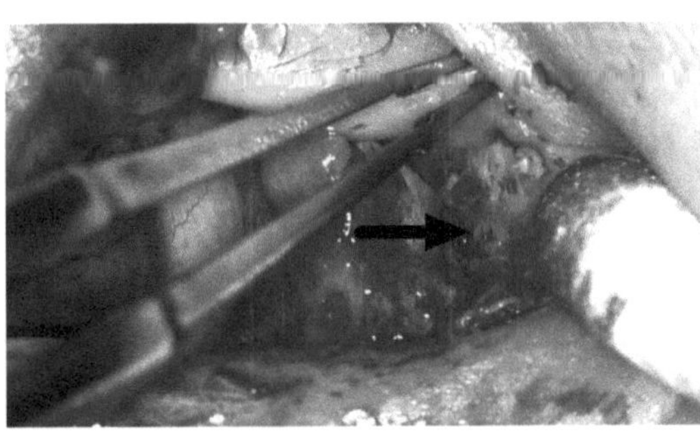

FIGURE 1.—Identification of the proximal torn canaliculus (arrow). (Reprinted from Örge FH, Dar SA. Canalicular laceration repair using a viscoelastic injection to locate and dilate the proximal torn edge. *J AAPOS*. 2015;19:217-219, with permission from the American Association for Pediatric Ophthalmology and Strabismus.)

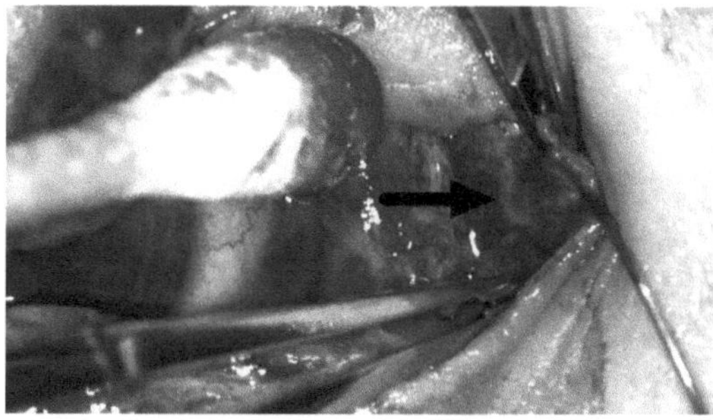

FIGURE 2.—Proximal torn edge with injected viscoelastic (arrow). (Reprinted from Örge FH, Dar SA. Canalicular laceration repair using a viscoelastic injection to locate and dilate the proximal torn edge. *J AAPOS.* 2015;19:217-219, with permission from the American Association for Pediatric Ophthalmology and Strabismus.)

and nasolacrimal duct, and avoids iatrogenic injury to an uninjured canaliculus (Figs 1 and 2).

▶ This article introduces a technique for locating and repairing a canalicular laceration, which is unique, to my knowledge. Viscoelastic is applied over the canalicular laceration area (Figs 1 and 2). This helps separate tissues, controls any bleeding, and, according to the authors, makes finding the cut end of the canaliculus easier. They do not inject it into the intact canaliculus, which I have tried a few times as a last resort with variable success. Once they find the distal cut end, they then inject a small amount into the distal cut end to help with the passage of the silicone tube.

I will definitely keep this in mind to help with repair of the next canalicular laceration. I will try to locate the cut end without the assistance of viscoelastic first because there is a cost associated with viscoelastic material. Any "trick" I can find to help locate the cut canaliculus more easily and make the repair easier I look forward to trying.

R. B. Penne, MD

Surgical outcomes of endoscopic dacryocystorhinostomy: analysis of 1083 consecutive cases

Jung S-K, Kim Y-C, Cho W-K, et al (Catholic Univ of Korea, Seoul)

Can J Ophthalmol 50:466-470, 2015

Objective.—We report on the surgical outcome of endoscopic dacryocystorhinostomy (DCR) and analyze factors that influence surgical failure.

Design.—Retrospective observational cases series.

Participants.—A total of 1083 cases who underwent endoscopic DCR with bicanalicular lacrimal stent insertion, performed by 1 surgeon between January 2007 and February 2013.

Methods.—A retrospective chart review of 1083 cases who underwent endoscopic DCR with bicanalicular lacrimal stent insertion was performed, focusing on factors that were expected to affect the surgical outcomes. Surgical outcomes were recorded as the resolution of symptoms and endoscopic evidence of ostium patency postoperatively.

Results.—The overall success rate of DCR was 92.7% (1004 cases). Of 79 cases with unsuccessful outcomes, the visualization of anatomical obstruction with endoscopy was possible in 68 cases (86%), whereas no anatomic evidence of obstruction was found in 11 cases (14%). In total, 64 cases underwent additional lacrimal intervention, and 12 cases underwent revision surgery twice after the initial DCR operation. Radioactive iodine ablation was associated with surgery failure by logistic regression analysis. However, other factors, such as sex, age, the presence of earlier accidental tube removal, indications for surgery, and Guardix injection, did not show statistically significant differences.

Conclusions.—Endoscopic DCR is a surgical technique that has a predictable, favourable success rate. It could be considered appropriate for the initial treatment of nasolacrimal duct obstruction (Tables 3 and 5).

▶ This is a large study looking at the success of endoscopic dacryocystorhinostomies (DCRs), and the authors found that they are successful in 92.7% of the cases. The study looks at 1083 cases (Table 3), which is a large number. Success was defined as lack of tearing. Previous studies of endoscopic DCR have shown a fair success rate but with smaller numbers (Tables 3 and 5). This is another study showing that endoscopic DCR is as successful as external DCR surgery, and other factors besides success rate should be used in patient selection.

The only 2 factors that correlated with failure were previous radioactive iodine (RAI) treatment for thyroid ablation and previous facial trauma. It makes sense that in cases with previous facial trauma with scarring, success may be lower. I have seen a significant number of patients with lacrimal obstruction after treatment with RAI for thyroid cancer, which is a much higher

TABLE 3.—Surgical Outcome of Initial Dacryocystorhinostomy After Silicone Tube Removal (n = 1083)

Surgical Outcome	Cases, n (%)
Disappearance of ocular discomfort, n (%)	1004 (92.7)
Persistence of ocular discomfort, n (%)	79 (7.3)
Large and patent ostium (diameter >10 mm), n (%)	11 (1.0)
Small ostium or granulation tissue development, n (%)	68 (6.3)
Management to resolve persistent discomfort	
Conservative care (large ostium: small ostium ratio)	11 (7:4)
Additional lower-lid correction(large ostium: small ostium ratio)	4 (3:1)
Lacrimal intervention, n (%)	64 (5.9)

Reprinted from Jung S-K, Kim Y-C, Cho W-K, et al. Surgical outcomes of endoscopic dacryocystorhinostomy: analysis of 1083 consecutive cases. *Can J Ophthalmol.* 2015;50:466-470, with permission from Canadian Ophthalmological Society.

TABLE 5.—Success Rates of Endoscopic Dacryocystorhinostomy in Previous Studies

	Yung and Hardman-Lea[5]	Nussbaumer et al.[6]	Fayet et al.[7]	Massegur et al.[8]	Horn et al.[9]	Karim et al.[10]	Yang and Oh[11]
Cases, n	191	201	300	96	108	105	102
Surgeons, n	2	Not mentioned	2	1	Not mentioned	1	1
Definition of success	Disappearance of epiphora	Disappearance of epiphora	Disappearance of epiphora and/or lacrimal irrigation	Disappearance of epiphora	Symptom relief and patent ostium	Symptom relief and patent ostium	Symptom relief and patent ostium
Success rate	89%	90%	87%	92%	90%	82.4%	90%
Follow-up (mo)	6	12	12	>6	3	>6	12

Editor's Note: Please refer to original journal article for full references.

Reprinted from Jung S-K, Kim Y-C, Cho W-K, et al. Surgical outcomes of endoscopic dacryocystorhinostomy: analysis of 1083 consecutive cases. *Can J Ophthalmol*. 2015;50:466-470, with permission from Canadian Ophthalmological Society.

dose of RAI than when the thyroid is ablated for hyperthyroidism. I will need to be more aware of DCR failure and RAI use.

R. B. Penne, MD

New Method for Removing Thermosensitive Acrylic Punctal Plugs From Lacrimal Puncta

Zhang M, Zhang X (Huazhong Univ of Science and Technology, Wuhan, China)

Cornea 34:1557-1559, 2015

Purpose.—This study explored a new method for removing thermosensitive acrylic punctal plugs from lacrimal puncta.

Methods.—A total of 14 dry eye patients (14 eyes), who required the removal of thermosensitive acrylic punctal plugs from the lacrimal puncta because of serious complications, were recruited. Among the 14 patients, lacrimal punctal granuloma formation occurred in 3 patients, tearing occurred in 6 patients, canaliculitis occurred in 3 patients, and chronic inflammation of the ocular surface occurred in 2 patients. The plugs were removed using a new method. Briefly, after local anesthesia was administered, a small lid clamp was used to flip the eyelid outward. After the application of the lid clamp, the plug could be removed without the use of any additional tools if the lacrimal punctum was large enough. If the lacrimal punctum was not large enough, microforceps were used to expand the lacrimal punctum before the application of the lid clamp. If the plug still could not be removed after the expansion of the lacrimal punctum, we moved the small lid clamp from the distal side of the lacrimal ductule to the lacrimal punctum.

Results.—Using this method, the plug was successfully removed in all of the patients.

Conclusions.—This is a simple and effective method for removing thermosensitive acrylic punctal plugs from lacrimal puncta.

Clinical Trial Registration—URL.—http://www.clinicaltrials.gov. Unique identifier: ChiCTR-IPR-14005476 (Fig 1).

▶ This article offers a simpler alternative to canaliculotomy for removal of thermosensitive punctal plugs that are causing a problem, such as canaliculitis, granuloma formation, tearing, and irritation. Most teaching has indicated that a canaliculotomy was required to remove these plugs. This article describes a much simpler procedure, which does not cut the punctum thus preventing the distortion and potential decreased function of the lacrimal pump possibly associated with punctal distortion. This procedure is described nicely in the article (Fig 1) and is something I will try the next time a need to remove a thermosensitive punctal plug. It does require injection of local anesthesia but is simple and only requires a chalazion clamp and jeweler's forceps.

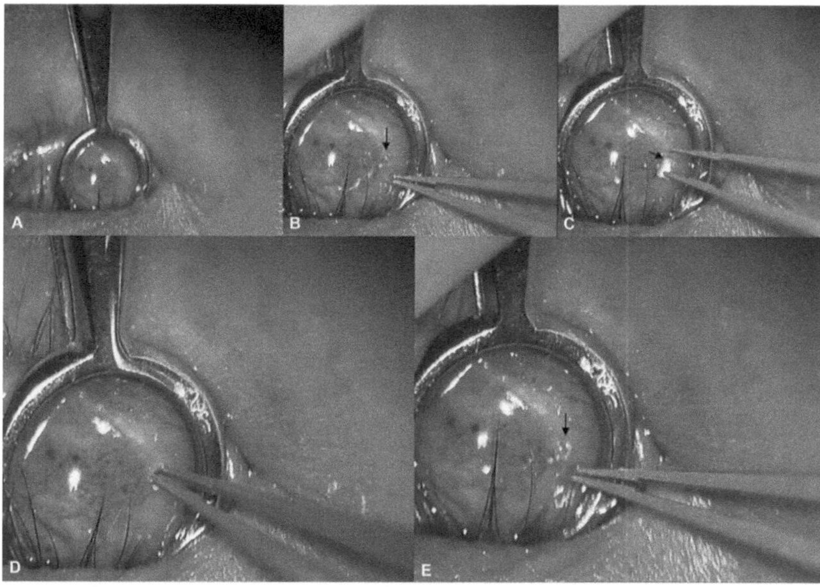

FIGURE 1.—The process for the new method for removing thermosensitive acrylic punctal plugs. A, Use a small lid clamp to flip the eyelid outward. B, Tap the tissue that surrounds the lacrimal point to facilitate plug removal. C, Remove the plug if the lacrimal point is large enough. D, Expand the lacrimal point. E, Remove the plug from the expanded lacrimal point.(Reprinted from Zhang M, Zhang X. New method for removing thermosensitive acrylic punctal plugs from lacrimal puncta. *Cornea.* 2015;34:1557-1559, with permission from Wolters Kluwer Health, Inc.)

If this does not work, it is simple to change over and do a canaliculotomy for plug removal.

R. B. Penne, MD

Risk Factors for Developing Thyroid-Associated Ophthalmopathy Among Individuals With Graves Disease

Stein JD, Childers D, Gupta S, et al (Univ of Michigan, Ann Arbor; et al)
JAMA Ophthalmol 133:290-296, 2015

Importance.—Thyroid-associated ophthalmopathy (TAO) is a common and debilitating manifestation of Graves disease (GD). Presently little is known about factors that may increase the risk of developing TAO among patients with GD.

Objective.—To identify risk factors associated with the development of TAO among individuals with newly diagnosed GD.

Design, Setting, and Participants.—In this longitudinal cohort study, all beneficiaries 18 years of age or older with newly diagnosed GD who were continuously enrolled in a large nationwide US managed care network and who visited an eye care professional 1 or more times from 2001 to 2009 were identified. *International Classification of Diseases, Ninth Revision, Clinical Modification* billing codes were used to identify those who developed manifestations of TAO. Multivariable Cox regression was used to determine the hazard of developing TAO among persons with newly diagnosed GD, with adjustment for sociodemographic factors, systemic medical conditions, thyrotropin levels, and medical and surgical interventions for management of hyperthyroidism.

Main Outcomes and Measures.—Manifestations of TAO measured by hazard ratios (HRs) with 95% CIs.

Results.—Of 8404 patients with GD who met the inclusion criteria, 740 (8.8%) developed TAO (mean follow-up, 374 days since initial GD diagnosis). After adjustment for potential confounders, surgical thyroidectomy, alone or in combination with medical therapy, was associated with a 74% decreased hazard for TAO (adjusted HR, 0.26 [95% CI, 0.12-0.51]) compared with radioactive iodine therapy alone. Statin use (for ≥60 days in the past year vs <60 days or nonuse) was associated with a 40% decreased hazard (adjusted HR, 0.60 [CI, 0.37-0.93]). No significant association was found for the use of nonstatin cholesterol-lowering medications or cyclooxygenase 2 inhibitors and the development of TAO.

Conclusions and Relevance.—If prospective studies can confirm our finding that a thyroidectomy and statin use are associated with substantially reduced hazards for TAO among patients with GD, preventive measures for this burdensome manifestation of GD may become a reality.

▶ This is a longitudinal cohort study looking at 8404 patients with the new diagnosis of Graves disease (GD), then looking at those who developed thyroid-associated ophthalmopathy (TAO) and determining factors that may make an individual at risk for developing TAO (Fig in the original article).

Seven hundred and forty GD patients (8.8%) developed TAO. Surgical thyroidectomy with or without medical treatment decreased the risk of developing TAO. The risk of TAO in this group when compared with patients treated with radioactive iodine (RAI) alone was 74% less. Statin use was associated with a 40% decreased risk of developing TAO. Another finding was that elevated levels of thyrotropin (T3) may be associated with an increased risk of developing TAO. This approached, but did not reach statistical significance in this study.

This is a study of a large group of GD patients looking for trends, and a few were found. Further prospective studies are required to confirm these. The decreased risk of developing TAO in patients undergoing thyroidectomy compared with RAI is not surprising and has been suggested in previous articles. The decreased risk of developing TAO in those patients on statins to lower cholesterol was surprising and is intriguing. This article suggests that the anti-inflammatory effects of statins may be the reason. Further study is needed to determine why. If the mechanism for this lower risk of developing TAO when taking statins can be determined, it may lead the way to new treatment to suppress or prevent TAO.

R. B. Penne, MD

Effects of Azithromycin on Gene Expression Profiles of Proinflammatory and Anti-inflammatory Mediators in the Eyelid Margin and Conjunctiva of Patients With Meibomian Gland Disease

Zhang L, Su Z, Zhang Z, et al (Baylor College of Medicine, Houston, TX)

JAMA Ophthalmol 133:1117-1123, 2015

Importance.—Topical application of azithromycin suppresses expression of proinflammatory mediators while restoring transforming growth factor β1 (TGF-β1) levels as evaluated by eyelid margin and conjunctival impression cytology.

Objective.—To explore the effects of azithromycin therapy on expression of proinflammatory and anti-inflammatory mediators in meibomian gland disease (MGD).

Design, Setting, and Participants.—Case-control study performed in a clinic setting from August 17, 2010, to December 31, 2010. Sixteen patients with posterior blepharitis and conjunctival inflammation due to MGD were treated with azithromycin, 1%, drops for 4 weeks. Impression cytology of the lower eyelid margin and tarsal conjunctiva to measure cytokine expression by quantitative real-time polymerase chain reaction as well as tear collection to measure matrix metalloproteinase 9 (MMP-9) activity were performed once in 8 asymptomatic healthy control participants and 5 times in the 16 symptomatic patients (every 2 weeks for 8 weeks), before, during, and after azithromycin treatment.

Exposure.—Azithromycin, 1%, drops for 4 weeks.

Main Outcomes and Measures.—Cytokine expression in the eyelid margin and conjunctiva, and MMP-9 activity in tears.

Results.—Compared with a 1-time measurement of 8 healthy participants, among 16 symptomatic patients, the mean (SD; 95% CI) fold change of expression of proinflammatory mediators interleukin 1β (IL-1β), IL-8, and MMP-9 increased to 13.26 (4.33; 11.14-15.38; $P < .001$), 9.38 (3.37; 7.73-11.03; $P < .001$), and 13.49 (4.92; 11.08-15.90; $P < .001$), respectively, in conjunctival cells and to 11.75 (3.96; 9.81-13.69; $P < .001$), 9.31 (3.28; 7.70-10.92; $P < .001$), and 11.52 (3.50; 9.81-13.24; $P < .001$), respectively, in the eyelid margin of patients with MGD. In contrast, the mean (SD; 96% CI) fold change of expression of TGF-β1 messenger RNA (mRNA) decreased to 0.58 (0.25; 0.46-0.70; $P = .02$) and 0.63 (0.14; 0.56-0.70; $P = .02$) in conjunctival and eyelid margin cells, respectively, of patients with MGD. Azithromycin, 1%, caused a change in the expression pattern of these mediators toward normal levels during 4 weeks of treatment. Levels of IL-1β, IL-8, and MMP-9 mRNA remained suppressed, although they rebounded toward pretreatment values 4 weeks after azithromycin withdrawal. Expression of TGF-β1 increased during treatment and remained at levels similar to the healthy controls after drug withdrawal. Change in tear MMP-9 activity was similar to the pattern of MMP-9 transcripts.

Conclusions and Relevance.—While the study did not control for potential confounding factors over time independent of the intervention that

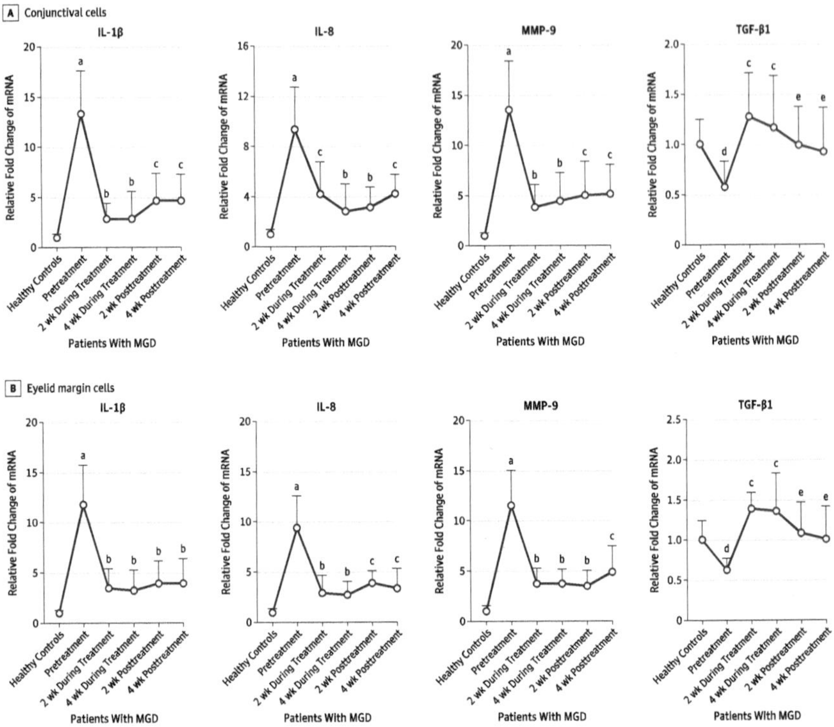

FIGURE 2.—Effects of azithromycin on cytokine profiles in meibomian gland disease (MGD). Messenger RNA (mRNA) levels of proinflammatory mediators interleukin 1β (IL-1β), IL-8, and matrix metalloproteinase 9 (MMP-9) and transforming growth factor β1 (TGF-β1) in conjunctival (A) and eyelid margin (B) cells, measured once in healthy controls and 5 times (every 2 weeks before, during, and after azithromycin treatment) in patients with MGD. Data points indicate mean; error bars, standard deviation. [a]$P < .001$ vs healthy controls. [b]$P < .001$ vs pretreatment levels. [c]$P < .01$ vs pretreatment levels. [d]$P < .05$ vs healthy controls. [e]$P < .05$ vs pretreatment levels. (Reprinted from Zhang L, Su Z, Zhang Z, et al. Effects of azithromycin on gene expression profiles of proinflammatory and anti-inflammatory mediators in the eyelid margin and conjunctiva of patients with meibomian gland disease. *JAMA Ophthalmol.* 2015;133:1117-1123, with permission from American Medical Association.)

may have contributed to the results, topical azithromycin suppressed expression of proinflammatory mediators and increased expression of TGF-β1 to normal levels. Increased TGF-β1 expression may contribute to the anti-inflammatory activity of azithromycin in MGD (Fig 2).

▶ This study showed the effects of azithromycin 1% drops at a cellular level in meibomian gland dysfunction (MGD). The authors showed an interesting gene expression profile in the conjunctival and eyelid margin cells with elevated expression of proinflammatory mediators interleukin (IL)-1β, IL-8, and matrix metallopeptidase-9 and reduced expression of anti-inflammatory cytokine transforming growth factor-β1 in patients with MGD compared with a younger healthy control group with no signs of MGD. They also demonstrated that the topical application of an azithromycin 1% ophthalmic solution altered this pattern by reversing the expression of these proinflammatory and anti-inflammatory mediators in patients with MGD (Fig 2).

I think this gives some hope for further advancement in the topical treatment of MGD. Azithromycin 1% has definite cellular effects, and I hope this type of research can lead to a model for further research and drug development for MGD. It also makes one think that azithromycin 1% should be helpful in the treatment of MGD.

R. B. Penne, MD

Long term patient-reported benefit from ptosis surgery

Maycock N, MacGregor C, Saunders DA, et al (Royal Bournemouth Hosp, United Kingdom)

Eye (Lond) 29:872-874, 2015

Purpose.—To assess the long term impact of ptosis surgery on health-related quality-of-life using the Glasgow Benefit Inventory (GBI) patient-reported outcome measure.

Patients and Methods.—A retrospective case note review was carried out on all patients who had undergone ptosis surgery (6 November 2008 to 5 December 2010) by one surgeon at Royal Bournemouth Hospital. Patient demographics, surgical technique, and complications were recorded. The GBI questionnaire data was obtained by telephone interview.

Results.—A total of 62 ptosis operations (33 right, 29 left, of which 18 were bilateral) on 44 patients; 20 male, 24 female were included. Median age 77 years (range: 17–95 years). One wound dehiscence occurred, but no redo ptosis procedures were required. GBI data was obtained on 32 patients (45 ptosis procedures) at a mean follow-up period of 42.8 months postoperatively (range 31–67 months). The mean total GBI score for

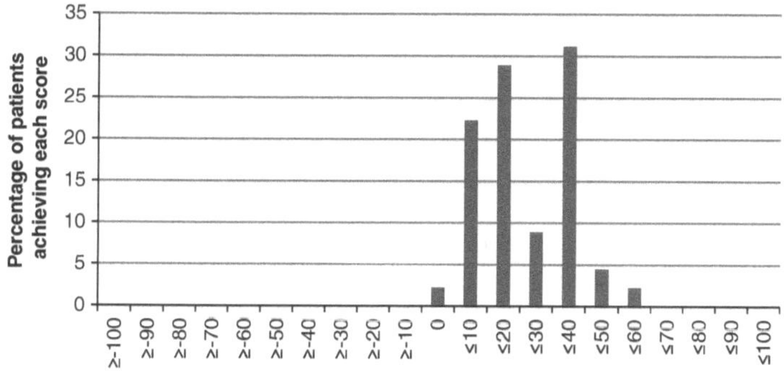

FIGURE 1.—Graph showing GBI scores following ptosis surgery. (Reprinted from Maycock N, MacGregor C, Saunders DA, et al. Long term patient-reported benefit from ptosis surgery. *Eye (Lond)*. 2015;29:872-874, with permission from Macmillan Publishers Limited.)

ptosis surgery was +21.36 (range 0–58.33; 95% confidence interval: 17.28–25.43, $P < 0.05$).

Conclusion.—Patients derived a highly significant benefit to their health-related quality-of-life from ptosis surgery measured by the GBI that was maintained for up to 5 years (Fig 1).

▶ The authors used the Glasgow Benefit Inventory (GBI) to evaluate the long-term quality-of-life benefits of ptosis surgery. This was a small study that ultimately looked at 35 patients (44 eyes) having undergone ptosis surgery an average of 42 months earlier. Their findings were that patients derive a highly significant benefit to their health-related quality of life from ptosis surgery measured by the GBI, and this was maintained for up to 5 years (Fig 1).

This is an example of what may be required more and more frequently in the health care market. Showing a quality-of-life benefit from an intervention will be important. There are many different tools available, and the GBI is just one. It is nice in that it does not need to be done preoperatively.

R. B. Penne, MD

Recurrent Thyroid Eye Disease

Patel P, Khandji J, Kazim M (Columbia Univ College of Physicians and Surgeons, New York)

Ophthal Plast Reconstr Surg 31:445-448, 2015

Purpose.—The natural history of thyroid eye disease follows a biphasic course featuring an initial active stage followed by a durable quiescent stage. Reactivation of thyroid eye disease is defined by recurrence of inflammatory signs and symptoms after a period of stability lasting at least 6 months. It is thought to be rare and is poorly studied. The goal of this study was to define the incidence and characteristics of recurrent thyroid eye disease.

Methods.—A retrospective chart review of 415 visits of patients with thyroid eye disease was performed between 2006 and 2012. Recurrent cases were identified by subjective historical accounts of disease recurrence, review of prior orbital imaging, and photographic evidence.

Results.—Among 415 cases of thyroid eye disease, 65 cases of recurrence (15.7%) were identified. Most cases of reactivation occurred within the first 10 years after the initial episode of thyroid eye disease. The mean age of patients at the first event was 42.2 years and 52.6 years at the second event. Eighteen patients had identifiable events that may have triggered disease recurrence. The recurrence rate was higher among patients that had been smokers during their first episode of thyroid eye disease (22%) compared with the nonsmokers (14.6%).

Conclusions.—Although uncommon, recurrence of thyroid eye disease does not appear to be as rare as previously believed. A better

TABLE 2.—Recurrent and Nonrecurrent TED Group Statistics

	Recurrent	Nonrecurrent
Average age at first TED event	42.2	50.6
Average age at second TED event	52.6	
Number of patients with multiple TED recurrences	6	
Average interval between first and second event (years)	10.3	
Average age at first thyroid disease diagnosis*	41.2	46.9
Thyroid state at first event		
Hyperthyroid	81.5%	80.8%
Euthyroid	10.8%	6.9%
Hypothyroid	7.7%	12%
Thyroid state at recurrence†		
Hyperthyroid	30.3%	
Euthyroid	66.7%	
Hypothyroid	3.0%	
Treatment of thyroid disease		
Oral medication only	50.8%	
Radioactive iodine	36.9%	
Thyroidectomy	12.3%	
Patients with TED family history	4.6%	6.8%

TED, thyroid eye disease.
*This average does not include those patients who were euthyroid.
†This does not include patients who underwent radioactive iodine or thyroidectomy.
Reprinted from Patel P, Khandji J, Kazim M. Recurrent thyroid eye disease. *Ophthal Plast Reconstr Surg.* 2015;31:445-448, with permission from The American Society of Ophthalmic Plastic and Reconstructive Surgery, Inc.

understanding of the natural history of thyroid eye disease is important as it impacts patient education and management (Table 2).

▶ The recurrence rate of thyroid eye disease (TED) is quoted as 5% based on a single study in 2004 by Selva.[1] This retrospective chart review finds a rate of 15.7%, which is much higher. However, when the study details are examined, the 2004 study used 5 years as the time the disease had to be stable before being considered inactive. This study uses 6 months. If this study were to use the 5-year cutoff, their rate of recurrence would be 7.7%, which is much closer to the 5%. I believe that 6 months of stability is currently accepted by most people as the amount of time needed to demonstrate motility. Thus, using that criterion, 15.7% is the best figure to use when discussing recurrence of TED.

A number of factors were looked at trying to find factors that would correlate with an increased chance of recurrence, including smoking, radioactive iodine, gender, and older age; none of these reached clinical significance. There is so much we still do not know about TED. Although this study showing a higher chance of recurrence of TED is not good news to a patient, it does allow us to tell patients more accurately what can happen in the future after their TED is stable.

R. B. Penne, MD

Reference

1. Selva D, Chen C, King G. Late reactivation of thyroid orbitopathy. *Clin Experiment Ophthalmol.* 2004;32:46-50.

Pathogenesis of thyroid eye disease: review and update on molecular mechanisms

Khong JJ, McNab AA, Ebeling PR, et al (Univ of Melbourne, St Albans, Victoria, Australia; Royal Victorian Eye and Ear Hosp, East Melbourne, Victoria, Australia; et al)

Br J Ophthalmol 100:142-150, 2016

Orbital changes in thyroid orbitopathy (TO) result from de novo adipogenesis, hyaluronan synthesis, interstitial oedema and enlargement of extraocular muscles. Cellular immunity, with predominantly CD4 + T cells expressing Th1 cytokines, and overexpression of macrophage-derived cytokines, perpetuate orbital inflammation. Orbital fibroblasts appear to be the major effector cells. Orbital fibroblasts express both thyrotropin receptor (TSHR) and insulin-like growth factor-1 receptor (IGF-1R) at higher levels than normal fibroblasts. TSHR expression increases in adipogenesis; TSHR agonism enhances hyaluronan production. IGF-1R stimulation leads to adipogenesis, hyaluronan synthesis and production of the chemokines, interleukin (IL)-16 and Regulated on Activation, Normal T Cell Expression and Secreted, which facilitate lymphocyte trafficking into the orbit. Immune activation uses a specific CD40:CD154 molecular bridge to activate orbital fibroblasts, which secrete pro-inflammatory cytokines including IL-1β, IL-1α, IL-6, IL-8, macrophage chemoattractant protein-1 and transforming growth factor-β, to perpetuate orbital inflammation. Molecular pathways including adenylyl cyclase/cyclic adenosine monophosphate, phophoinositide 3 kinase/AKT/mammalian target of rapamycin, mitogen-activated protein kinase are involved in TO. The emergence of a TO animal model and a new generation of TSHR antibody assays increasingly point towards TSHR as the primary autoantigen for extrathyroidal orbital involvement. Oxidative stress in TO resulting from imbalances of the oxidation-reduction state provides a framework of understanding for smoking prevention, achieving euthyroidism and the use of antioxidants such as selenium. Progress has been made in the understanding of the pathogenesis of TO, which should advance development of novel therapies targeting cellular immunity, specifically the CD40:CD40 ligand interaction, antibody-producing B cells, cytokines, TSHR and IGF-1R and its signalling pathways. Further studies in signalling networks and molecular triggers leading to burnout of TO will further our understanding of TO (Fig 1, Table 1).

▶ This article is the latest on what we know about thyroid eye disease at a cellular level. By the time this is published, things will have changed further. The value is as a resource in trying to understand the complicated paths that lead to TED (Fig 1). This knowledge will lead to better targeted treatment of TED. If we can treat the inflammation early with systemic, targeted medication (Table 1), we will prevent the secondary scarring and the need for surgery. This is likely years away, but for now I would encourage anyone who treats TED to read this summary of the pathogenesis of TED. It goes through the pathway of

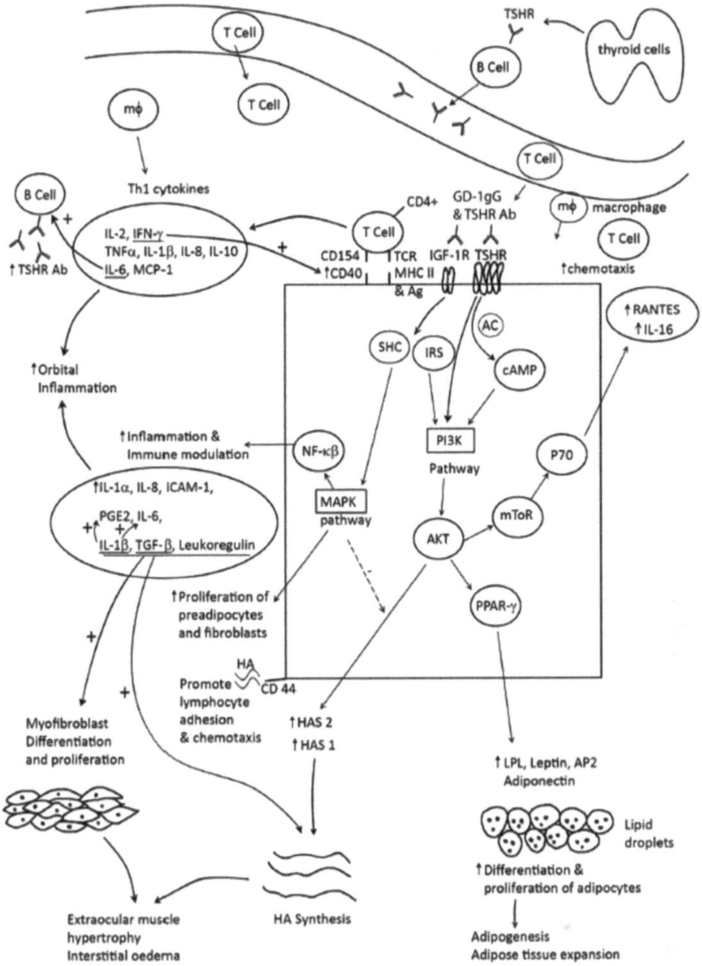

FIGURE 1.—Model of pathogenesis of thyroid orbitopathy (TO). T cell interacts with orbital fibroblast via CD40:CD154 ligation, and interaction of Major histocompatibility complex class II (MHC II), autoantigen and T cell receptor activate orbital fibroblast with increase secretion of intercellular adhesion molecule-1 (ICAM-1), nuclear translocation of nuclear factor (NF)-κβ, interleukin (IL)-1, IL-6, IL-8, macrophage chemoattractant and prostaglandin E2 (PGE2) secretion. Cytokines showed Th1 dominance with increase IL-1β, interferon (IFN)-γ, tumour necrosis factor (TNF)-α and IL-6. IFN-γ increases CD40 expression, IL-6 modulates B cell immunoglobulin (Ig) secretion. Orbital fibroblast upregulates pro-inflammatory cytokines IL-1β, transforming growth factor (TGF)-β, leukoregulin that perpetuate orbital inflammation and increase hyaluronan (HA) synthesis. TGF-β induces myofibroblast proliferation and differentiation and promotes lymphocyte adhesion and chemotaxis by CD44 and HA interaction. IgG from Graves' disease (GD) and insulin-like growth factor-1 (IGF-1) upregulates secretion of Regulated on Activation, Normal T Cell Expression and Secreted (RANTES) and IL-16, which increase T cell migration into the orbit; the AKT/mammalian target of rapamycin (mTOR)/P70 pathway seems involve in IL-16 upregulation. Activating thyrotropin receptor (TSHR) increases hyaluronan synthase (HAS) via adenyl cyclase/cyclic adenosine monophosphate (cAMP) and AKT/phophoinositide 3 kinase (PI3K) pathway. IGF-1 can also induce HAS and HA synthesis, the effect is unmasked by mitogen activated protein kinase (MAPK) inhibitor. Both TSHR and IGF-1R activate PI3K/AKT pathway to upregulate peroxisome proliferator-activated receptor-γ (PPAR-γ) expression, differentiation and proliferation of adipocytes and enhance adipogenesis. IGF-1R uses Src homology 2 domaincontaining (SHC)/insulin receptor substrate (IRS)/MAPK signalling to increase proliferation of pre-adipocytes. Switching off proximal SHC signalling on MAPK in turn permit differentiation of pre-adipocyte to adipocytes and enhance adipogenesis. (Reprinted from Khong JJ, McNab AA, Ebeling PR, et al. Pathogenesis of thyroid eye disease: review and update on molecular mechanisms. *Br J Ophthalmol.* 2016;100:142-150.)

TABLE 1.—Novel and Potential Immunotherapies in Clinical and Preclinical Trials for TO

Class of Drugs	Mechanism of Action	Example
CD20 monoclonal antibody	Deplete B cells and precursor by recognising surface CD20 marker	Rituximab[110–112]
IL-6 receptor monoclonal antibody	Binding to soluble and membrane bound IL-6 receptor and inhibit pro-inflammatory cytokine IL-6	Tocilizumab[57]
TNF-α monoclonal antibody	Bind and block TNF-α from interacting with cell surface TNF receptors.	Adalimumab[118] Infliximab[117]
Soluble TNF receptor	A soluble TNF-α receptor-Fc protein that prevent TNF-α and TNF-β from binding to membrane bound TNF receptors	Etanercept[116]
Small-molecule TSHR antagonist	Binding within transmembrane region of TSHR, blocking signalling of TSH either as allosteric inverse agonist or neutral antagonist	Org 274179-0[113] NCGC00229600[114] NCGC00242595[60]
IGF-1R monoclonal antibody	IGF-1R blocking, reduces both IGF-1R and TSHR expression	Teprotumumab[115]
Antioxidant	Increase reserve for selenoproteins involve in oxidation reduction activity, eg, glutathione peroxidase, thioredoxin reductase, iodothyronine deiodinases	Sodium selenite[121]

Editor's Note: Please refer to original journal article for full references.

IGF-1R, insulin-like growth factor-1 receptor; IL, interleukin; TNF, tumour necrosis factor; TO, thyroid orbitopathy; TSHR, thyrotropin receptor.

Reprinted from Khong JJ, McNab AA, Ebeling PR, et al. Pathogenesis of thyroid eye disease: review and update on molecular mechanisms. *Br J Ophthalmol.* 2016;100:142-150.

inflammation and the potential targets for treatment from our current knowledge.

R. B. Penne, MD

Age and Dose Are Major Risk Factors for Liver Damage Associated with Intravenous Glucocorticoid Pulse Therapy for Graves' Orbitopathy

Sisti E, Coco B, Menconi F, et al (Univ Hosp of Pisa, Italy)

Thyroid 25:846-850, 2015

Background.—High-dose intravenous glucocorticoid (ivGC) pulse therapy, which is commonly used for Graves' orbitopathy (GO), has been associated with acute liver damage (ALD), resulting in a fatal outcome in a few cases. No certain risk factors for ALD have been established. Consequently, a large retrospective cohort study was performed.

Methods.—The relationship between ALD and several potential risk factors was assessed in 1076 consecutive patients with GO given ivGC. ALD was defined as an increase of alanine aminotransferase ≥300 IU/L.

Results.—Fourteen cases of ALD were recorded, resulting in a morbidity of 1.3%. Thirteen patients recovered and one died, resulting in a mortality of 0.09%. There was a significant, positive correlation of ALD with age and methylprednisolone acetate (MPA) cumulative dose, and ALD was more common (relative risk [RR] = 2.8; $p = 0.05$) in patients aged ≥53 years (9/420; 2.14%) than in those aged <53 years (5/656; 0.76%). In patients aged ≥53 years, there was a significant positive correlation of ALD with MPA cumulative dose, and with MPA dose per infusion. Thus, the frequency of ALD in this age group was greater (RR = 3.48; $p = 0.04$) in patients with a MPA dose per infusion ≥0.7 g (5/111, 4.5% vs. 4/308, 1.29%). Regardless of age, no cases of ALD were observed for MPA doses per infusion <0.57 g.

Conclusions.—Age and MPA dose are significant risk factors for ALD, with the following practical implications. First, the total MPA cumulative dose should not exceed 8.5 g (the average dose in patients without ALD). Second, in patients aged ≥53 years, selection and observation should be quite strict. However, being aged ≥53 years should not be seen as an absolute contraindication to ivGC, especially in patients with severe GO, considering that the risk of ALD, although statistically significant, was relatively low. Third, the MPA dose should not exceed 0.57 g per infusion, a measure to be applied regardless of age.

▶ The use of intravenous corticosteroids for treatment of active Graves orbitopathy has become much more common. One large risk of this treatment is liver damage. This study looks at 1076 patients who were treated with intravenous corticosteroids and found 14 who developed acute liver damage (ALD). The authors then looked at these patient and made recommendations for safe treatment.

They found no cases of ALD if infusion dose of methylprednisolone acetate (MPA) was less than 570 mg. A cumulative dose not to exceed 8.5 grams of MPA was also safe. They also found a higher change of ALD in patients 53 years of age or older. They made the point that using intravenous steroids in patients 53 or older was not contraindicated but needed to be done with greater caution. These standards are a good start for guidelines on how to be safe with the use of system MPA. They may be modified with time as our experience with this treatment increases.

R. B. Penne, MD

Are You Missing an Entropion? The Test of Induced Entropion 2

Kennedy AJ, Chowdhury H, Athwal S, et al (Western Sussex Hosps NHS Trust, Worthing, United Kingdom)

Ophthal Plast Reconstr Surg 31:437-439, 2015

Purpose.—Entropion is the inward turning of the eyelid. The most common type of entropion is involutional, a combination of eyelid laxity, lower eyelid retractor weakness, and orbicularis oculi override. Unfortunately, the condition can be intermittent and remain undiagnosed, leading to

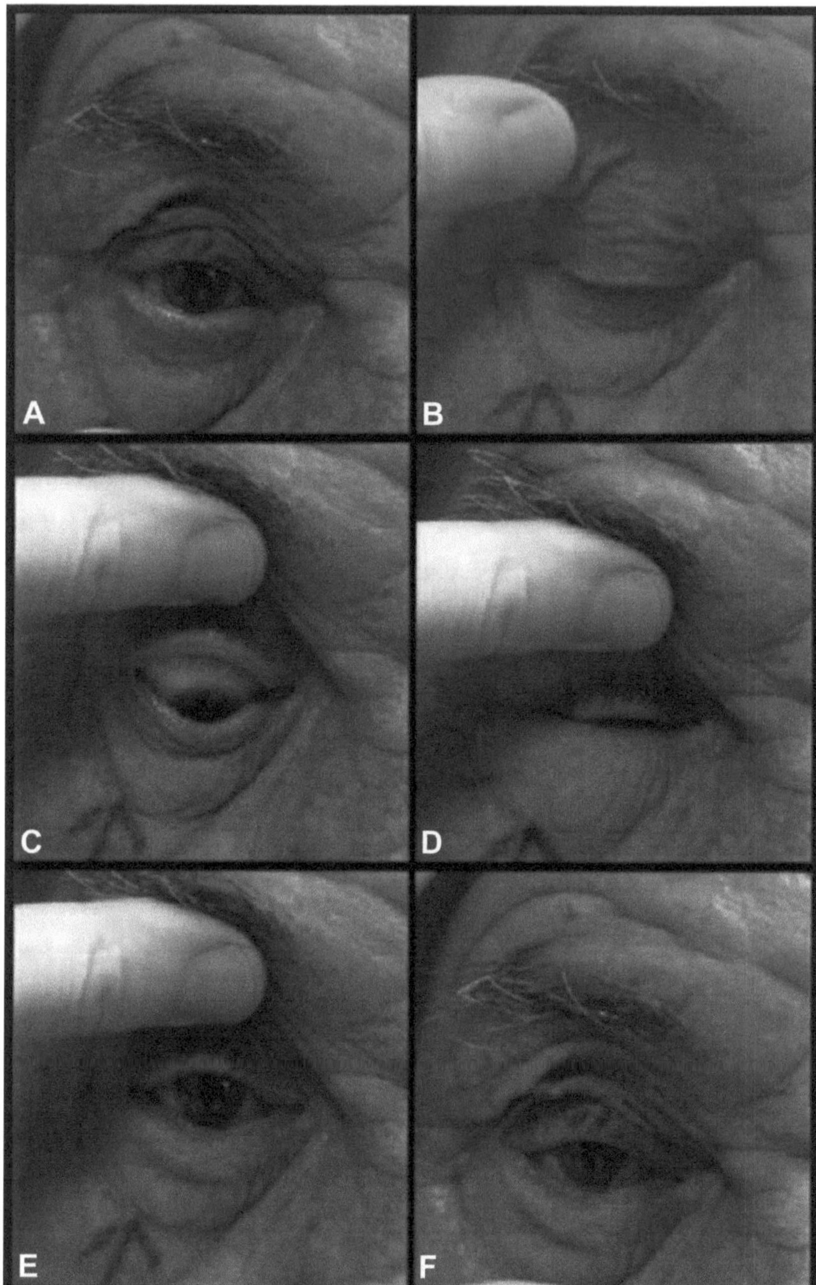

FIGURE 2.—The TIE-2 test being performed on the same patient as in Figure 1 (**A**). The 3 steps are illustrated: the patient is asked to look down (**B**), the eyelid is held up high (**C**) and the patient is asked to close their eyelids tightly (**D**). The patient is then asked to relax (**E**). This time, an entropion has been provoked (**F**). *Editor's Note*: Please refer to original journal article for full references. (Reprinted from Kennedy AJ, Chowdhury H, Athwal S, et al. Are you missing an entropion? The test of induced entropion. *Ophthal Plast Reconstr Surg*. 2015;31:437-439, with permission from The American Society of Ophthalmic Plastic and Reconstructive Surgery, Inc.)

ocular surface damage. In suspected cases, clinicians can use provocation techniques to elicit the condition. These include the forced closure of the eyelids, the tetracaine provocation test, and the test of induced entropion (TIE). The authors present an alternative diagnostic test: the TIE-2.

Methods.—The TIE-2 test is performed by asking the patient to look down while the examiner holds the upper eyelid open and high to prevent downward movement. The patient is then asked to close their eyelids as tightly as possible. An entropion will then be induced. To illustrate the technique, the authors present 2 patients seen in the oculoplastics clinic with symptoms and signs suggestive of intermittent entropion, in whom conventional provocation tests were unsuccessful.

Results.—In both cases, conventional methods did not provoke an entropion. However, the TIE-2 test successfully induced an entropion, leading to the correct diagnosis and appropriate management.

Conclusion.—When there is suspicion of intermittent entropion that is not revealed with existing provocation tests, the TIE-2 is a simple and useful diagnostic tool (Fig 2).

► Most of the time, an entropion presents with an obviously inwardly turned lower eyelid. Rarely a patient presents with a history that is consistent with an entropion or clinical findings (inferior corneal superficial punctate keratitis and an unstable lower eyelid) of an entropion, but there is no evidence of the entropion on clinical examination. There are a few things to try to produce the entropion in the office. I place tetracaine in the eye and have the patient close his or her eyes with force to try and bring out the entropion. This often works.

This article demonstrates a simple procedure that can be used if this does not work (Fig 2). This is worth remembering as an alternative to try and bring out an intermittent entropion. This technique will probably not be used often, but I did use it once, and it worked. It offers another trick to keep in your toolbox of examination techniques.

R. B. Penne, MD

8 Pediatric Ophthalmology

Outcomes of an Inner-City Vision Outreach Program: Give Kids Sight Day

Dotan G, Truong B, Snitzer M, et al (Wills Eye Hosp, Philadelphia, PA; et al)

JAMA Ophthalmol 133:527-532, 2015

Importance.—Low-socioeconomic urban children often do not have access to ophthalmic care.

Objective.—To characterize the demographic characteristics and ophthalmic conditions in children attending Give Kids Sight Day (GKSD), an outreach ophthalmic care program held annually in Philadelphia, Pennsylvania, providing vision screening and immediate treatment when needed.

Design, Setting, and Participants.—Retrospective case-series study of children attending GKSD in 2012 (GKSD 2012) at an ophthalmology center in Philadelphia. Registration forms and records of all children attending GKSD 2012 were reviewed.

Main Outcomes and Measures.—Demographic characteristics, insurance status, spoken languages, reasons for attending, prior failure of vision screening, and attendance pattern of previous events were analyzed. The ophthalmological findings of these children were examined, including refractive errors, need for optical correction, and diagnoses for which continuous ophthalmic care was necessary. For children who needed ophthalmic follow-up, the rate of return to clinic and barriers for continuous care were analyzed.

Results.—We studied 924 children (mean age, 9 years; age range, 0-18 years; 51% female; 25% speaking a non-English language) coming from 584 families who attended GKSD 2012, of whom 27% were uninsured and 10% were not aware of their insurance status. Forty-two percent of participants had public insurance, which covered vision care and glasses, but 35% did not know their benefits and did not realize vision care was covered. Forty-nine percent of children attended because they failed community vision screening. Provision of free glasses and failure of previous vision screening were the most common reasons families elected to attend GKSD (64% and 49%, respectively). Eighty-five percent of children attended GKSD 2012 for the first time, whereas 15% attended prior events. Glasses were provided to 61% of attendees. Ten percent of the attendees needed continuous ophthalmic care, most commonly for amblyopia. Ten children needed ocular surgery for cataract, strabismus, nystagmus, ptosis, or nasolacrimal duct obstruction. With the assistance of a social worker, 59% of children requiring continuous treatment returned to the clinic, compared with 2% in prior years before social worker intervention.

Conclusions and Relevance.—Programs such as GKSD can bridge the gap between successful vision screening and ophthalmic treatment, a gap that often occurs in low-socioeconomic urban populations. Those with public insurance coverage for vision services may not realize these services are covered. Social worker intervention is useful in overcoming common barriers to follow-up care.

▶ Vision loss, especially amblyopia, is common in the pediatric population and is often asymptomatic. Prompt treatment is often necessary to prevent long-term vision loss. Even with vision screening, many children, especially those from urban, low-income families do not receive adequate follow-up ophthalmic care. Ophthalmic care, such as Give Kids Sight Day, in which I have personally participated, provides an excellent method to reach many children. It is not only necessary to make the proper ophthalmic diagnosis; equally important is the follow-up. Involving social workers is vital to provide many of these families guidance to follow the direction the ophthalmologist has provided and ensure better follow-up care.

L. B. Nelson, MD, MBA

Evaluation of Temporal Association Between Vaccinations and Retinal Hemorrhage in Children

Binenbaum G, Christian CW, Guttmann K, et al (The Children's Hosp of Philadelphia, PA; et al)

JAMA Ophthalmol 133:1261-1265, 2015

Importance.—Vaccinations have been proposed as a cause of retinal hemorrhage in children, primarily as part of a defense strategy in high-stakes abusive head trauma cases. If vaccination injections cause retinal hemorrhage, this consideration would affect the evaluation of children for suspected child abuse.

Objectives.—To describe the prevalence and causes of retinal hemorrhage among infants and young children in an outpatient ophthalmology clinic and to test the hypothesis that, if vaccination injections cause retinal hemorrhage, then retinal hemorrhage would be seen frequently and be temporally associated with immunization.

Design, Setting, and Participants.—Retrospective cohort study between June 1, 2009, and August 30, 2012, at The Children's Hospital of Philadelphia pediatric ophthalmology clinics among 5177 children 1 to 23 months old undergoing a dilated fundus examination as an outpatient for any reason. Children with intraocular surgery or active retinal neovascularization were excluded from the study.

Main Outcomes and Measures.—The prevalence and causes of retinal hemorrhage, as well as the temporal association between vaccination injection within 7, 14, or 21 days preceding examination and retinal hemorrhage.

Results.—Among 7675 outpatient fundus examinations, 9 of 5177 children had retinal hemorrhage for a prevalence of 0.17% (95% CI, 0.09%-0.33%). All 9 had abusive head trauma diagnosable with nonocular findings. Among a subset of 2210 children who had complete immunization records and underwent 3425 fundoscopic examinations, 163 children had an eye examination within 7 days of vaccination, 323 within 14 days, and 494 within 21 days. No children had retinal hemorrhage within 7 days of vaccination, 1 child had hemorrhage within 14 days, and no additional child had hemorrhage within 21 days. There was no temporal association between vaccination injection and retinal hemorrhage in the prior 7 days ($P > .99$), 14 days ($P = .33$), or 21 days ($P = .46$).

Conclusions and Relevance.—Retinal hemorrhage was rare among outpatients younger than 2 years. Considering both immediate and delayed effects, no temporal association existed between vaccination injection and retinal hemorrhage. Vaccination injections should not be considered a potential cause of retinal hemorrhage in children, and this unsupported theory should not be accepted clinically or in legal proceedings. Ophthalmologists noting incidental retinal hemorrhage on an outpatient examination should consider a child abuse evaluation in the absence of other known ocular or medical disease.

► Retinal hemorrhages are rare in children under age 2 years. One hypothesis that has been proposed is the association with vaccinations and hemorrhages in young children. The authors found that retinal hemorrhages are extremely rare in infants and young children undergoing ophthalmologic examinations. Any young child with retinal hemorrhage needs to be carefully evaluated by a number of health care providers to document child abuse as the most likely etiology.

L. B. Nelson, MD, MBA

The long-term outcomes in children who are not compliant with spectacle treatment for accommodative esotropia

Hussein MA, Weakley D, Wirazka T, et al (Texas Children's Hosp, Dallas; UT Southwestern Med Ctr, Dallas; et al)

J AAPOS 19:169-171, 2015

Purpose.—To evaluate the long-term motor and sensory outcomes of children who have refractive accommodative esotropia and are noncompliant with spectacle wear.

Methods.—The medical records of patients diagnosed with pure refractive accommodative esotropia between 1999 and 2004 were retrospectively reviewed. All patients had hyperopia of at least 3 D and at least 1 year's follow-up. Patients were classified according to degree of compliance with spectacle wear as good, fair, and poor. The main outcome measures were sensory and motor outcomes.

Results.—A total of 92 patients were included. The mean follow-up period was 61.4 months (range, 12-200 months). Compared to patients with good compliance, those with fair compliance had a significantly higher risk for poor sensory outcome (odds ratio [OR] = 4.56; 95% CI 2.1-24.7; $P = 0.0003$) and poor motor outcome (OR = 4.1; 95% CI, 1.44-11.75; $P = 0.0065$). Patients with poor compliance likewise had a higher risk for poor sensory outcome (OR = 12.3; 95% CI, 1.29-96.79; $P = 0.0061$) and poor motor outcome (OR = 11.7; 95% CI, 2.38-74.19; $P = 0.0006$).

Conclusions.—Fair and poor compliance with spectacle use greatly increases the risk of poor sensory and motor outcomes in children with pure refractive accommodative esotropia.

▶ Accommodative esotropia usually develops at an average age of 2 to 3 years and is characterized by moderate to high hyperopia. Prompt treatment usually results in successful binocular sensory functions and motor alignment. Most children will comply with the wearing of their appropriate optical correction. However, occasionally children will not comply with the constant wearing of these glasses, which will ultimately cause a nonaccommodative esotropia, often requiring surgery. It is imperative for the child's caretaker to be adequately explained the importance of the full-time wearing of the optical correction to avoid the adverse effects of loss of binocular function.

L. B. Nelson, MD, MBA

Comparative study of lateral rectus recession versus recession-resection in unilateral surgery for intermittent exotropia

Suh SY, Choi J, Kim S-J (Univ of California-Los Angeles; Inje Univ Sanggye Paik Hosp, Seoul, Korea; Seoul Natl Univ College of Medicine, Korea; et al)
J AAPOS 19:507-511, 2015

Purpose.—To compare the outcomes of unilateral lateral rectus recession to unilateral recession-resection in the treatment of patients with intermittent exotropia.

Methods.—The medical records of patients with intermittent exotropia with exodeviation of 20^{Δ} to 25^{Δ} who underwent unilateral lateral rectus recession or recession-resection at a single center from 2002 to 2010 were retrospectively reviewed, and surgical outcomes between groups were compared.

Results.—Of 70 patients, 37 underwent lateral rectus recession; 33, recession-resection. The mean preoperative exodeviation was $22.2^{\Delta} \pm 2.1^{\Delta}$

at distance and $22.3^{\Delta} \pm 3.3^{\Delta}$ at near in the lateral rectus group and $24.5^{\Delta} \pm 1.4^{\Delta}$ at distance and $26.4^{\Delta} \pm 3.6^{\Delta}$ at near in the recession-resection group. Successful surgical outcome was defined as esodeviation of $\leq 5^{\Delta}$ to exodeviation of $\leq 10^{\Delta}$ at distance in primary position. The mean follow-up period was 37.1 months in the lateral rectus group and 44.6 months in the recession-resection group ($P = 0.078$). The surgical success did not differ significantly between groups at the final follow-up (45.9% in the lateral rectus group and 39.4% in the recession-resection group; $P = 0.215$). However, posteroperative overcorrection was less common in the lateral rectus group through 12 months' follow-up.

Conclusions.—Surgical outcomes at a mean of 3.4 years did not differ significantly between groups. In our study cohort, unilateral lateral rectus recession showed a low risk of overcorrection in the treatment of mild to moderate angle exotropia.

▶ Unilateral lateral rectus recession is a very effective treatment for moderate intermittent exotropia. The authors found the surgical outcome did not differ significantly between the unilateral rectus recession versus recession-resection groups. Unilateral-lateral rectus recession has a lower rate of overcorrection, the surgery is limited to 1 horizontal muscle, has shorter anesthesia time, and is easier surgery. The success of unilateral lateral rectus recession has been confirmed by other investigators as well. Therefore, the unilateral lateral rectus recession should be considered the primary surgical option for the treatment of moderate-angle intermittent exotropia.

L. B. Nelson, MD, MBA

Ocular Complications in Children with Diabetes Mellitus

Geloneck MM, Forbes BJ, Shaffer J, et al (The Children's Hosp of Philadelphia, PA; Perelman School of Medicine at the Univ of Pennsylvania, Philadelphia; et al)

Ophthalmology 122:2457-2464, 2015

Purpose.—The effectiveness of annual eye examinations in diabetic children is unclear. We sought to determine the prevalence and onset of ocular pathology in children with diabetes mellitus (DM), identify risk factors for ocular disease, and recommend a screening regimen for asymptomatic children.

Design.—Retrospective, consecutive cohort study.

Participants.—Children aged less than 18 years with type 1 or 2 DM examined over a 4-year period.

Methods.—All children underwent a complete eye examination, including dilated fundoscopy and cycloplegic refraction. A literature review was performed, identifying the youngest reported age and shortest reported duration of DM before the diagnosis of diabetic retinopathy (DR).

Main Outcome Measures.—Prevalence of DR, cataract, high refractive error, and strabismus.

Results.—A total of 370 children (mean age, 11.2 years; range, 1-17.5 years) had 693 examinations, with a mean DM duration of 5.2 years (range, 0.1-16.2 years) and a mean hemoglobin A_{1c} (HbA_{1c}) of 8.6 (range, 5-≥14). No children had DR. A total of 12 children had cataract; 5 required extraction but were identified by decreased vision, not diabetic screening. A total of 19 children had strabismus; only 1 was microvascular paralytic strabismus. A total of 41 children had high refractive error. There were no associations between these conditions and duration or control of DM. In the literature, the youngest age at diagnosis of severe DR was 15 years, and the shortest duration of disease was 5 years.

Conclusions.—Diabetic retinopathy is rare in children regardless of duration and control of DM. On the basis of our study and literature review, screening examinations for type 1 diabetes could begin at age 15 years or at 5 years after the diagnosis of DM, whichever occurs later, unless the child is judged by the endocrinologist as being at unusually high risk. Other ocular complications are identifiable through existing amblyopia screening methods.

► In many typical pediatric ophthalmology practices, children recently diagnosed with diabetes are referred for yearly ophthalmological exams. Most of these children have no ophthalmological symptoms. It is rare for any of these children, regardless of their diabetic cataract, to have any signs of diabetic retinopathy. No children in this study were diagnosed with retinopathy. The earliest documented age of severe diabetic retinopathy has been age 15 years, and the shortest duration of diabetes before the development was 5 years. Severe vision-threatening diabetic retinopathy is extremely rare in children regardless of the duration or control of their diabetes, and new guidelines need to be established. Current screening guidelines are inadequate and create an unnecessary financial burden on families with a child with diabetes. Further collaborative studies need to be performed to establish better guidelines.

L. B. Nelson, MD, MBA

Prevalence of Amblyopia in School-Aged Children and Variations by Age, Gender and Ethnicity in a Multi-Country Refractive Error Study

Xiao O, for the Refractive Error Study in Children Study Group (Sun Yat-sen Univ, Guangzhou, China; et al)

Ophthalmology 122:1924-1931, 2015

Purpose.—To estimate the age-, gender-, and ethnicity-specific prevalence of amblyopia in children aged 5 to 15 years using data from the multi-country Refractive Error Study in Children (RESC).

Design.—Population-based, cross-sectional study.

Participants.—Among 46 260 children aged 5 to 15 years who were enumerated from 8 sites in the RESC study, 39 551 had a detailed ocular examination and a reliable visual acuity (VA) measurement in 1 or both eyes. Information on ethnicity was available for 39 321 of these participants. This study focused on findings from the 39 321 children.

Methods.—The examination included VA measurements, evaluation of ocular alignment and refractive error under cycloplegia, and examination of the external eye, anterior segment, media, and fundus.

Main Outcome Measures.—The proportion of children aged 5 to 15 years with amblyopia in different ethnic cohorts. Amblyopia was defined as best-corrected visual acuity (BCVA) of ≤20/40 in either eye, with tropia, anisometropia (≥2 spherical equivalent diopters [D]), or hyperopia (≥+6 spherical equivalent D), after excluding children with fundus or anterior segment abnormalities.

Results.—The overall prevalence of amblyopia was 0.74% (95% confidence interval, 0.64-0.83) with significant ($P < 0.001$) variation across ethnic groups: 1.43% in Hispanic, 0.93% in Chinese, 0.62% in Indian, 0.52% in Malay, 0.35% in Nepali, and 0.28% in African children. Amblyopia was not associated with age or gender. The most common cause of amblyopia was anisometropia.

Conclusions.—In this study, the prevalence of amblyopia varied with ethnicity and was highest in Hispanic children and lowest in African children. Most cases were unilateral and developed before the age of 5 years. The impact of changes of definitions on prevalence estimates is discussed.

▶ Amblyopia is the most common cause of unilateral visual loss in young children. The authors found that most of the children in this study developed amblyopia by age 5. However, refractive errors can change beyond that age, and some cases of amblyopia actually develop before age 9 but older than age 5. The finding of the prevalence of amblyopia being highest in the Hispanic children and lowest in African children was probably based on genetics and not necessarily socioeconomics. It is not surprising that the authors found a very low incidence of bilateral amblyopia, which is consistent with other studies.

L. B. Nelson, MD, MBA

Effectiveness of strabismus surgery on the health-related quality of life assessment of children with intermittent exotropia and their parents: a randomized clinical trial

Wang X, Gao X, Xiao M, et al (Central South Univ, Changsha, Hunan, China)

J AAPOS 19:298-303, 2015

Purpose.—To evaluate the ability of strabismus surgery to improve the health-related quality of life (HRQOL) assessment scores of children with intermittent exotropia and their parents.

Methods.—For this prospective, randomized, parallel group study, 130 children (8-17 year of age) with intermittent exotropia were recruited and randomized to undergo either corrective strabismus surgery or active monitoring without surgery. Each child was accompanied by a parent. HRQOL was assessed with 3 intermittent exotropia questionnaires (IXTQ)–the child self-report, parental proxy report, and parental self-report–administered at enrollment and 3 months after intervention. The primary outcome was change in IXTQ score after 3 months for both groups.

Results.—At enrollment the scores of the surgery group (n = 63) and monitoring group (n = 57) did not differ significantly ($P > 0.05$). The sex of the reporting parent had no significant influence on the proxy or parental scores at enrollment or at 3 months ($P > 0.05$, multivariate analysis). Strabismus surgery significantly improved all parts of the IXTQ scores ($P < 0.0001$, repeated measures analysis of variance). No significant changes were found for the child scores at 3 months in the monitoring group ($P = 0.33$). However, the parental and proxy scores were significantly decreased ($P < 0.0001$).

Conclusions.—Corrective strabismus surgery significantly improved the HRQOL scores of the children with intermittent exotropia and their parents.

► Children with intermittent exotropia experience intermittent periods of diplopia, lack of focus, closing 1 eye indoors, and the psychosocial aspects of strabismus. Parents of children with intermittent exotropia are often aware of these symptoms as well. Therefore, it is not surprising that the authors found that surgery for intermittent exotropia improved the health-related quality-of-life assessment of the affected children and their parents. At the same time, this quality of life assessment worsened for the affected children and their parents in those children who were not operated on during the time period of the study.

L. B. Nelson, MD, MBA

Role of Educational Exposure in the Association Between Myopia and Birth Order

Guggenheim JA, for the UK Biobank Eye and Vision Consortium (Cardiff Univ, Wales; et al)

JAMA Ophthalmol 133:1408-1414, 2015

Importance.—Visual impairment due to myopia is an important public health issue. A prior analysis of population-based cohorts aged 15 to 22 years recruited from the United Kingdom and Israel suggested myopia and high myopia were approximately 10% more common in first-born compared with later-born children.

Objective.—To examine whether myopia was associated with birth order in an earlier generation than studied previously and, if so, whether the association was attenuated after adjusting for education exposure, as predicted by the hypothesis that the education of children with later birth orders is less intense.

Design, Setting, and Participants.—Cross-sectional study of UK Biobank participants recruited from 2006 to 2010. Analysis was restricted to participants aged 40 to 69 years who had a vision assessment, self-reported white ethnicity, and no history of eye disorders (N = 89 120). Myopia and high myopia were defined as autorefraction of −0.75 diopters (D) or less and −6.00 D or less, respectively.

Exposures.—Birth order and information on potential confounders including highest educational qualification ascertained using a structured questionnaire.

Main Outcomes and Measures.—Odds ratios (ORs) for myopia and high myopia by birth order, using logistic regression and adjusting for age and sex (model 1) or age, sex, and highest educational qualification (model 2).

Results.—In model 1 (no adjustment for education), birth order was associated with both myopia and high myopia (eg, comparing first- vs second-born individuals; OR, 1.12; 95% CI, 1.08-1.16; $P = 1.40E\text{-}11$ and OR, 1.21; 95% CI, 1.11-1.30; $P = 3.60E\text{-}06$ for myopia and high myopia, respectively). The risk for myopia became progressively lower for later birth orders, suggesting a dose response. In model 2 (after adjusting for education), the effect sizes were attenuated by approximately 25% (OR, 1.09; 95% CI, 1.05-1.12; $P = 1.30E\text{-}06$ and OR, 1.15; 95% CI, 1.06-1.25; $P = 4.60E\text{-}04$ for myopia and high myopia, respectively) and the apparent dose response was abolished.

Conclusions and Relevance.—These data suggest that the association between birth order and myopia is not due to a new environmental pressure in the last 30 to 40 years. The attenuated effect size after adjusting for educational exposure supports a role for reduced parental investment in education of children with later birth orders in their relative protection from myopia.

▶ The data from this study suggest that there is an association in firstborn individuals having a higher incidence of myopia than later-born individuals. The authors suggested that increasing parental investment in education to earlier-born children may be a potential factor in these individual's higher incidence of myopia.

One weakness of this study is the self-reporting, which may not adequately document the educational experience of the participants. Other factors, such as genetics, gender, and time spent outdoors, need further investigation.

L. B. Nelson, MD, MBA

Instructions to Patients and Families Following Strabismus Surgery

Dotan G, Qureshi HM, Nelson LB (Tel Aviv Univ, Israel; Wills Eye Hosp, Philadelphia, PA)

J Pediatr Ophthalmol Strabismus 52:142-146, 2015

Purpose.—To analyze postoperative instructions provided to patients and families after strabismus surgery.

Methods.—In April 2012, a 12-question electronic survey was sent to all members of the American Association for Pediatric Ophthalmology and Strabismus (AAPOS) regarding their instructions to patients undergoing strabismus surgery. The questions specifically addressed patients' daily activities, such as their resumption of school and work, sports, swimming, normal showering and bathing, and contact lens use.

Results.—One hundred two responses were completed; 96% were from pediatric ophthalmologists regularly performing strabismus surgery. Participation was greater by North American members (86%) and respondents with more than 10 years of experience (75%). Fifty percent of the respondents advised patients to resume normal showering and bathing 24 hours after surgery. Conversely, respondents recommended that children wait 3 to 4 days before resuming schoolwork (52%) and at least 2 weeks before playing in a sandbox (47%). Furthermore, respondents indicated that patients should refrain from participating in sports-related activities for at least 1 week (43%) and should not go swimming for at least 2 weeks (56%). Finally, 47% advised their patients not to wear contact lenses for 2 weeks after surgery.

Conclusions.—Overall, the responses indicated a high regard among AAPOS members for promoting normal healing and prevention of infection and other postoperative complications; however, certain trends, such as the recommendation regarding normal showering, may intimate a lack of further infection prevention.

▶ Postoperative recommendations provided to parents and their families after strabismus surgery generally lack consensus regarding the need for and duration of these instructions. Variability of these instructions are often based on a surgeon's personal experience, training, institutional policies, patient age, procedure performed, and individual factors that may differ from patient to patient. However, these postoperative instructions are necessary to avoid any possible complication caused by the direct result of patient's or family's behavior (eg, excessive eye rubbing or poor hygiene). In the study, I am surprised that only 47% of respondents suspended sandbox play for 2 weeks, considering that sand and dirt are often contaminated with potentially disease-causing organisms. Swimming pool water has been widely recognized as a medium of infection transmission, yet 28% of respondents recommended swimming resumption after 1 week. Is that too early after strabismus surgery? Perhaps all of the variability in the respondents demonstrated by this survey will result in a committee at the American Association for Pediatric

Ophthalmology and Strabismus to create some new guidelines and policies in response to postoperative instructions after strabismus surgery.

L. B. Nelson, MD, MBA

Improvement in Fusion and Stereopsis Following Surgery for Intermittent Exotropia

Feng X, Zhang X, Jia Y (Shanxi Med Univ, China)

J Pediatr Ophthalmol Strabismus 52:52-57, 2015

Purpose.—To evaluate fusion stereopsis in patients with intermittent exotropia before and after strabismus surgery.

Methods.—Fifty-three patients (mean age: 11.8 years, range: 5 to 25 years) with intermittent exotropia were enrolled. Fusion was measured with the Worth 4-dot test. Near stereopsis was examined with Titmus and stereoscopic test charts (created in China by Shao-Ming Yan). Distance stereopsis was tested with random-dot stereograms produced by Tianjin Eye Hospital. All patients completed the tests preoperatively and 2 and 6 weeks postoperatively.

Results.—There were no statistically significant differences in stereoscopic test charts among groups preoperatively ($P > .05$) and postoperatively ($P > .05$) or on Titmus tests preoperatively ($P > .05$) and postoperatively ($P > .05$). Among 53 patients, the percentage of distance stereoscopic improvement was 49% after 2 weeks and 77% after 6 weeks compared to 13% preoperatively. Six weeks postoperatively, random-dot stereograms were significantly different in those younger than 7 years and older than 13 years ($P < .05$), as well as those 7 to 13 years and older than 13 years ($P < .05$). Fifty (94%) demonstrated peripheral fusion and only 21 (40%) demonstrated central fusion preoperatively. Six weeks postoperatively, all patients exhibited peripheral fusion and 52 (98%) demonstrated central fusion. Central fusion in patients with intermittent exotropia significantly increased after 6 weeks (chi-square = 42.29, $P < .01$).

Conclusions.—Patients with intermittent exotropia have good near stereoacuity preoperatively and postoperatively. Even if surgery is postponed until adolescence, distance stereopsis can still be recovered. Surgical intervention can restore central fusion and stereoacuity in patients with intermittent exotropia.

► There are a number of reasons that children with intermittent exotropia have strabismus surgery. If one eye drifts out on a regular basis, one eye stays out through blinking and there is a reasonable amount of exotropia measured then surgery is indicated. Once the criteria for surgery for intermittent exotropia are present, the shorter the duration before surgery will often improve the long-term success rate for the functional and mechanical features.

L. B. Nelson, MD, MBA

Strabismus Surgical Subspecialization: A Population-Based Analysis

Campbell RJ, Gill SS, ten Hove M, et al (Queen's Univ, Kingston, Ontario, Canada; Queen's Univ site, Kingston, Ontario, Canada; et al)

JAMA Ophthalmol 133:555-559, 2015

Importance.—The growing complexity of medical and surgical care has resulted in increasing subspecialization. To date, data have been lacking regarding the degree to which subspecialization has affected the provision of strabismus surgical services. This gap is important to address given the implications for health care human resources planning and educational programs.

Objective.—To investigate the effect of subspecialization on the provision of strabismus surgery services.

Design, Setting, and Participants.—Population-based study in Ontario, Canada, which provides universal health care coverage to the provincial population. Participants included all ophthalmologists in Ontario and the provincial population of approximately 12 million persons from January 1, 1994, through December 31, 2011.

Main Outcomes and Measures.—Surgeon-level rates of strabismus surgery.

Results.—From January 1, 1994, through December 31, 2011, the percentage of ophthalmologists who provided strabismus surgery decreased from 37.7% (156 of 414 surgeons) to 12.5% (54 of 432 surgeons; difference, 25.2%; 95% CI, 19.3%-30.9%; $P < .001$), a 66.8% decline from the baseline level. Of ophthalmologists who provided strabismus surgery during the same period, the mean number of strabismus procedures per surgeon grew from 16.2 to 55.3 per year, a 241.4% increase (95% CI, 20.4%-461.6%; $P < .001$). These trends occurred at all career stages.

Conclusions and Relevance.—Strabismus surgery has evolved into a subspecialized field of ophthalmology during the past 15 years. These findings may have important implications for health care professionals and health care system leaders, including the need to account for subspecialization in physician human resources decisions to ensure access to quality strabismus surgery across regions. Furthermore, residency education programs and their governing organizations may need to account for strabismus subspecialization when designing curriculum and accreditation requirements.

▶ As medical and surgical care have become more complex, resulting in increasing specialization and subspecialization, the authors have documented a steady decrease in the proportion of ophthalmologists who provide strabismus surgical care. At the same time, strabismus surgical volumes have increased significantly among a subset of ophthalmologists. Recently, the number of pediatric ophthalmology fellowship applicants has decreased to the point that fellowship programs are having a difficult time filling their programs. If this trend continues, we may reach a point when there will be a shortage of pediatric ophthalmologists. The American Association of Pediatric Ophthalmology and Strabismus is presently evaluating the situation.

L. B. Nelson, MD, MBA

The Clinical Course of Intermittent Exotropia With Small Initial Deviation

Lee BJ, Kim S-J, Yu YS (Seoul Natl Univ College of Medicine, Korea; et al)

J Pediatr Ophthalmol Strabismus 52:206-212, 2015

Purpose.—To address the clinical course of patients who initially presented with small exodeviation (≥ 10 and ≤ 18 prism diopters [PD]) and to investigate the risk factors associated with progression.

Methods.—The clinical records of patients who were first diagnosed as having intermittent exotropia of small initial deviation from August 2008 to March 2011 and were followed up for 2 or more years were reviewed retrospectively. The initial clinical features associated with the risk of disease progression and surgical intervention were analyzed.

Results.—Among 86 patients who met the inclusion criteria, 37 reached a distance deviation of 20 PD or greater and 51 underwent surgical correction for exodeviation during the follow-up. Cumulative percentages of patients whose distance deviation reached 20 PD or greater and who underwent surgery at 24 months were 47.5% and 47.7%, respectively. Mean initial stereoacuity was significantly worse in patients whose final exodeviation progressed to 20 PD or greater. The cumulative probability of surgery was significantly higher in patients who showed constant deviation at the initial examination.

Conclusions.—Nearly half of patients with small exodeviation are expected to reach a final distance deviation of 20 PD or greater or to undergo surgery after 2 years of follow-up. Initial constant deviation was associated with increased cumulative probability of surgical intervention.

▶ In patients with intermittent exotropia of 15 prism diopters or greater, the decision to operate should be based on the frequency and recovery of the deviation along with reduced stereoacuity and increased symptoms. This is one of the first studies that provides specific information about the clinical course in a small-angle subgroup (10-18 prism diopters) of patients with intermittent exotropia. The authors found that the mean distant deviation increased during the follow-up period, and the angle of deviation reached 20 prism diopters or greater in approximately half of the patients at 2 years after diagnosis. Surgical treatment was also inevitable in nearly half of the patients at the 2-year follow-up. The data presented in this study delineate the probable result of treatment or observation in young children with multiangle intermittent exotropia. This information may ultimately result in better treatment decisions and improved outcomes for these patients.

L. B. Nelson, MD, MBA

Beyond Screening for Risk Factors: Objective Detection of Strabismus and Amblyopia

Jost RM, Yanni SE, Beauchamp CL, et al (Retina Foundation of the Southwest, Dallas, TX; the Ctr for Adult Strabismus, Dallas, TX; et al)
JAMA Ophthalmol 132:814-820, 2014

Importance.—Commercially available automated vision screening devices assess refractive risk factors, not amblyopia or strabismus, underreferring affected children and overreferring healthy children. Nearly half of affected children are not identified until after age 5 years, when treatment is less effective.

Objectives.—To determine the diagnostic accuracy of the Pediatric Vision Scanner (PVS), a binocular retinal birefringence scanner, to objectively identify strabismus and amblyopia, and to compare retinal birefringence screening with a widely used automated pediatric screening device.

Design, Setting, and Participants.—Three hundred consecutive preschool children (aged 2-6 years) were screened using the PVS and the SureSight Autorefractor at 2 pediatric ophthalmology private practices. A masked comprehensive pediatric ophthalmic examination provided the gold standard for determining sensitivity and specificity for each screening device.

Main Outcomes and Measures.—The primary outcome was sensitivity and specificity of the PVS for detecting the targeted conditions, strabismus and amblyopia, in children aged 2 to 6 years. Secondary outcomes included the positive and negative likelihood ratios of the PVS for identifying the targeted conditions. In addition, sensitivity, specificity, and positive and negative likelihood ratios of the SureSight Autorefractor for the targeted conditions were assessed in the same cohort of children.

Results.—Of the 300 patients, 188 had strabismus only, amblyopia only, or both, and 112 had no strabismus or amblyopia. The sensitivity of the PVS to detect strabismus and amblyopia (0.97; 95% CI, 0.94-1.00) was significantly higher than that of the SureSight Autorefractor (0.74; 95% CI, 0.66-0.83). Specificity of the PVS for strabismus and amblyopia (0.87; 95% CI, 0.80-0.95) was significantly higher than that of the SureSight Autorefractor (0.62; 95% CI, 0.50-0.73).

Conclusions and Relevance.—The PVS identified children with strabismus and/or amblyopia with high sensitivity, outperforming the SureSight Autorefractor. Accurate, early detection of these conditions could improve long-term vision outcomes of affected preschool children.

▶ Amblyopia is the most common cause of monocular vision loss in childhood. Regular pediatric visits may not always identify amblyopia and strabismus mostly because the findings may be subtle and the child may be uncooperative. Commonly available automated screening devices detect refractive errors but may miss children with amblyopia and strabismus.

A device, a binocular retinal birefringence scanner, has become available that detects whether fixation of a target is foveal and steady in each eye. The authors have found that this device has a high sensitivity and specificity for detecting amblyopia and strabismus. Additional studies in a primary care setting are necessary to assess its true clinical value.

L. B. Nelson, MD, MBA

Stability of the Functional Cure in Congenital Esotropia
Ing MR
J Pediatr Ophthalmol Strabismus 52:335-338, 2015

Purpose.—To report the stability of the functional cure in a chart review of patients with congenital esotropia.

Methods.—The charts of 31 patients with congenital esotropia, encountered in 2007-2012 with functional cure, were studied. The stability of the cure and duration of follow-up were determined by comparing the first recorded date of cure with the date of the last examination. The mean age of the patients analyzed was 19.5 years.

Results.—Two patients decompensated in the subgroup of 24 patients who did not require hyperopic correction and 1 patient decompensated in the subgroup of 7 patients who required hyperopic correction. All patients with decompensation were realigned by secondary surgery. A small subgroup of 4 patients demonstrated gradual improvement of stereoacuity to 60 arc seconds or better.

Conclusions.—The functional cure of congenital esotropia is relatively stable in patients within the first 20 years. The secondary use of hyperopic correction and secondary surgery increased this stability.

▶ In this article, Dr. Ing reviews his results in 31 patients with infantile esotropia who were surgically aligned before 2 years of age and diagnosed as having monofixation syndrome. The findings showed that the majority (28 of 31: 90%) of patients with monofixation syndrome examined during a 5-year period continued to have this form of binocularity. Only 2 of the 24 patients who required or responded to hyperopic correction decompensated. Both of these patients responded to secondary surgery. One-quarter of the patients with infantile esotropia later developed the need for hyperopic correction to stabilize the alignment achieved by surgery.

The retention of monofixation syndrome was relatively stable during the first 2 decades of life, with most remaining unchanged. A small percentage of patients were recorded as improving their sensory binocular status by developing their stereoacuity to a relatively higher grade over time. A second small percentage of patients showed decompensation, and this group of patients required secondary surgery to restore their limited binocularity. These findings indicate that surgically aligned patients with the monofixation syndrome need to be monitored for the possibility of decompensation. Furthermore, the patients who developed misalignments greater than 8 prism diopters did not complain of diplopia and so would likely go unrecognized until the deviation become cosmetically unacceptable. In those postoperative patients in whom the decompensation of their alignment is recognized, the surgeon should consider hyperopic correction or secondary surgery to reestablish monofixation syndrome binocularity.

L. B. Nelson, MD, MBA

9 Neuro-ophthalmology

Positive Auto-Antibody Activity With Retina and Optic Nerve in Smokers and Non-Smokers: The Controversy Continues
Chin EK, Almeida DR, Lam KV, et al
Ophthalmic Surg Lasers Imaging Retina 46:106870, 2015

Auto-antibodies assist with the diagnosis of ocular paraneoplastic syndromes and autoimmune ocular conditions however, the frequency of positive test results as a possible precursor to future disease is unknown. The frequency of positive antibodies in heavy smokers who may be at risk for autoimmune-related retinopathy and optic neuropathy was evaluated. Serum antibody activity was evaluated through the use of Western blot reactions from pig retina and optic nerve extract. Fifty-one patients were included: 35 patients were smokers (average: 40.9 pack-year history) and 26 patients had no past smoking history. None of the patients had any visual complaints or known eye disease. Of the patients studied, 76.5% (39 patients: 18 smokers, 21 non-smokers) had positive antiretinal antibodies, and 19.6% (10 patients: 3 smokers, 7 non-smokers) had positive antioptic nerve antibodies. Anti-retinal antibodies were seen in a majority of randomly selected patients with and without a past smoking history. Anti-optic nerve bodies were less common, but more prevalent in those who never smoked. The specificity of these antibodies remains greatly uncertain and clinical correlation is warranted.

▶ This is a very sobering article. When we suspect a patient has autoimmune retinopathy, we obtain and rely on the finding of antiretinal antibodies to support the diagnosis. A positive finding often leads to treatment, which is associated with high risk, including steroids, immunosuppression, plasma exchange, and intravenous immunoglobulin.

This study, which was performed in one of the main go-to labs for the diagnosis of autoimmune retinopathy, found that 46% of smokers and 81% of non-smokers without visual symptoms had antibodies to retinal antigens. The authors conclude "the detection of autoimmune reactions using Western blot reactions may for now be only a supplement to clinical findings." This is a study on a small population sample. If borne out on further study, it would make the very costly and complicated process of obtaining retinal and optic nerve antibodies obsolete.

M. L. Moster, MD

Cardiovascular Risk Factors in Central Retinal Artery Occlusion: Results of a Prospective and Standardized Medical Examination

Callizo J, for the European Assessment Group for Lysis in the Eye (Georg-August Univ, Goettingen, Germany; et al)

Ophthalmology 122:1881-1888, 2015

Purpose.—To analyze the underlying risk factors in patients with nonarteritic central retinal artery occlusion (CRAO) in a well-defined and homogenous group of patients enrolled in the European Assessment Group for Lysis in the Eye (EAGLE) study.

Design.—Analysis of the cardiovascular risk factors in a prospective, randomized clinical trial.

Participants.—Seventy-seven EAGLE patients with nonarteritic CRAO.

Methods.—Analysis of vascular risk factors and underlying diseases detected by questionnaire and standardized physical examination within 1 month after occlusion.

Main Outcome Measures.—The standardized physical examination included carotid Doppler ultrasonography, echocardiography, electrocardiography, blood pressure monitoring, pulse rate, urine analysis, body mass index analysis, and laboratory tests.

Results.—Seventy-seven of 84 patients had complete datasets for analysis. Fifty-two (67%) patients had cardiovascular risk factors in their medical history, and comprehensive phenotyping identified at least 1 new risk factor in 60 patients (78%; 95% confidence interval, 67%–87%). Thirty-one (40%) had carotid artery stenosis of at least 70%. Eleven patients experienced a stroke, 5 of those within 4 weeks after the CRAO occurred. Arterial hypertension was found in 56 (73%) patients and was newly diagnosed in 12 (16%) study participants. Cardiac diseases were also highly prevalent (22% coronary artery disease, 20% atrial fibrillation, and 17% valvular heart disease).

Conclusions.—Previously undiagnosed vascular risk factors were found in 78% of all CRAO patients. The most meaningful risk factor was ipsilateral carotid artery stenosis. A comprehensive and prompt diagnostic work-up is mandatory for all CRAO patients.

▶ Although many articles have reviewed risk factors for central retinal artery occlusion (CRAO), this study benefits from having a standardized evaluation process for a homogeneous study population of acute, angiographically proven CRAO patients. They had carotid Doppler ultrasonography (more than 70% stenosis was deemed to be clinically relevant), echocardiography (transthoracic or transesophageal, depending on the cardiologist's decision), electrocardiography, blood pressure monitoring, pulse rate, urinalysis, body mass index (BMI), and laboratory tests.

The evaluations were completed for 77 of the 84 patients in the EAGLE study. Fifty-four patients were men, and 23 were women; the mean age was 62.2 years old. In 25% with no known risk factors at baseline, a newly diagnosed risk factor was found. In 53% with known risk factors, at least 1 new risk factor was found. In 14% with known risk factors, no new risk factors were found. In total, 71 (92%) patients had cardiovascular risk factors or events, and 60 (78%) patients had more than 1 risk factor or event.

The most common new diagnoses were hypercholesterolemia and carotid artery stenosis. Only in 1 patient with carotid artery stenosis was it known before, and 29 patients had it newly diagnosed. Six patients (8%) reported a previous stroke, and 5 patients (6%) had a stroke newly diagnosed in MRI during follow-up. One of those had experienced a silent stroke, 2 patients experienced a stroke immediately after local intraarterial fibrinolysis, and 2 others experienced a stroke a few days after conservative treatment. Of those 5 patients, 4 had an ipsilateral carotid artery stenosis. Three patients (4%) had a history of transient ischemic attack (TIA), and a TIA was newly diagnosed in 1 patient. Taken together, 9 patients had a history of stroke or TIA, and 15 patients had a stroke or TIA diagnosis before or after the CRAO event.

Although not a surprise, the findings verify frequent cardiovascular risk factors and stroke in CRAO patients, which are often not known until after the presentation of CRAO.

M. L. Moster, MD

Intravenous Fibrinolytic Therapy in Central Retinal Artery Occlusion: A Patient-Level Meta-analysis

Schrag M, Youn T, Schindler J, et al (Yale Univ, New Haven, CT; et al)

JAMA Neurol 72:1148-1154, 2015

Importance.—Central retinal artery occlusion (CRAO) is an ophthalmologic emergency that can result in blindness. At present, no proven therapy for CRAO exists. Treatment with fibrinolytic agents has shown promise but remains of unproven benefit.

Objectives.—To assess the efficacy of systemic fibrinolytic therapy for patients with CRAO and to define a time window of efficacy.

Data Sources.—We systematically queried PubMed,Web of Science, and Scopus using the following index terms: "retinal artery occlusion" OR "retinal ischemia" AND "thrombolysis" OR "fibrinolysis" OR "tissue plasminogen activator" OR "streptokinase" OR "urokinase." Search was not limited by year of publication or language and was conducted in August 2014. In addition, we evaluated the references from relevant review articles.

Study Selection.—We assembled observational studies reporting on visual acuity outcomes after CRAO. Inclusion criteria were complete reporting of visual outcomes after CRAO (with or without fibrinolytic therapy) and a series of more than 5 patients for fibrinolysis treatment or more than 20 cases when untreated or treated with conservative modalities.

Data Extraction and Synthesis.—Patient-level datawere sought for studies reporting outcomes of treatment with fibrinolysis. Summary statistics were obtained for conservative treatment and natural history studies.

The studies were weighted by the inverse of variance and merged in a random-effects model.

Main Outcomes and Measures.—Rate of visual recovery (defined as improvement of visual acuity from 20/200 or worse at presentation to 20/100 or better) was calculated for patients treated with fibrinolytic and conservative therapies and those who received no treatment.

Results.—We obtained summary statistics from 7 studies that included 396 patients who received no treatment after CRAO and from 8 studies that included 419 patients treated with ocular massage, anterior chamber paracentesis, and/or hemodilution (conservative treatment). Patient-level data were obtained for 147 patients treated with systemic fibrinolysis. We found that fibrinolysis was beneficial at 4.5 hours or earlier after symptom onset compared with the natural history group (17 of 34 [50.0%] vs 70 of 396 [17.7%]; odds ratio, 4.7 [95% CI, 2.3-9.6]; $P < .001$). Absolute risk reduction was 32.3%, with a number needed to treat of 4.0 (95% CI, 2.6-6.6). We also found that conservative treatment significantly worsened visual acuity outcomes and recovery rates after CRAO compared with the natural history group (31 of 419 [7.4%; 95% CI, 3.7%-11.1%] vs 70 of 396 [17.7%; 95% CI, 13.9%-21.4%]; $P < .001$; number needed to harm, 10.0 [95% CI, 6.8-17.4]).

Conclusions and Relevance.—Our analysis suggests that a clinical trial of early systemic fibrinolytic therapy for CRAO is warranted and that conservative treatments are futile and may be harmful.

▶ This meta-analysis of available studies for 3 approaches to treatment of central retinal artery occlusion compared the rate of visual recovery for no treatment, conservative therapy, and with intravenous fibrinolytic treatment (t-PA, streptokinase, or urokinase). Conservative therapies included any combination of sublingual isosorbide dinitrate, topical timolol maleate, systemic inhalation of 10% carbon dioxide, hyperbaric oxygen, ocular massage, intravenous acetazolamide, mannitol, anterior chamber paracentesis, hemodilution, and corticosteroids.

The rate of recovery was defined as the percent of patients who presented with 20/200 or worse visual acuity who improved to 20/100 or better. The first surprise was that patients with conservative therapies had a decreased rate of recovery compared with no treatment (7.4% vs 17.7%). The most important finding was a higher rate of recovery with IV fibrinolysis within 4.5 hours of symptom onset than no treatment (50% vs 17.7%). Subgroup analysis of the tPA group showed similar findings. Fibrinolysis at later time points was not associated with improvement. Hemorrhagic complications occurred, but only in the streptokinase group, not in the more commonly used tPA.

As a meta-analysis, there are the usual methodologic concerns. Studies were all performed differently and analyzed differently. Visual recovery was assessed at the end of an acute hospitalization or "shortly thereafter" without longer term follow-up. Time of entry is likely delayed for the some of the "no treatment" groups because there was no time pressure to enter early for treatment. Despite these limitations, it appears that intravenous fibrinolysis within 4.5 hours is likely beneficial and a prospective study assessing this is warranted. This is the same time frame for benefit in most stroke studies and easier to achieve than intraarterial therapy because of the lack of requirement of mobilization of an interventional team.

Finally, we should consider abandoning our conservative therapies because our assumption ("it can't hurt") may be wrong.

M. L. Moster, MD

Acute nonarteritic anterior ischemic optic neuropathy and exposure to phosphodiesterase type 5 inhibitors

Campbell UB, Walker AM, Gaffney M, et al

J Sex Med 12:139-151, 2015

Introduction.—Nonarteritic anterior ischemic optic neuropathy (NAION), a rare visual disorder, has been reported in men using phosphodiesterase type 5 inhibitors (PDE5i) for erectile dysfunction.

Aim.—We examined whether intermittent use of PDE5i is associated with acute NAION onset within approximately five half-lives following drug ingestion.

Methods.—One hundred two ophthalmology centers in the United States and Europe identified potential cases of NAION. An expert adjudication committee conducted a blind review of the records of those with recent PDE5i use to classify cases as Definite, Possible, or not NAION. Subjects provided information on PDEi use via telephone interview. Each NAION case's PDE5i exposure immediately prior to onset was compared against his recent patterns of use in an observational case-crossover design. A sample size of 40 cases with intermittent PDE5i exposure in the 30 days prior to NAION onset was needed to detect an odds ratio (OR) of 3.0 with 80% power.

Main Outcome Measures.—The daily relative risk for **acute** NAION on days within five half-lives of PDE5i use vs. other days was estimated via an OR obtained from conditional logistic regression.

Results.—Among 43 Definite NAION cases with PDE5i **exposure** in the prior 30 days, the OR was 2.15 (95% confidence interval [CI]: 1.06, 4.34). When 21 Possible NAION cases were included (n = 64), the OR was 2.36 (95% CI: 1.33, 4.19).

Conclusions.—We found an approximately twofold increased risk of **acute** NAION within five half-lives of PDE5i use compared with use in a more prior time period. Bias from inaccurate recall of **exposure** was unlikely to have substantially affected the results. Based on our results, we estimate that weekly use of PDE5i adds three NAION cases per 100,000 men 50 years and older annually.

▶ This study found that there is an increased risk of nonarteritic anterior ischemic optic neuropathy (NAION) temporally related to phosphodiesterase type 5 inhibitor (PDE5i) use. This case-crossover design trial came up with 2 estimates of the number of additional cases of NAION expected from PDE5i use. Estimating a use of 1 in 5 days yields a risk of an additional 3 annual cases of definite NAION per 100 000 patients. However, daily use yields a risk of an additional 34 annual probable or definite cases of NAION per 100 000 patients.

The authors claim that bias from inaccurate recall of exposure was not likely to affect the results. This is likely true because the control group was not patients claiming not to have used PDE5i but having used it more than 1 day before the NAION.

Some previous reports claim that NAION is coincidental to PDE5i use and the association is because men with erectile dysfunction have vascular disease. However, this study clearly shows an association of NAION with PDE5i use.

M. L. Moster, MD

Association of Nonarteritic Ischemic Optic Neuropathy With Obstructive Sleep Apnea Syndrome: Consequences for Obstructive Sleep Apnea Screening and Treatment

Aptel F, Khayi H, Pépin J-L, et al (Université Grenoble Alpes, Grenoble, France; et al)

JAMA Ophthalmol 133:797-804, 2015

Importance.—The prevalence of obstructive sleep apnea syndrome (OSAS) in patients with nonarteritic anterior ischemic optic neuropathy (NAION) and its influence on second eye involvement is not well known.

Objective.—To evaluate the prevalence of OSAS in patients with NAION and risk factors of second eye involvement.

Design, Setting, and Participants.—In this cohort study, we examined 118 patients with anterior ischemic optic neuropathy referred to a tertiary care center from January 1, 2003, through December 31, 2010.

Exposures.—Patients underwent polysomnography to detect OSAS and were prospectively followed up to assess the risk of second eye involvement.

Main Outcomes and Measures.—The prevalence of OSAS in patients with NAION and the risk of second eye involvement using survival analysis based on the presence of OSAS, indication for ventilation treatment with continuous positive airway pressure, and other potential ocular and systemic confounders.

Results.—In 89 patients with NAION who underwent polysomnography, 67 (75%) had OSAS. Second eye involvement was found in 10 (13.7%) of 73 patients at 3 years: 8 (15.4%) of 52 patients with OSAS at 3 years and 2 (9.5%) of 21 patients without OSAS at 3 years; $P = .04$. In multivariate analysis, nonadherence to ventilation treatment with continuous positive airway pressure in patients with severe OSAS increased the risk of second eye involvement (hazard ratio, 5.54; 95% CI, 1.13-27.11; $P = .04$).

Conclusions and Relevance.—These results suggest that OSAS is common in patients with NAION and that polysomnography should be considered in these patients. These findings also suggest that patients with severe OSAS who are nonadherent to ventilation treatment with continuous positive airway pressure have an increased risk of second eye involvement.

▶ Four findings of this study strike me. First, the prevalence of obstructive sleep apnea syndrome (OSAS) in nonarteritic anterior ischemic optic neuropathy (NAION) is higher than we thought—75%; and even though there was no non-NAION control population in this study, the authors quote studies of an 18% prevalence in the over 50-year-old population. Second, although numbers are small, the risk of second eye involvement is greater in those with OSAS. Third, patients with severe OSAS who do not treat with CPAP have a much greater risk of second eye involvement. Finally, this study suggests that sleep questionnaires are not sensitive enough to pick up all patients who have OSAS.

So how does this change my practice? Instead of my current discussion with the patient (and preferably the patient's roommate) about whether the patient snores, I will order polysomnography on all NAION patients. I realize it is only 1 study and the number with second eye involvement is small, but with the devastating consequences of second eye involvement, I want to err on the side of being overly protective.

M. L. Moster, MD

Predictors of relapse and treatment outcomes in biopsy-proven giant cell arteritis: a retrospective cohort study

Labarca C, Koster MJ, Crowson CS, et al (Universidad del Desarrollo, Santiago, Chile; Mayo Clinic, Rochester, MN)

Rheumatology (Oxford) 55:347-356, 2016

Objective.—To evaluate characteristics of relapse, relapse rates, treatment and outcomes among patients with biopsy-proven GCA in a large, single-institution cohort.

Methods.—We conducted a retrospective review of all patients with biopsy-proven GCA from 1998 to 2013. Demographic, clinical, laboratory and treatment data at presentation and during follow-up were collected. Comparisons by relapse rate were performed using chi-square tests. Prednisone discontinuation by initial oral dose ≤440 and >40 mg/day was compared using Cox models.

Results.—The cohort included 286 patients [74% female, mean age at diagnosis 75.0 years (S.D. 7.6), median follow-up 5.1 years). During follow-up, 73 patients did not relapse, 80 patients had one relapse and 133 had two or more relapses. The first relapse occurred during the first year in 50% of patients, by 2 years in 68% and by 5 years in 79%. More patients with established hypertension ($P = 0.007$) and diabetes ($P = 0.039$) at GCA diagnosis were in the high relapse rate group (≥0.5 relapses/year) and more females were in the low or high relapse groups than in the no relapse group ($P = 0.034$). Patients receiving an initial oral prednisone dose >40 mg/day were able to reach a dose of <5 mg/day [hazard ratio (HR) 1.46 (95% CI 1.09, 1.96)] and discontinue prednisone [HR 1.56 (95% CI 1.09, 2.23)] sooner than patients receiving 440 mg/day without an increase in observed glucocorticoid-associated adverse events.

Conclusion.—Females and patients with hypertension or diabetes at GCA diagnosis have more relapses during follow-up. Patients treated with an initial oral prednisone dose >40 mg/day achieved earlier prednisone discontinuation.

▶ This article addressing the treatment of giant cell arteritis (GCA) patients with steroids found that 74% had a relapse, and 50% had it within the first year. Relapse in this report represented 29% with laboratory elevations and 24% with symptoms. Findings associated with an increased risk of relapse were diabetes or hypertension at onset. Also, women were more likely to have a relapse.

I think one of the reasons for the high relapse rate is the loose definition of relapse. They included patients whose C-reactive protein or erythrocyte sedimentation rate rose but do not stipulate whether they repeated the testing to verify the rise in value. To me, this would include many patients that are tapering a steroid but have tapered a bit too rapidly and have to raise the steroid dose for a short period. I would not consider that a true relapse.

In neuro-ophthalmology, we see severe cases of GCA and anecdotally do not have nearly the percentage of relapse as this cohort did. It is likely because we are slower to taper the steroids in our population. This population, with only 5.7% with permanent visual loss, likely was tapered a lot more quickly than we would.

Nonetheless, the take home message for me is that I have to be a bit more careful in tapering steroids in women and patients with hypertension or diabetes.

M. L. Moster, MD

Prevalence and distribution of VZV in temporal arteries of patients with giant cell arteritis

Gilden D, White T, Khmeleva N, et al (Univ of Colorado School of Medicine, Aurora; et al)

Neurology 84:1948-1955, 2015

Objective.—Varicella-zoster virus (VZV) infection may trigger the inflammatory cascade that characterizes giant cell arteritis (GCA).

Methods.—Formalin-fixed, paraffin-embedded GCA-positive temporal artery (TA) biopsies (50 sections/TA) including adjacent skeletal muscle and normal TAs obtained postmortem from subjects >50 years of age were examined by immunohistochemistry for presence and distribution of VZV antigen and by ultrastructural examination for virions.

Adjacent regions were examined by hematoxylin & eosin staining. VZV antigen–positive slides were analyzed by PCR for VZV DNA.

Results.—VZV antigen was found in 61/82 (74%) GCA-positive TAs compared with 1/13 (8%) normal TAs ($p < 0.0001$, relative risk 9.67, 95% confidence interval 1.46, 63.69). Most GCA-positive TAs contained viral antigen in skip areas. VZV antigen was present mostly in adventitia, followed by media and intima. VZV antigen was found in 12/32 (38%) skeletal muscles adjacent to VZV antigen–positive TAs. Despite formalin fixation, VZV DNA was detected in 18/45 (40%) GCA-positive VZV antigen–positive TAs, in 6/10 (60%) VZV antigen–positive skeletal muscles, and in one VZV antigen–positive normal TA. Varicella-zoster virions were found in a GCA-positive TA. In sections adjacent to those containing VZV, GCA pathology was seen in 89% of GCA-positive TAs but in none of 18 adjacent sections from normal TAs.

Conclusions.—Most GCA-positive TAs contained VZV in skip areas that correlated with adjacent GCA pathology, supporting the hypothesis that VZV triggers GCA immunopathology. Antiviral treatment may confer additional benefit to patients with GCA treated with corticosteroids, although the optimal antiviral regimen remains to be determined.

▶ This is an intriguing article demonstrating evidence that varicella-zoster virus (VZV) triggers giant cell arteritis (GCA). As noted, not all patients had evidence of VZV, suggesting that VZV may be one of numerous causes of GCA.

The study was done in specimens that were deidentified, so no clinical information is available about a clinical history of zoster, medications, or zoster vaccination.

The authors propose that the spread of VZV is from transaxonal spread to arteries, infecting the adventitia with subsequent transmural spread and primarily affecting the temporal artery. They do not speculate on how the disease spreads to all the other arteries typically involved in GCA. Presumably, there would be a systemic inflammatory response that affects arteries remote from the TA.

The authors advocate addition of antiviral treatment with intravenous acyclovir to corticosteroids in GCA patients and suggest it may shorten the length of treatment with steroids. This is likely a premature recommendation but one certainly worth further study. Until then corticosteroids remains the mainstay of treatment of GCA.

M. L. Moster, MD

The cost-effectiveness of different strategies to evaluate optic disk drusen in children

Leon M, Hutchinson AK, Lenhart PD, et al (Emory Univ, Atlanta, GA)
J AAPOS 18:449-452, 2014

Purpose.—To compare the costs of diagnostic work-up for optic disk drusen where ophthalmic ultrasound was performed prior to imaging and invasive studies with those where ophthalmic ultrasound was performed after such studies.

Methods.—The medical records of patients <18 years of age evaluated at a tertiary referral center between 2007 and 2012 for "swollen" optic nerves were retrospectively reviewed. The main outcome measure was cost of diagnostic work-up according to Georgia Medicaid global reimbursement rates.

Results.—A total of 46 children with a B-scan ultrasound–confirmed diagnosis of calcified optic disk drusen were included. Neuroimaging was performed in 23 patients, of whom 20 had the study prior to ophthalmic ultrasound. The mean cost of evaluations for patients undergoing ancillary testing prior to ophthalmic ultrasound was $1,173; for those undergoing ancillary testing after, $305.

Conclusions.—Because optic disk drusen can mimic the appearance of papilledema, it is more cost-effective to perform ophthalmic ultrasonography prior to neuroimaging, especially when the patient is asymptomatic. If ophthalmic ultrasonography confirms the presence of drusen, it is more cost-effective to reassess the clinical picture before proceeding with further tests.

▶ This study found that when patients with calcified optic disk drusen found on ultrasound (US) had the US before other studies (eg, MRI, lumbar puncture [LP]), the cost was much lower. Possible reasons they provide for why neuroimaging and/or lumbar puncture were ordered before US include lack of access to US, shortage of staff trained to detect drusen, and medicolegal reasons.

The findings show money savings, and I actually think the savings are underestimated in this study. First, they used Georgia Medicaid reimbursement rates for the calculations, which are likely lower than private insurers. Additionally, they used an LP cost of $107, which I doubt includes all the studies that the cerebrospinal fluid is sent for.

The findings of money savings are no surprise, and I think the authors make reasonable recommendations to perform the US first if the suspicion of true elevation of intracranial pressure based on clinical history and funduscopic exam is low. One can always do the further workup after US if there is still suspicion of elevated intracranial pressure, as indeed was done in 3 patients in this study.

M. L. Moster, MD

SSRI-associated optic neuropathy

Lochhead J (St Mary's Hosp, Newport, Isle of Wight, United Kingdom)
Eye 29:1233-1235, 2015

Purpose.—We report five cases of optic neuropathy (ON) identified over a 2-year period within an island population of 140 000. These cases display characteristics possibly related to long-term treatment with selective serotonin reuptake inhibitors (SSRIs).

Methods.—Retrospective analysis of casenotes. Each case has been assessed using the Naranjo algorithm to indicate likelihood of adverse drug reaction (ADR).

Results.—Clinical assessment and investigation confirmed ON in all cases with a vascular origin suspected. SSRI cessation may help protect the unaffected eye and in some cases recovery of vision seems possible. The Naranjo scores indicated possible ADR in four cases and probable ADR in one case.

Conclusions.—In 2004, ~7% of the UK adult population was receiving SSRI treatment for a range of 4.8–7.7 years. The most common ophthalmic side effect is acute glaucoma. Currently, there remain no reports of SSRI associated ON, although papilloedema has been reported. A potential mechanism for ischaemic optic neuropathy (ION) has been described in relation to raised serotonin levels. A single case of central retinal vein occlusion exists along with reports of deep vein thrombosis (DVT) and ischaemic stroke. We recommend a review of SSRI treatment in cases of acute ON.

▶ This article reports 5 cases of optic neuropathy occurring in patients taking selective serotonin reuptake inhibitors (SSRIs). The authors suggest that in 4 cases, there was a possible adverse drug reaction (ADR), and in 1 case a probable ADR based on the Naranjo algorithm.[1] They propose a possible contribution of SSRIs to ischemia and decreased perfusion and quote prior reports of increased serotonin being associated with decreasing optic nerve perfusion.

I have a few problems with this article. First, the clinical presentations were quite varied, including 1 with a simultaneous bilateral anterior ischemic optic neuropathy, 2 with gradually progressive bilateral visual loss without disc edema, and 2 with a sudden unilateral visual loss with normal disc appearance. Three different presentations of optic neuropathy would be unusual as an ADR.

Second, when I perform an independent calculation of the Naranjo score, in most of the cases, I got a lower score than reported. All of the cases fall into the "possible" ADR rather than the "probable" ADR range for me.

Despite these criticisms, it appears that an extensive workup for other etiologies was performed as described: "MRI scan, CXR, FBC, U and E, serum B12, coagulopathies, autoimmune serology, ESR, CRP, serum ACE, fundus fluorescein angiography, optical coherence tomography, visual fields, electroretinogram, and visual evoked potentials. Leber's mutation and serology for lyme, syphilis and bartonella were also performed where appropriate." However, 4 of the 5 cases had either diabetes, a smoking history, or both.

The bottom line for me is that in a patient with an optic neuropathy with no clear diagnosis after evaluation who is on an SSRI, we should consider whether the SSRI might be playing a role.

M. L. Moster, MD

Reference

1. Naranjo CA, Busto U, Sellers EM, et al. A method for estimating the probability of adverse drug reactions. *Clin Pharmacol Ther.* 1981;30:239-245.

Optical coherence tomography reflects brain atrophy in multiple sclerosis: A four-year study

Saidha S, Al-Louzi O, Ratchford JN, et al (Johns Hopkins Univ, Baltimore, MD; et al)

Ann Neurol 78:801-813, 2015

Objective.—The aim of this work was to determine whether atrophy of specific retinal layers and brain substructures are associated over time, in order to further validate the utility of optical coherence tomography (OCT) as an indicator of neuronal tissue damage in patients with multiple sclerosis (MS).

Methods.—Cirrus high-definition OCT (including automated macular segmentation) was performed in 107 MS patients biannually (median follow-up: 46 months). Three-Tesla magnetic resonance imaging brain scans (including brain-substructure volumetrics) were performed annually. Individual-specific rates of change in retinal and brain measures (estimated with linear regression) were correlated, adjusting for age, sex, disease duration, and optic neuritis (ON) history.

Results.—Rates of ganglion cell + inner plexiform layer (GCIP) and whole-brain ($r = 0.45$ $p < 0.001$), gray matter (GM $r = 0.37$ $p < 0.001$), white matter (WM $r = 0.28$ $p = 0.007$), and thalamic ($r = 0.38$ $p < 0.001$) atrophy were associated. GCIP and whole-brain (as well as GM and WM) atrophy rates were more strongly associated in progressive MS ($r = 0.67$ $p < 0.001$) than relapsing-remitting MS (RRMS $r = 0.33$ $p = 0.007$). However, correlation between rates of GCIP and whole-brain (and additionally GM and WM) atrophy in RRMS increased incrementally with stepwise refinement to exclude ON effects excluding eyes and then patients (to account for a phenotype effect), the correlation increased to 0.45 and 0.60, respectively, consistent with effect modification. In RRMS, lesion accumulation rate was associated with GCIP ($r = -0.30$ $p = 0.02$) and inner nuclear layer ($r = -0.25$ $p = 0.04$) atrophy rates.

Interpretation.—Over time GCIP atrophy appears to mirror whole-brain, and particularly GM, atrophy, especially in progressive MS, thereby reflecting underlying disease progression. Our findings support OCT for clinical monitoring and as an outcome in investigative trials.

▶ OCT has become an invaluable clinical tool in ophthalmology and neuro-ophthalmology, often localizing the abnormality and actually confirming particular diagnoses. In neurology, OCT does not have this clinical importance, but is becoming extremely worthwhile in the study of neurodegenerative disorders. It is the only place where neurons and axons can be visualized noninvasively in patients.

This study is part of a growing literature supporting the notion that neurodegeneration may be studied with retinal OCT as a biomarker.

The study found that the rate of ganglion cell + inner plexiform layer (GCIP) thinning is associated with whole brain, gray matter, white matter, and thalamic atrophy in patients with progressive MS, more so than patients with relapsing MS over an approximately 4-year time period. After adjusting for multiple comparisons, peripapillary retinal nerve fiber layer thinning was only associated with brainstem and caudate atrophy. Therefore, GCIP thinning may be a marker of disease activity and disability progression, representing a global neurodegenerative process.

The correlation of GCIP with brain atrophy is important, and I wonder whether future studies may find that when the GC layer is segmented separately, it may correlate even more with brain atrophy in the GCIP segment.

M. L. Moster, MD

Oligoclonal bands predict multiple sclerosis in children with optic neuritis

Heussinger N, Kontopantelis E, Gburek-Augustat J, et al (Children's Hosp Aschaffenburg, Germany; Univ of Manchester, United Kingdom; Univ Children's Hosp Tübingen, Germany; et al)

Ann Neurol 77:1076-1082, 2015

We retrospectively evaluated predictors of conversion to multiple sclerosis (MS) in 357 children with isolated optic neuritis (ON) as a first demyelinating event who had a median follow-up of 4.0 years. Multiple Cox proportional-hazards regressions revealed abnormal cranial magnet resonance imaging (cMRI hazard ratio [HR] = 5.94, 95% confidence interval [CI] = 3.39–10.39, $p < 0.001$), presence of cerebrospinal fluid immunoglobulin G oligoclonal bands (OCB HR = 3.69, 95% CI = 2.32–5.86, $p < 0.001$), and age (HR = 1.08 per year of age, 95% CI = 1.02–1.13, $p = 0.003$) as independent predictors of conversion, whereas sex and laterality (unilateral vs bilateral) had no influence. Combined cMRI and OCB positivity indicated a 26.84-fold higher HR for developing MS compared to double negativity (95% CI = 12.26–58.74, $p < 0.001$). Accordingly, cerebrospinal fluid analysis may supplement cMRI to determine the risk of MS in children with isolated ON.

▶ This report is a retrospective, multicenter study that included 357 children (< 18 years of age) with optic neuritis to determine the prognostic indicators for the conversion to McDonald criteria MS (MCMS). At a median follow-up of 4 years, 40.6% of the patients developed MCMS and 1.4% developed neuromyelitis optica (NMO). Higher age, abnormal cranial magnet resonance imaging (cMRI) and presence of oligoclonal bands (OCB) were predictors for the development of MS. The presence of an abnormal cMRI and OCB had a higher predictive value than each factor alone. With both OCB and MRI negative, 8% went on to MS, with both positive 95% went on to MS. With OCB positive and MRI negative, 35% went on to MS; with MRI positive and OCB negative, the number was 49%.

The findings contrast with those of the Optic Neuritis Treatment Trial (ONTT)[1,2] in adults, which found the MRI to be a strong predictor of conversion to MS but the addition of positive OCB on top of a positive MRI did not convey a further increase in risk. Among the 39 patients with normal brain MRI, CDMS developed in 3 of 11 patients (27%) with OCB present but in only I of 28 (4%) without OCB ($P = .06$). In contrast, among the 37 patients with abnormal brain MRI, CDMS developed in 13 of 27 (48%) with OCB and in 5 of 10 (50%) without oligoclonal bands ($P = 1.00$). The reason for this difference is not clear to me.

Additionally, the conversion rate to MS was much higher in this group than in the ONTT. One of the reasons for the high rate of conversion to MS in this study compared with older studies is likely that the criteria for developing MS were McDonald criteria, allowing for the diagnosis of MS based on MRI demonstration of dissemination in time and space and not requiring a second clinical event.

This study would suggest to me that, at least in children, we obtain a cerebrospinal fluid examination at the time of diagnosis if finding OCBs will move us toward an earlier treatment with disease modifying therapy.

M. L. Moster, MD

References

1. Optic Neuritis Study Group. The 5-year risk of MS after optic neuritis. Experience of the optic neuritis treatment trial. *Neurology.* 1997;49:1404-1413.
2. Cole SR, Beck RW, Moke PS, Kaufman DI, Tourtellotte WW. The predictive value of CSF oligoclonal banding for MS 5 years after optic neuritis. Optic Neuritis Study Group. *Neurology.* 1998;51:885-887.

International consensus diagnostic criteria for neuromyelitis optica spectrum disorders

Wingerchuk DM, Banwell B, Bennett JL, et al (Mayo Clinic, Scottsdale, AZ; Children's Hosp of Philadelphia, PA; Univ of Colorado Denver, Aurora; et al)
Neurology 85:177-189, 2015

Neuromyelitis optica (NMO) is an inflammatory CNS syndrome distinct from multiple sclerosis (MS) that is associated with serum aquaporin 4 immunoglobulin G antibodies (AQP4-IgG). Prior NMO diagnostic criteria required optic nerve and spinal cord involvement but more restricted or more extensive CNS involvement may occur. The International Panel for NMO Diagnosis (IPND) was convened to develop revised diagnostic criteria using systematic literature reviews and electronic surveys to facilitate consensus. The new nomenclature defines the unifying term NMO spectrum disorders (NMOSD), which is stratified further by serologic testing (NMOSD with or without AQP4-IgG). The core clinical characteristics required for patients with NMOSD with AQP4-IgG include clinical syndromes or MRI findings related to optic nerve, spinal cord, area postrema, other brainstem, diencephalic, or cerebral presentations. More stringent clinical criteria, with additional neuroimaging findings, are required for diagnosis of NMOSD without AQP4-IgG or when serologic testing is unavailable. The IPND also

TABLE 1.—NMOSD Diagnostic Criteria for Adult Patients

Diagnostic criteria for NMOSD with AQP4-IgG
1. At least 1 core clinical characteristic
2. Positive test for AQP4-IgG using best available detection method (cell-based assay strongly recommended)
3. Exclusion of alternative diagnoses[a]

Diagnostic criteria for NMOSD without AQP4-IgG or NMOSD with unknown AQP4-IgG status
1. At least 2 core clinical characteristics occurring as a result of one or more clinical attacks and meeting all of the following requirements:
   a. At least 1 core clinical characteristic must be optic neuritis, acute myelitis with LETM, or area postrema syndrome
   b. Dissemination in space (2 or more different core clinical characteristics)
   c. Fulfillment of additional MRI requirements, as applicable
2. Negative tests for AQP4-IgG using best available detection method, or testing unavailable
3. Exclusion of alternative diagnoses[a]

Core clinical characteristics
1. Optic neuritis
2. Acute myelitis
3. Area postrema syndrome: episode of otherwise unexplained hiccups or nausea and vomiting
4. Acute brainstem syndrome
5. Symptomatic narcolepsy or acute diencephalic clinical syndrome with NMOSD-typical diencephalic MRI lesions (figure 3)
6. Symptomatic cerebral syndrome with NMOSD-typical brain lesions (figure 3)

Additional MRI requirements for NMOSD without AQP4-IgG and NMOSD with unknown AQP4-IgG status
1. Acute optic neuritis: requires brain MRI showing (a) normal findings or only nonspecific white matter lesions, OR (b) optic nerve MRI with T2-hyperintense lesion or T1-weighted gadoliniumenhancing lesion extending over >1/2 optic nerve length or involving optic chiasm (figure 1)
2. Acute myelitis: requires associated intramedullary MRI lesion extending over ≥3 contiguous segments (LETM) OR ≥3 contiguous segments of focal spinal cord atrophy in patients with history compatible with acute myelitis (figure 1)
3. Area postrema syndrome: requires associated dorsal medulla/area postrema lesions (figure 2)
4. Acute brainstem syndrome: requires associated periependymal brainstem lesions (figure 2)

Editor's Note: Please refer to original journal article for full references.

Abbreviations: AQP4 = aquaporin-4; IgG = immunoglobulin G; LETM = longitudinally extensive transverse myelitis lesions; NMOSD = neuromyelitis optica spectrum disorders.

[a]See table 2 and text discussion on serologic considerations for recommendations regarding interpretation of clinical and serologic testing.

Reprinted from Wingerchuk DM, Banwell B, Bennett JL, et al. International consensus diagnostic criteria for neuromyelitis optica spectrum disorders. *Neurology.* 2015;85:177-189, with permission from American Academy of Neurology.

proposed validation strategies and achieved consensus on pediatric NMOSD diagnosis and the concepts of monophasic NMOSD and opticospinal MS (Table 1).

▶ As time goes on, the diagnostic criteria for neuromyelitis optica (NMO) are evolving. Originally a clinical diagnosis, requiring bilateral optic neuritis and transverse myelitis, with the advent of the aquaporin 4 immunoglobulin G antibody (AQP4-IgG) assay, the clinical criteria have been less stringent and diagnosis likely more accurate. Table 1 outlines the clinical criteria with or without a positive AQP4-IgG.

Clinical presentations highly suggestive of NMO include simultaneous bilateral optic neuritis, posterior optic nerve and chiasmal involvement, severe visual loss with poorer recovery, extensive lengthy enhancement of the optic nerve on MRI, and an altitudinal visual field defect.

The continued refinement of the diagnostic criteria will improve our diagnostic accuracy and allow the appropriate therapy. Remember that some MS treatments may be harmful in patients with NMO.

M. L. Moster, MD

Longitudinally extensive optic neuritis as an MRI biomarker distinguishes neuromyelitis optica from multiple sclerosis

Mealy MA, Whetstone A, Orman G, et al (Johns Hopkins Univ, Baltimore, MD)
J Neurol Sci 355:59-63, 2015

Objective.—To differentiate MRI characteristics of optic neuritis associated with neuromyelitis optica (NMO) and relapsing remitting multiple sclerosis (RRMS).

Background.—Optic neuritis is a common presenting feature of both neuromyelitis optica and multiple sclerosis. Distinguishing between NMO and RRMS is important in guiding treatment, but biomarkers of NMO and MS can be absent early in the disease process. We looked for differences in MRI characteristics of optic neuritis associated with NMO and MS that provide an early clue in the diagnostic workup.

Design/Methods.—We conducted a retrospective analysis of 26 NMO and 26 RRMS patients presenting to the Johns Hopkins Hospital with MRI-confirmed acute optic neuritis. MRIs were assessed to identify the location and longitudinal extent of each contrast enhancing lesion. For the purposes of this study, the optic nerve was divided into intraorbital, canalicular, pre-chiasmal, chiasmal, and optic tract.

Results.—There are distinct differences in MRI characteristics between NMO- and RRMS-associated optic neuritis. The majority of NMO lesions were longitudinally extensive measuring at least 17.6 mm in length and involving at least three optic nerve segments. At a cutoff of 17.6 mm lesion length, the specificity for NMO is 76.9% with a sensitivity of 80.8% and positive likelihood ratio of 3.50. Conversely, MS lesions were more commonly focal in one optic nerve segment localized anteriorly.

Conclusions.—Optic neuritis in NMO has a distinct pattern on MRI as compared with RRMS and can help differentiate these two neuroinflammatory diseases at presentation.

▶ One of the challenges in the acute optic neuritis patient is deciding when to be concerned about neuromyelitis optica (NMO). This study found that, similar to lesions of the spinal cord, extensive optic nerve lesions are highly suggestive of but not exclusive to NMO. Additionally, lesions that are bilateral, involving the optic tract or chiasm are more likely NMO than multiple sclerosis (MS).

One limitation of the study is that only approximately half of the patients had dedicated orbital MRIs. Another issue is that with bilateral lesions (25% of the time with NMO), the lengths of the 2 lesions were added together. This might be a confounding factor because bilateral disease by itself increases the likelihood of NMO even with a short lesion. Finally, the radiologist was "unblinded" in this study, which makes little sense to me.

Despite the limitations, it is clear that a lengthy lesion, particularly posteriorly in the optic nerve, increases the likelihood of a diagnosis of NMO rather than MS.

M. L. Moster, MD

Oral versus intravenous high-dose methylprednisolone for treatment of relapses in patients with multiple sclerosis (COPOUSEP): a randomised, controlled, double-blind, non-inferiority trial

Le Page E, for the COPOUSEP investigators, the West Network for Excellence in Neuroscience (Clinical Neuroscience Centre, Rennes, France; et al)

Lancet 386:974-981, 2015

Background.—High doses of intravenous methylprednisolone are recommended to treat relapses in patients with multiple sclerosis, but can be inconvenient and expensive. We aimed to assess whether oral administration of high-dose methylprednisolone was non-inferior to intravenous administration.

Methods.—We did this multicentre, double-blind, randomised, controlled, non-inferiority trial at 13 centres for multiple sclerosis in France. We enrolled patients aged 18–55 years with relapsing-remitting multiple sclerosis who reported a relapse within the previous 15 days that caused an increase of at least one point in one or more scores on the Kurtzke Functional System Scale. With use of a computer-generated randomisation list and in blocks of four, we randomly assigned (1:1) patients to either oral or intravenous methylprednisolone, 1000 mg, once a day for 3 days. Patients, treating physicians and nurses, and data and outcome assessors were all masked to treatment allocation, which was achieved with the use of saline solution and placebo capsules. The primary endpoint was the proportion of patients who had improved by day 28 (decrease of at least one point in most affected score on Kurtzke Functional System Scale), without need for retreatment with corticosteroids, in the per-protocol population. The trial was powered to assess non-inferiority of oral compared with intravenous methylprednisolone with a predetermined non-inferiority margin of 15%. This trial is registered with ClinicalTrials.gov, number NCT00984984.

Findings.—Between Jan 29, 2008, and June 14, 2013, we screened 200 patients and enrolled 199. We randomly assigned 100 patients to oral methylprednisolone and 99 patients to intravenous methylprednisolone with a mean time from relapse onset to treatment of 7·0 days (SD 3·6) and 7·4 days (3·9), respectively. In the per-protocol population, 66 (81%) of 82 patients in the oral group and 72 (80%) of 90 patients in the intravenous group achieved the primary endpoint (absolute treatment difference 0·5%, 90% CI −9·5 to 10·4). Rates of adverse events were similar, but insomnia was more frequently reported in the oral group (77 [77%]) than in the intravenous group (63 [64%]).

Interpretation.—Oral administration of high-dose methylprednisolone for 3 days was not inferior to intravenous administration for improvement of disability scores 1 month after treatment and had a similar safety profile. This finding could have implications for access to treatment, patient comfort, and cost, but indication should always be properly considered by clinicians.

▶ To test the hypothesis that 1000 mg/day of oral methylprednisolone is not inferior to 1000 mg/day of intravenous (IV) methylprednisolone in treating a relapse of multiple sclerosis, a double-blind, randomized controlled trial was performed comparing the 2 treatments. The primary end point of the study was the proportion of patients who improved by day 28, and the results were that oral methylprednisolone was not inferior to IV methylprednisolone (81% vs 80%, respectively).

Although these findings are reassuring, 2 important results from the Optic Neuritis Treatment Trial are not addressed by this study. First is the evidence that IV methylprednisolone postpones further demyelinating events in the first 2 years after treatment. Second is that oral steroids in more standard doses (1 mg/kg/day) is associated with twice the recurrence rate of optic neuritis.

M. L. Moster, MD

The Driving Visual Field and a History of Motor Vehicle Collision Involvement in Older Drivers: A Population-Based Examination

Huisingh C, McGwin G Jr, Wood J, et al (Univ of Alabama at Birmingham; Queensland Univ of Technology, Brisbane, Australia; et al)

Invest Ophthalmol Vis Sci 56:132-138, 2014

Purpose.—We designed a visual field test focused on the field utilized while driving to examine associations between field impairment and motor vehicle collision involvement in 2000 drivers aged 70 years or older.

Methods.—The "driving visual field test" involved measuring light sensitivity for 20 targets in each eye, extending 15° superiorly, 30° inferiorly, 60° temporally, and 30° nasally. The target locations were selected on the basis that they fell within the field region utilized when viewing through the windshield of a vehicle or viewing the dashboard while driving. Monocular fields were combined into a binocular field based on the more sensitive point from each eye. Severe impairment in the overall field or a region was defined as average sensitivity in the lowest quartile of sensitivity. At-fault collision involvement for 5 years prior to enrollment was obtained from state records. Poisson regression was used to calculate crude and adjusted rate ratios (RRs) examining the association between field impairment and at-fault collision involvement.

Results.—Drivers with severe binocular field impairment in the overall driving visual field had a 40% increased rate of at-fault collision involvement (RR, 1.40; 95% confidence interval [CI]: 1.07–1.83). Impairment in the lower and left fields was associated with elevated collision rates (RR, 1.40; 95% CI: 1.07–1.82 and RR, 1.49; 95% CI: 1.15–1.92, respectively), whereas impairment in the upper and right field regions was not.

Conclusions.—Results suggest that older drivers with severe impairment in the lower or left region of the driving visual field are more likely to have a history of at-fault collision involvement.

► Previous studies of visual field (VF) defects in relation to motor vehicle collisions (MVCs) have had varying results. Some of the differences relate to the method of testing (monocular vs binocular, threshold vs screening etc). Moreover, the rules related to driving vary from state to state in the United States and from country to country. The range in the United States is from no rules related to visual field testing to up to 140 degrees of binocular VF required. Presumably each state's rule is based on some available scientific evidence.

This study correlated VF results in 2000 subjects over age 70 with their past 5-year driving record, looking at MVCs where the subject was considered to be at fault. The findings were that VF defects were associated with a 40% increased risk of at-fault collision involvement. The locations of VF defect associated with increased risk include the horizontal meridian, lower VF, and left VF but not the upper and right VF.

This study is more useful than many previous studies. First, the authors developed a threshold VF based on the actual parts of the VF used in driving situations and eliminated points that are not involved. This improves the validity of the test results. Second, they adjusted for confounding variables, including age, sex, race, visual acuity, contrast sensitivity, mental status (Mini-Mental Status Exam), visual processing speed, and number of medical conditions the subject had. Third, it was conducted in Alabama, where drivers do not undergo repeat visual testing after receiving their initial driving license, and despite the requirement for 110 degrees of VF along the horizontal meridian, there is no routine testing.

One limitation of this study might be related to one of the confounding factors corrected for. The number of medical conditions is not the same as the actual medical condition. For instance, if 1 patient has hypertension but another has had a stroke with hemiparesis, those are not equal. Another limitation the authors point out is that subjects with VF defects may have self-selected not to drive, which would contribute to underestimating the risk in this study.

An interesting finding is that the impairment in the left VF was more important than the right VF. One wonders whether this is related to oncoming traffic and whether the results might be the opposite in countries where one drives on the left side of the road.

Finally, it is surprising that 14% of this randomly selected sample had an at-fault MVC in the previous 5 years. Whether this is really higher than younger Alabama subjects is not known from this study but raises some interesting questions.

Studies such as this one might lead to improved testing of the VF like the Estermann program and more useful guidelines.

M. L. Moster, MD

Risk Factors for Developing Thyroid-Associated Ophthalmopathy Among Individuals With Graves Disease

Stein JD, Childers D, Gupta S, et al (Univ of Michigan, Ann Arbor; et al)
JAMA Ophthalmol 133:290-296, 2015

Importance.—Thyroid-associated ophthalmopathy (TAO) is a common and debilitating manifestation of Graves disease (GD). Presently little is known about factors that may increase the risk of developing TAO among patients with GD.

Objective.—To identify risk factors associated with the development of TAO among individuals with newly diagnosed GD.

Design, Setting, and Participants.—In this longitudinal cohort study, all beneficiaries 18 years of age or older with newly diagnosed GD who were continuously enrolled in a large nationwide US managed care network and who visited an eye care professional 1 or more times from 2001 to 2009 were identified. *International Classification of Diseases, Ninth Revision, Clinical Modification* billing codes were used to identify those who developed manifestations of TAO. Multivariable Cox regression was used to determine the hazard of developing TAO among persons with newly diagnosed GD, with adjustment for sociodemographic factors, systemic medical conditions, thyrotropin levels, and medical and surgical interventions for management of hyperthyroidism.

Main Outcomes and Measures.—Manifestations of TAO measured by hazard ratios (HRs) with 95% CIs.

Results.—Of 8404 patients with GD who met the inclusion criteria, 740 (8.8%) developed TAO (mean follow-up, 374 days since initial GD diagnosis). After adjustment for potential confounders, surgical thyroidectomy, alone or in combination with medical therapy, was associated with a 74% decreased hazard for TAO (adjusted HR, 0.26 [95% CI, 0.12-0.51]) compared with radioactive iodine therapy alone. Statin use (for ≥60 days in the past year vs <60 days or nonuse) was associated with a 40% decreased hazard (adjusted HR, 0.60 [CI, 0.37-0.93]). No significant association was found for the use of nonstatin cholesterol-lowering medications or cyclooxygenase 2 inhibitors and the development of TAO.

Conclusions and Relevance.—If prospective studies can confirm our finding that a thyroidectomy and statin use are associated with substantially reduced hazards for TAO among patients with GD, preventive measures for this burdensome manifestation of GD may become a reality.

▶ One of the most frustrating conditions we treat is thyroid-associated ophthalmopathy (TAO), related to the complexity of the symptoms and the limited efficacy of our treatments. Optimally patients with Graves disease

(GD) could be treated in a way that would decrease the risk of developing TAO. This study found that 8.8% of patients who were diagnosed with GD and were followed for a mean of 374 days went on to develop TAO. Associated with a higher risk of TAO were treatment with radioactive iodine (RAI), elevated thyroid-stimulating hormone (TSH), and an elevated thyroid-stimulating immunoglobulin. Associated with a lower risk were treatment with thyroidectomy and use of statins.

The study has the limitation of lack of clinical information, merely using coding from a billing database. For instance, it is possible that the risk of TAO may be modified by the lipid abnormalities rather than the treatment with a statin, but lipid levels and diagnoses were not assessed. Additionally, there is no information available on smoking status in this study.

Interestingly in addition to verifying our prior understanding of RAI increasing the risk of TAO, this study provides evidence that thyroidectomy decreases the risk. Further study is warranted to determine whether thyroidectomy, statin use, and avoidance of posttreatment elevations of TSH will result in fewer patients developing TAO.

M. L. Moster, MD

Clinical Utility of Acetylcholine Receptor Antibody Testing in Ocular Myasthenia Gravis

Peeler CE, De Lott LB, Nagia L, et al (Harvard Med School, Boston, MA; Univ of Michigan, Ann Arbor; Michigan State Univ, East Lansing)

JAMA Neurol 72:1170-1174, 2015

Importance.—The sensitivity of acetylcholine receptor (AChR) antibody testing is thought to be lower in ocular myasthenia gravis (OMG) compared with generalized disease, although estimates in small-scale studies vary. There is little information in the literature about the implications of AChR antibody levels and progression from OMG to generalized myasthenia gravis.

Objectives.—To test the hypothesis that serum AChR antibody testing is more sensitive in OMG than previously reported and to examine the association between AChR antibody levels and progression from OMG to generalized myasthenia gravis.

Design, Setting, and Participants.—A retrospective, observational cohort study was conducted of 223 patients (mean [SD] age, 59.2 [16.4] years; 139 [62.3%] male) diagnosed with OMG between July 1, 1986, and May 31, 2013, at 2 large, academic medical centers.

Main Outcomes and Measures.—Baseline characteristics, OMG symptoms, results of AChR antibody testing, and progression time to generalized myasthenia gravis (if this occurred) were recorded for each patient. Multiple logistic regression was used to measure the association between all clinical variables and antibody result. Kaplan-Meier survival analysis was performed to examine time to generalization.

Results.—Among the 223 participants, AChR antibody testing results were positive in 158 participants (70.9%). In an adjusted model, increased age at diagnosis (odds ratio [OR], 1.03; 95% CI, 1.01-1.04; $P=.007$) and progression to generalized myasthenia gravis (OR, 2.92; 95% CI, 1.18-7.26; $P=.02$) were significantly associated with positive antibody test results. Women were less likely to have a positive antibody test result (OR, 0.36; 95% CI, 0.19-0.68; $P=.002$). Patients who developed symptoms of generalized myasthenia gravis had a significantly higher mean (SD) antibody level than those who did not develop symptoms of generalized myasthenia gravis (12.7 [16.5] nmol/L vs 4.2 [7.9] nmol/L; $P=.002$).

Conclusions and Relevance.—We demonstrate a higher sensitivity of AChR antibody testing than previously reported in the largest cohort of patients with OMG available to date. Older age, male sex, and progression to generalized myasthenia gravis were significantly associated with a positive antibody test result. In addition, to our knowledge, this is the first report of an association between high AChR antibody levels and progression from OMG to generalized disease.

▶ This study found a higher percentage of positive acetylcholine receptor antibody (AchRAb) in ocular myasthenia gravis (OMG) patients than previous reports (70.9%). There is difficulty in estimating this percentage because of the lack of a "gold standard" in identifying those antibody-negative patients who truly have MG. This study's standard was "the clinical impression of 1 of 4 experienced neuro-ophthalmologists who followed up each patient longitudinally for a mean of 60 months." It is difficult to tell how many antibody-negative patients who truly had OMG were excluded because they did not fit the standard. Nonetheless, I am not suggesting that I have a better way of making the diagnosis than 5-year follow-up of an experienced neuro-ophthalmologist. So the bottom line is that we are probably diagnosing more of our patients with +AchRAb and sending fewer for single-fiber electromyography, which is good.

Finding both that AchRAb positivity and that a higher level of antibody were associated with an increased risk of progression to generalized MG is also helpful if borne out in further studies.

One of the explanations from the authors for the increased positivity is that over time the assay has been improved. This study includes patients seen between 1986 and 2013, and I wonder whether the percentage of positivity is even greater with today's assays.

What do I change next Monday based on this article? I am more comfortable that I am missing fewer diagnoses of OMG than before when the AchRAb is negative, and I will pay more attention to the antibody level as a possible predictor for developing generalized MG.

M. L. Moster, MD

Prevalence and distribution of VZV in temporal arteries of patients with giant cell arteritis

Gilden D, White T, Khmeleva N, et al (Univ of Colorado School of Medicine, Aurora; et al)

Neurology 84:1948-1955, 2015

Objective.—Varicella-zoster virus (VZV) infection may trigger the inflammatory cascade that characterizes giant cell arteritis (GCA).

Methods.—Formalin-fixed, paraffin-embedded GCA-positive temporal artery (TA) biopsies (50 sections/TA) including adjacent skeletal muscle and normal TAs obtained postmortem from subjects >50 years of age were examined by immunohistochemistry for presence and distribution of VZV antigen and by ultrastructural examination for virions. Adjacent regions were examined by hematoxylin & eosin staining. VZV antigen–positive slides were analyzed by PCR for VZV DNA.

Results.—VZV antigen was found in 61/82 (74%) GCA-positive TAs compared with 1/13 (8%) normal TAs ($p < 0.0001$, relative risk 9.67, 95% confidence interval 1.46, 63.69). Most GCA-positive TAs contained viral antigen in skip areas. VZV antigen was present mostly in adventitia, followed by media and intima. VZV antigen was found in 12/32 (38%) skeletal muscles adjacent to VZV antigen–positive TAs. Despite formalin fixation, VZV DNA was detected in 18/45 (40%) GCA-positive VZV antigen–positive TAs, in 6/10 (60%) VZV antigen–positive skeletal muscles, and in one VZV antigen–positive normal TA. Varicella-zoster virions were found in a GCA-positive TA. In sections adjacent to those containing VZV, GCA pathology was seen in 89% of GCA-positive TAs but in none of 18 adjacent sections from normal TAs.

Conclusions.—Most GCA-positive TAs contained VZV in skip areas that correlated with adjacent GCA pathology, supporting the hypothesis that VZV triggers GCA immunopathology. Antiviral treatment may confer additional benefit to patients with GCA treated with corticosteroids, although the optimal antiviral regimen remains to be determined.

▶ In this thorough investigation, the authors hypothesize that varicella-zoster virus (VZV) may contribute to the pathogenesis of giant cell arteritis (GCA). GCA clinically presents with headache, scalp tenderness, and jaw claudication in patients over age 50 years. Vision loss occurs frequently, which requires immediate, time-sensitive administration of corticosteroid treatment to prevent vision loss in the contralateral eye. Often, definitive diagnosis is dependent on microscopic examination. Histologically, GCA-positive temporal arteries (TAs) typically exhibit intramural chronic inflammation, intimal hyperplasia, interruption of the internal elastic lamina, and at times multinucleated giant cells and epithelioid macrophages. Skip lesions are common, which complicates the diagnosis. Previous studies have disclosed the presence of VZV antigen and DNA in skipped sections, both in positive and negative TA biopsy specimens. The aim of this study is to further investigate the prevalence and distribution of VZV in TA in patients with GCA.

The authors retrospectively inspected 86 deidentified formalin-fixed, paraffin-embedded TAs with adjacent skeletal muscle from patients greater than 50 years of age with histopathologically confirmed GCA and 16 control TAs from postmortem subjects greater than 50 years of age. Fifty 5-μm sections per TA were immunostained with anti-VZV glycoprotein E antibody. If a section was found to be positive, an adjacent section was stained with hematoxylin and eosin for microscopic examination. In addition, each antigen-positive TA underwent polymerase chain reaction analysis for VZV DNA and ultrastructural examination with transmission electron microscopy.

Immunohistochemical analysis of 4100 sections from 82 histologically verified GCA-positive TA revealed VZV antigen in 74% TA compared with 8% normal TA. Furthermore, VZV antigen was found in 89% of adjacent sections in VZV antigen-positive TA but not in any of the 18 adjacent sections from normal TAs. The adventitia demonstrated highest positivity for VZV antigen, followed by media and intima layers. In addition, VZV antigen was found in 38% of surrounding skeletal muscle adjacent to VZV antigen-positive TA. This pattern of distribution, specifically affecting predominantly outer layers more than inner layers, appears to correlate with the anatomy and route of VZV infection; specifically, reactivation of VZV from the cranial nerve ganglia travels along the outside of the artery, invading then transmurally.

Based on the evidence from this study, the authors infer that VZV may present a possible cause for GCA, primarily affecting the TA. The high incidence of VZV-positive GCA TA specimens, compared with other previous studies, is believed to have been achieved by a more extensive and thorough sectioning and examination of specimens. Therefore, the authors propose the value of staining more than 10 sections when trying to uncover VZV antigen. Ultimately, the question remains whether patients would benefit from antiviral therapy when diagnosed with GCA. Proof of antiviral benefit, in addition to specific treatment regimen, will need further investigation.

P. M. Buch, MD
V. Lee, MD

Evaluation and neuroimaging of the Horner syndrome

Chen Y, Morgan ML, Barros Palau AE, et al (Baylor College of Medicine, Houston, TX; Houston Methodist Hosp, Houston, TX; et al)
Can J Ophthalmol 50:107-111, 2015

Objective.—To define the efficacy, safety, and cost-effectiveness of a single centre's approach to evaluating Horner syndrome (HS) including a simplified single neuroimaging protocol.

Design.—Case series study.

Participants.—Medical records of 34 patients diagnosed with HS at Houston Methodist Hospital (HMH) were reviewed after obtaining Institutional Review Board approval.

Methods.—A retrospective chart review was performed for all patients presenting with the diagnosis of HS at the HMH from January 2010 to November 2013. All patients had diagnostic imaging with contrast-enhanced brain magnetic resonance imaging (MRI) extending to the T2 level in the chest. They had either documented causative diagnosis for HS or were "idiopathic." Efficacy and cost-effectiveness of the proposed neuroimaging technique were analyzed compared with other recommended protocols.

Results.—We initially reviewed 34 charts with presumed diagnosis of HS; 27 charts were included in the analysis. The average age of patients was 46.6 years. Eleven patients (41%) had a final diagnosis of HS secondary to a proven cause, and 16 patients (59%) were diagnosed as "idiopathic." Ten patients (63%) in the idiopathic group had follow-up, and none of those with follow-up had an alternative cause. The estimated cost of our recommended MRI protocol was US$667.76 without magnetic resonance angiography (MRA) or US$1501.71 with MRA.

Conclusions.—A single contrast-enhanced brain MRI extending to the T2 level in the chest is an effective and simple means of ruling out life-threatening and other causative factors of HS. Compared with previous imaging recommendations, this proposed protocol may be simpler for clinicians to use and more cost-effective.

▶ The authors describe their approach to evaluating patients with Horner syndrome (HS), noting that prior literature has proposed various approaches. They use standard clinical criteria, selective use of apraclonidine and then imaging with a single MRI scan extending from the brain to T2 with an magnetic resonance angiogram (MRA) of the neck. They have found the approach to be effective and lower cost than many others. As the authors note, there are limitations to this study, including not knowing the true cost of studies (they used Medicare reimbursement rates), a small number of patients, limited follow-up, and the retrospective nature of the study.

So why review this study? The reason is that, as the subspecialty with the most expertise in HS, I think we have to come up with the best way to evaluate these patients and propose some changes to our radiology departments and institutions, as well as within insurance companies. With this in mind, I think the approach in this study makes a lot of sense.

Currently what I order on patients with nonlocalizable isolated HS depends on the office in which I see them (Wills Eye vs Suburban Philadelphia vs South Jersey), at which institution they are studied, and what insurance they have. The orders might include a combination of the following: MRI brain, MRI neck, MRI chest, MRA neck, CT brain, CT neck, CT chest, or CT angiogram. Sometimes the decision of what to obtain depends on my conversation with the medical reviewer at the insurance company. Even so, occasionally I am not confident that I have adequately imaged the entire sympathetic pathway.

If we can come up with an agreed on guideline along the lines recommended in this article, perhaps in partnership with American Academy of

Ophthalmology and the American Academy of Neurology, we can get appropriate imaging, easier insurance approvals, and not have to order up to 4 studies. Additionally, when I've seen patients who have been evaluated by neurologists or ophthalmologists, often a portion of the sympathetic pathway has been overlooked. Because many or most HS patients do not make it to a neuro-ophthalmologist, a simplified recommendation such as proposed here will lead to a more appropriate evaluation. As the authors note, their protocol is likely faster to perform, simpler for clinicians to order and less costly while adequately assessing all areas of concern in HS than most current protocols.

M. L. Moster, MD

10 Imaging

International consensus diagnostic criteria for neuromyelitis optica spectrum disorders

Wingerchuk DM, Banwell B, Bennett JL, et al (Mayo Clinic, Scottsdale, AZ; Children's Hosp of Philadelphia, PA; Univ of Colorado Denver, Aurora; et al)

Neurology 85:1-13, 2015

Neuromyelitis optica (NMO) is an inflammatory CNS syndrome distinct from multiple sclerosis (MS) that is associated with serum aquaporin-4 immunoglobulin G antibodies (AQP4-IgG). Prior NMO diagnostic criteria required optic nerve and spinal cord involvement but more restricted or more extensive CNS involvement may occur. The International Panel for NMO Diagnosis (IPND) was convened to develop revised diagnostic criteria using systematic literature reviews and electronic surveys to facilitate consensus. The new nomenclature defines the unifying term NMO spectrum disorders (NMOSD), which is stratified further by serologic testing (NMOSD with or without AQP4-IgG). The core clinical characteristics required for patients with NMOSD with AQP4-IgG include clinical syndromes or MRI findings related to optic nerve, spinal cord, area postrema, other brainstem, diencephalic, or cerebral presentations. More stringent clinical criteria, with additional neuroimaging findings, are required for diagnosis of NMOSD without AQP4-IgG or when serologic testing is unavailable. The IPND also proposed validation strategies and achieved consensus on pediatric NMOSD diagnosis and the concepts of monophasic NMOSD and opticospinal MS.

▶ Traditionally, neuromyelitis optica (NMO) was considered a monophasic illness with bilateral optic neuritis and myelitis. Greater recognition of heterogeneity and variability of the disease process has led to creation of the term NMO spectrum disorders (NMOSD). The International Panel for Neuromyelitis Optica Diagnosis (IPND) has recently proposed revised diagnostic criteria for NMOSD incorporating typical clinical presentations and MRI imaging features.

The panel has described 6 core clinical characteristics that include (1) optic neuritis, (2) acute myelitis, (3) area postrema syndrome (episode of otherwise unexplained hiccups or nausea and vomiting), (4) acute brainstem syndrome, (5) symptomatic narcolepsy or acute diencephalic clinical syndrome with NMOSD-typical diencephalic MRI lesions and (6) symptomatic cerebral syndrome with NMOSD-typical brain lesions.

They also describe typical MRI findings associated with NMOSD in spinal cord (acute and chronic phases), optic nerves and brain. Spinal cord involvement in NMOSD is typically LETM (longitudinally extensive transverse myelitis), involving greater than 3 vertebral segments (vs multiple sclerosis [MS] that typically involves only 1 or 2 vertebral segments) and greater involvement of the central gray of the cord (vs MS that typically involves peripheral aspects of the cord). Acute involvement may additionally demonstrate contrast enhancement and chronic phases may demonstrate long segment atrophy. Optic nerve MRI may demonstrate unilateral or bilateral optic neuritis. Compared with MS, NMOSD optic nerve lesions tend to be longer (those extending more than half the distance from orbit to chiasm), involve posterior parts of the nerve and have greater propensity to involve the optic chiasm. Seven typical signs of NMOSD-related brain involvement has been described by the panel: (1) lesions involving the dorsal medulla (especially the area postrema); (2) periependymal surfaces of the fourth ventricle in the brainstem/cerebellum; (3) lesions involving the hypothalamus, thalamus, or periependymal surfaces of the third ventricle; (4) large, confluent, unilateral, or bilateral subcortical or deep white matter lesions; (5) long (half the length of the corpus callosum or greater), diffuse, heterogeneous, or edematous corpus callosum lesions; (6) long corticospinal tract lesions, unilateral or bilateral, contiguously involving internal capsule and cerebral peduncle; and (7) Extensive periependymal brain lesions, often with gadolinium enhancement.

Seropositivity for AQP4-IgG is highly specific for NMOSD. In the presence of seropositivity, as per the IPND diagnostic criteria, only 1 core clinical characteristic is needed to confirm the diagnosis. However, even in the absence of AQP4-IgG seropositivity, the diagnosis can be confirmed in presence of at least 2 core characteristics that are disseminated in space and presence of typical MRI features congruent with NMOSD as detailed here. Many of the observations to construct these criteria were derived from relatively small case series. The IPND recommends several large-scale prospective validation and assessment strategies for future refinement of the diagnostic criteria.

R. Hegde, MD
K. S. Talekar, MD

Brain Imaging in Idiopathic Intracranial Hypertension

Bidot S, Saindane AM, Peragallo JH, et al (Emory Univ School of Medicine, Atlanta, GA; et al)

J Neuroophthalmol 35:400-411, 2015

Background.—The primary role of brain imaging in idiopathic intracranial hypertension (IIH) is to exclude other pathologies causing intracranial hypertension. However, subtle radiologic findings suggestive of IIH have emerged with modern neuroimaging. This review provides a detailed description of the imaging findings reported in IIH and discusses their possible roles in the pathophysiology and the diagnosis of IIH.

Evidence Acquisition.—References were identified by searches of PubMed from 1955 to January 2015, with the terms “idiopathic

TABLE 2.—Neuroimaging findings described in idiopathic intracranial hypertension (IIH)

Presumed Mechanism	Findings	Pooled Sensitivity [95% CI]	Pooled Specificity [95% CI]
Bony erosion from IIH	Empty sella	80% [71–89] (11,12)	83% [76–90] (8–10)
	CSF leak	NA	NA
	Meningocele/meningoencephalocele	11% [4–18]* (39)	0% [NA]* (39)
	Foramen ovale widening	50% [36–64]* (20)	80% [69–91]* (20)
Mechanical deformation from IIH	Posterior flattening of the posterior poles	66% [60–72] (8–10,12,19,20)	98% [96–100] (8–10,20)
	Optic nerve head protrusion	36% [28–44] (8–10,12,19,20)	99% [98–100] (8–10,20)
	Distention of the optic nerve sheath	58% [48–68] (9,10,12)	89% [85–95] (9,10)
	Vertical tortuosity of the optic nerve	43% [37–50] (8–10,12,19,20)	90% [85–95] (8–10,20)
	Transverse sinus venous stenosis	97% [93–100] (55,64,66)	93% [84–97]* (55)
Papilledema	Enhancement of the optic nerve head	17% [11–23] (8–10,19)	99% [97–100] (8–10)
Uncertain	Tonsillar herniation ≥5 mm	16% [10–22] (9,34,37)	95% [91–100] (9,34)

Pooled sensitivity and specificity were obtained from at least 2 studies using the same criteria to define the findings.
CSF, cerebrospinal fluid; NA, not available.
*Obtained from one single study (provided by the authors or recalculated).
Reprinted from Bidot S, Saindane AM, Peragallo JH, et al. Brain imaging in idiopathic intracranial hypertension. *J Neuroophthalmol.* 2015;35:400-411, with permission from North American Neuro-Ophthalmology Society.

intracranial hypertension," "pseudotumor cerebri," "intracranial hypertension," "benign intracranial hypertension," "magnetic resonance imaging," "magnetic resonance venography," "computed tomography (CT)," "CT venography," "imaging," and "cerebrospinal fluid (CSF) leak." Additional references were identified by hand search of relevant articles. When possible, we extracted the number of patients and control subjects from each study for each radiological finding. When at least 2 studies used the same criteria to define a radiological finding, all patients from these studies were pooled to obtain a mean sensitivity and specificity with 95% confidence interval.

Results.—Specific neuroimaging findings may suggest longstanding IIH, including empty sella, flattening of the posterior globes, optic nerve head protrusion, distention of the optic nerve sheaths, tortuosity of the optic nerve, cerebellar tonsillar herniation, meningoceles, CSF leaks, and transverse venous sinus stenosis.

Conclusion.—Although IIH remains a diagnosis of exclusion, the most recently proposed diagnostic criteria have included neuroimaging findings to suggest IIH when major diagnostic criteria are not fulfilled. However, these findings are not diagnostic of IIH, and their presence is not required for the diagnosis of definite IIH. Their incidental discovery on brain imaging should not prompt invasive procedures, unless other signs of IIH, such as papilledema, are present (Table 2).

▶ Idiopathic Intracranial Hypertension (IIH) is typically a diagnosis of exclusion with imaging used to rule out other causes of raised intracranial pressure, such as a space-occupying lesion, hydrocephalus, and venous sinus thrombosis. However, recently proposed diagnostic criteria[1] have included neuroimaging findings to suggest IIH when major diagnostic criteria are not fulfilled. Bidot et al, in this review of the literature, describe the neuroimaging findings that have been reported in IIH. They discuss their possible roles in the pathophysiology and diagnosis of this disorder. The various findings addressed in this review are empty sella, flattening of the posterior globes, distention of the optic nerve sheaths, cerebellar tonsillar herniation, meningoceles, widening of foramen ovale, cerebrospinal fluid leak, and transverse venous sinus stenosis (Table 2). None of the findings, they found, have both high sensitivity and specificity. Finally, they addressed the utility of combination of the various findings as a diagnostic tool. Because some of these findings are common in the normal population, they must therefore be interpreted with caution.

K. S. Talekar, MD

Reference

1. Friedman DI, Liu GT, Digre KB. Revised diagnostic criteria for the pseudotumor cerebri syndrome in adults and children. *Neurology*. 2013;81:1159-1165.

Quantitative Magnetic Resonance Venography is Correlated With Intravenous Pressures Before and After Venous Sinus Stenting: Implications for Treatment and Monitoring

Esfahani DR, Stevenson M, Moss HE, et al (Univ of Illinois at Chicago)

Neurosurgery 77:254–260, 2015

Background.—Endovascular stenting is an effective treatment for patients with clinically significant cerebral venous sinus stenosis. Traditionally, stenting is indicated in elevated intravenous pressures on conventional venography; however, noninvasive monitoring is more desirable. Quantitative magnetic resonance angiography is an imaging modality that measures blood flow noninvasively. Established in the arterial system, applications to the venous sinuses have been limited.

Objective.—To examine quantitative magnetic resonance venography (qMRV) in the measurement of venous sinus flow in patients undergoing endovascular stenting and to identify a relationship with intravenous pressures.

Methods.—Five patients with intracranial hypertension secondary to venous sinus stenosis underwent cerebral venous stenting between 2009 and 2013 at a single institution. Preoperatively, venous sinus flow was determined by using qMRV, and intravenous pressure was measured during venography. After stenting, intravenous pressure, qMRV flow, and clinical outcomes were assessed and compared.

Results.—A mean prestenotic intravenous pressure of 45.2 mm Hg was recorded before stenting, which decreased to 27.4 mm Hg afterward (Wilcoxon signed rank test $P = .04$). Total jugular outflow on qMRV increased by 260.2 mL/min. Analysis of the change in intravenous pressure and qMRV flow identified a linear relationship (Pearson correlation $r = 0.926$). All patients displayed visual improvement at 6 weeks.

Conclusion.—Venous outflow by qMRV increases after endovascular stenting and correlates with significantly improved intravenous pressures. These findings introduce qMRV as a potential adjunct to measure venous flow after stenting, and as a plausible tool in the selection and postoperative surveillance of the patient who has cerebral venous sinus stenosis.

► Stenosis of the distal transverse sinus has been shown to be associated with idiopathic intracranial hypertension.[1] Endovascular stenting is a treatment suggested for patients with intracranial hypertension associated with venous sinus stenosis.[2] Catheter venography and intravenous pressure measurement via femoral venous catheter is the current gold standard for characterizing venous sinus pathology. Noninvasive studies, including time-of-flight technique magnetic resonance venography (MRV) and contrast-enhanced MRV, are limited by lack of quantitative information. Quantitative magnetic resonance angiography has been evaluated, but its application in vein imaging has not been widely studied. In this small retrospective study, the authors explore the utility of quantitative MRV to examine flow rates in patients with idiopathic intracranial hypertension. They have reported a linear correlation between venous flow measured by quantitative MRV and intravenous sinus pressures measured by catheter angiography.

R. Hegde, MD
K. S. Talekar, MD

References

1. Johnston I, Kollar C, Dunkley S, Assaad N, Parker G. Cranial venous outflow obstruction in the pseudotumour syndrome: incidence, nature and relevance. *J Clin Neurosci*. 2002;9:273-278.
2. Puffer RC, Mustafa W, Lanzino G. Venous sinus stenting for idiopathic intracranial hypertension: a review of the literature. *J Neurointerv Surg*. 2013;5:483-486.

Orbital color Doppler ultrasound as noninvasive tool in the diagnosis of anterior-draining carotid-cavernous fistula

Venturini M, Cristel G, Marzoli SB, et al (San Raffaele Scientific Inst, Milan, Italy; et al)
Radiol Med 121(4):301-307, 2016

Purpose.—To investigate the role of orbital color Doppler ultrasound (OCDUS) in the diagnosis of carotid-cavernous fistula (CCF) with anterior drainage and particularly whether a negative OCDUS could avoid an invasive diagnostic cerebral angiography (DSA).

Materials and Methods.—Twenty-two consecutive patients with ophthalmic signs suspecting CCF were submitted to ophthalmologic examination, OCDUS and DSA. CCF diagnosis with OCDUS was based on the finding of a reversed, arterialized and low-resistive-index (RI <0.5) blood flow in the superior ophthalmic vein (SOV). Sensibility, specificity, PPV, NPV, and accuracy of OCDUS were calculated considering both patients and eyes, using DSA as gold standard.

Results.—DSA demonstrated 20 CCFs in 18 patients. Considering the patients, in 18/22 CCF diagnosis was positive at OCDUS and DSA while 4/22 were negative at both. Considering the eyes, in 24/43 CCF diagnosis was positive at both DSA and OCDUS (total eyes = 43, due to one case of SOV thrombosis). In 19/43 eyes diagnosis was negative at both OCDUS and DSA. So sensitivity, specificity, PPV, NPV, and accuracy of OCDUS in the patients and eyes analysis were all 100%.

Conclusions.—OCDUS is a reliable, noninvasive tool in the diagnosis of CCF; a negative OCDUS could avoid an invasive DSA in patients suspected for anterior-draining CCF.

▶ Carotid-cavernous fistulas (CCFs) are abnormal communications between the carotid arterial system and the cavernous sinus. They can be direct or indirect fistulas based on the source of feeder vessels. Diagnostic cerebral angiography (DSA) is considered the gold standard for the diagnosis and characterization of carotid-cavernous fistula. However, DSA is an invasive procedure. In cases of clinically suspect CCF, CT and magnetic resonance angiography usually lack hemodynamic information, in addition to other specific limitations. Because Doppler ultrasound evaluation of the superior ophthalmic vein reflects the intracranial venous hemodynamics, it serves as an excellent noninvasive tool. Typical findings on Doppler ultrasound are dilated superior ophthalmic vein with reversed, arterialized, low-resistance blood flow.[1] In the current retrospective study, the authors evaluated the sensitivity, specificity, and positive and negative predictive values of Doppler ultrasound compared with DSA. A small patient population and the retrospective nature of the study are obvious limitations. However, the study emphasizes the role of Doppler ultrasound imaging, which is noninvasive and cost-effective, serving as a reliable screening tool to detect the presence of CCF.

R. Hegde, MD

Reference

1. Flaharty P, Lieb WE, Sergott RC, Bosley TM, Savino PJ. Color doppler imaging: a new non-invasive technique to diagnose and monitor carotid-cavernous sinus fistulas. *Arch Ophthalmol.* 1991;109:522-526.

Subperiosteal orbital abscess: volumetric criteria for surgical drainage

Tabarino F, Elmaleh-Bergès M, Quesnel S, et al (Université Paris 7 Denis Diderot, France; et al)

Int J Pediatr Otorhinolaryngol 79:131-135, 2015

Objective.—To investigate predictive factors of surgical management of subperiosteal orbital abscess in children.

Methods.—A retrospective monocentric study was conducted between 2000 and 2011 with children hospitalized for acute pediatric orbital cellulitis (APOC). Clinical, biological and radiological data as well as medical and surgical management were collected and analyzed. All patients received intravenous antibiotics and underwent a CT-scan. Orbit and subperiosteal intraorbital abscess dimensions were measured on axial and coronal planes and the abscess volume was calculated using a spheroid model.

Results.—Eighty-three children with APOC (mean age: 4.5 years) were included, 53 were boys (63.9%). Thirty-two children (38.6%) presented with a subperiosteal orbital abscess. Mean abscess volume was 570 mm^3 and mean exophthalmos was 4.7 mm. Twenty patients were treated surgically, 11 of which by an endoscopic approach. A positive correlation was observed between the volume of the abscess or exophthalmos and surgical drainage: 57.9% of patients underwent surgery when exophthalmos was >4 mm, 29.4% between 2 and 4 mm, and none when <2 mm. All patients with an abscess volume >500 mm^3 or >5% of orbital volume were operated on whereas only 30% or 39% of patients, respectively, in case of smaller volumes ($P < 0.05$).

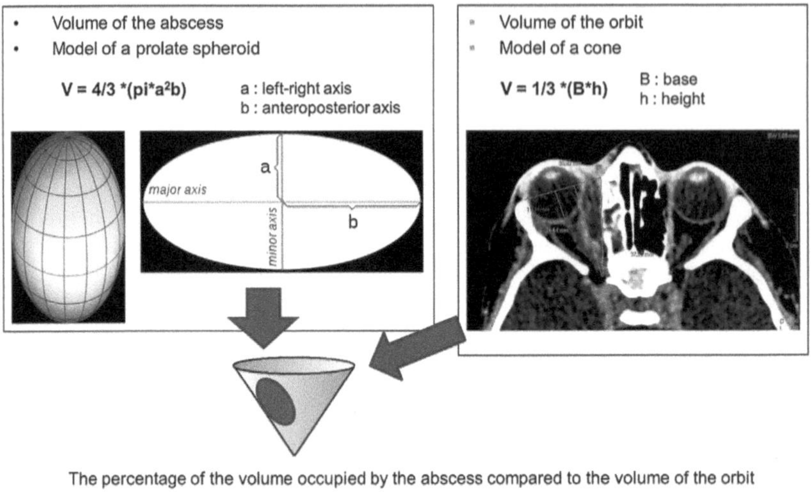

FIGURE 1.—Method for calculating the volume of the orbit and of the abscess. (Reprinted from Tabarino F, Elmaleh-Bergès M, Quesnel S, et al. Subperiosteal orbital abscess: volumetric criteria for surgical drainage. *Int J Pediatr Otorhinolaryngol.* 2015;79:131-135, with permission from Elsevier Ireland Ltd.)

Conclusion.—Surgery for subperiosteal orbital abscess is usually performed in case of visual complications or unfavorable medical outcome. The importance of the exophthalmos and the volume of the abscess measured on the CT-scan are predictive factors of surgery in children with subperiosteal orbital abscess without visual complications (Fig 1).

▶ In this retrospective study, the authors aim to determine the prognostic factors of the surgical management of subperiosteal orbital abscess in the case of acute pediatric orbital cellulitis considering the volume of the orbit. Measures of the abscess and of the orbit used in the study are demonstrated in Fig 1. The authors report that mean volume of the abscess and mean percentage of the orbital volume occupied by the abscess were significantly greater in the surgical group than in the group without surgery. They found that when abscess measured more than 500 mm^3 or more than 5% of the orbital volume, the patients underwent surgery in 100% of cases, as opposed to 30% ($P < .001$) or 39% ($P < .003$), respectively, in cases of smaller volume. Previous studies determining a threshold for the size or the volume of an abscess requiring surgery have not considered the orbital volume; they report a positive correlation between the volume of the abscess in percentage of the orbital volume and the risk of surgical management. These studies have also reported that when the volume of the abscess was greater than 5%, surgical management was necessary in 100% of patients.

K. S. Talekar, MD

11 Ocular Oncology

Decadelong Profile of Women in Ophthalmic Publications

Franco-Cardenas V, Rosenberg J, Ramirez A, et al (David Geffen School of Medicine, Los Angeles, CA; Albert Einstein College of Medicine, Bronx, NY; et al)

JAMA Ophthalmol 133:255-259, 2015

Importance.—In recent decades, there has been an increase in the number of women practicing medicine. We believe this shift may be reaching academic publications in ophthalmology and changing gender trends.

Objective.—To determine whether there has been an increase in women publishing academic articles and editorials in ophthalmology during the past decade.

Design, Setting, and Participants.—In this observational retrospective study, 3 ophthalmology journals were sampled from 2000 and 2010 for at least 100 articles per journal, per year, and all editorials published in both years. Data reviewed included the authors' gender, number of authors, number of references, subspecialty, and country of origin.

Exposure.—Publication by women authors.

Main Outcomes and Measures.—The primary outcome measure was an increase in women publishing in ophthalmology. The hypothesis was formulated before data collection.

Results.—Our analysis included 671 original articles (336 from 2000 and 335 from 2010) and 89 editorials. The percentage of original articles with a woman as first author increased from 23.2% in 2000 to 32.5% in 2010, a difference of 9.3% (95% CI, 23.3%-32.5%; $P = .005$). The percentage of original articles with a woman last author increased from 16.4% in 2000 to 24.2% in 2010, a difference of 7.8% (95% CI, 16.4%-24.2%; $P = .01$). The percentage of original articles with a woman first author increased in Asia from 1.2% in 2000 to 8.4% in 2010, a difference of 7.2% (95% CI, 1.2%-8.4%; $P < .001$). The percentage of articles with a woman last author increased in Europe from 2.2% in 2000 to 7.5% in 2010, a difference of 5.3% (95% CI, 2.2%-7.5%; $P < .001$) and in Asia from 0% in 2000 to 6.0% in 2010, a difference of 6.0% (95% CI, 0%-6%; $P < .001$). Editorials were written predominantly by men: 33 of 38 editorials (87%) in 2000 and 46 of 51 (90%) in 2010, a difference of 3% (95% CI, 87%-90%; $P = .62$), showing a trend toward decreased editorial authorship by women during the past decade.

Conclusions and Relevance.—Our data suggest an increase in women publishing original investigations in ophthalmic literature, but no increase in editorial authorship.

▶ In the medical profession, women have historically been fewer in number compared with men. However, over the past 50 years, there has been a refreshingly noticeable change in this trend.[1,2] The proportion of women being awarded MD degrees in the United States has steadily risen from 26.8% in 1983 to 48.3% in 2010.[1] This translates to a commensurate increase in women entering the field of ophthalmology, in which a 10-fold increase from 3.6% in 1969 to 37.7% in 1999 was observed.[1] According to Mansour et al, of the 3 major ophthalmology journals, including *Archives of Ophthalmology* (*JAMA Ophthalmology*), *American Journal of Ophthalmology*, and *Ophthalmology*, the rate of female first authorship in the past 5 decades had increased dramatically from 5.2% in 1969 to 29.2% in 2009 with the peak rise observed after 1989. The number of female senior authors, reviewers, and editorial board members also increased over the years.[1] This evolution is parallel to the rise in number of US female physicians. Despite this, it was noted that none of the 3 journals have ever had a female editor in chief.[1]

There are several reasons for the increase in participation of women in the domain of medicine, from greater opportunity for education to desire for independence and personal career, high academic goals, women's rights and health movement, political laws in the United States, and the interesting fact that there is a notable reduced drive of young men into the academic arena.[1,2] However, to serve on the editorial board of a leading journal, an individual must demonstrate discipline as an unwavering leading contributor. The underrepresentation of women as editors of ophthalmology journals could be attributed to the "pipeline phenomenon."[1,3] This has been described as insufficient time given to the newly increased number of female medical students to reach a senior rank at a point where one might be considered for an editorial board membership.[1,3] In addition, women must strike a balance between career and family life, hence shortening their work life.[1] At the higher levels of academic medicine, women remain in the minority because they tend to have a predilection to enter primary care medicine as a more "family-friendly" specialty with a flexible work schedule.[1] Also, the lack of female surgical mentors and exposure to possible gender discrimination during surgical rotations has lead women to seek nonsurgical specialties.[1]

In this report, Franco-Cardenas et al analyzed the decade-long profile of women involved in writing ophthalmic publications and reported an increase in female first authorship from 23.2% in 2000 to 32.5% in 2010, and an increase in female last authorship from 16.4% in 2000 to 24.2% in 2010, reflecting a proportionate increase in practicing women ophthalmologists. However, they reported a decrease in editorial authorship by women. As previously noted, women have only recently gained prominence in this field and have not yet attained seniority as a group, which could represent a time lag rather than discrimination. According to the American Medical Association, 35.2% of total ophthalmologists are aged 55 years and older, and of this group, 94% are men. To determine whether the decrease in editorial authorship is due to time bias or true gender bias, a longer study period is required. In addition, subgroup analysis has revealed an increase in retina and cataract publications from both men and women authors, reflecting rapid advancements in the field. These authors concluded that examination and discussion of gender trends in authorship could promote gender equality and motivation. They also identified that women lend a thoughtful and appropriate viewpoint in academic discussions and could act as role models to the younger generation.

C. L. Shields, MD

Chloe T. L. Khoo, BS contributed to the writing of this review under the direction of Carol L. Shields, MD, Co-Director of the Ocular Oncology Service of Wills Eye Hospital, Philadelphia, PA.

References

1. Mansour AM, Shields CL, Maalouf FC, et al. Five-decade profile of women in leadership positions at ophthalmic publications. *Arch Ophthalmol.* 2012;130: 1441-1446.
2. Jeffe DB, Whelan AJ, Andriole DA. Primary care specialty choices of United States medical graduates, 1997–2006. *Acad Med.* 2010;85:947-958.
3. Wilkes MS, Kravitz RL. Policies, practices, and attitudes of North American medical journal editors. *J Gen Intern Med.* 1995;10:443-450.

Retinal Vascular Layers Imaged by Fluorescein Angiography and Optical Coherence Tomography Angiography

Spaide RF, Klancnik JM Jr, Cooney MJ (Macula Consultants of New York)
JAMA Ophthalmol 133:45-50, 2015

Importance.—The retinal vasculature is involved in many ocular diseases that cause visual loss. Although fluorescein angiography is the criterion standard for evaluating the retina vasculature, it has risks of adverse effects and known defects in imaging all the layers of the retinal vasculature. Optical coherence tomography (OCT) angiography can image vessels based on flow characteristics and may provide improved information.

Objective.—To investigate the ability of OCT angiography to image the vascular layers within the retina compared with conventional fluorescein angiography.

Design, Setting, and Participants.—In this study, performed from March 14, 2014, through June 24, 2014, a total of 5 consecutive, overlapping B-scan OCT angiography images composed of 216 A-scans were obtained at 216 discrete positions within a region of interest, typically a 2 × 2-mm area of the retina. The flow imaging was based on split-spectrum amplitude decorrelation angiography (SSADA), which can dissect layers of vessels in the retina. These distinct layers were compared with the fluorescein angiograms in 12 healthy eyes from patients at a private practice retina clinic to evaluate the ability to visualize the radial peripapillary capillary network. The proportion of the inner vs outer retinal vascular layers was estimated by 3 masked readers and compared with conventional fluorescein angiograms of the same eyes.

Main Outcomes and Measures.—Outcome measures were visualization of the radial peripapillary capillary network in the fluorescein and SSADA scans and the proportion of the inner retinal vascular plexus vs the outer retinal capillary plexus as seen in SSADA scans that would match the fluorescein angiogram.

Results.—In none of the 12 eyes could the radial peripapillary capillary network be visualized completely around the nerve head by fluorescein angiography, whereas the network was readily visualized in the SSADA scans. The fluorescein angiograms were matched, with a mean proportion of the inner vascular plexus being 95.3% (95% CI, 92.2%-97.8%) vs 4.7% (95% CI, 2.6%-5.7%) for the outer capillary plexus from the SSADA scans.

Conclusions and Relevance.—Fluorescein angiography does not image the radial peripapillary or the deep capillary networks well. However, OCT angiography can image all layers of the retinal vasculature without dye injection. Therefore, OCT angiography, and the findings generated, have the potential to affect clinical evaluation of the retina in healthy patients and patients with disease.

▶ Since its introduction in 1961,[1] fundus fluorescein angiography (FFA) has contributed to our understanding of many retinal diseases. This technology allows accurate delineation of large and medium-sized retinal vessels. Despite its importance, FFA remains a relatively invasive procedure requiring intravenous dye injection with potential adverse effects, especially if dye allergy is found.

Histopathologically, the retina is nourished by multilayered capillary networks, which can be broadly divided into the radial peripapillary capillary network and superficial and deep plexus layers. Mendes and colleagues have indicated that although FFA provides excellent imaging of the superficial vascular plexus, there is little imaging information regarding the superficial capillary layer and the deep capillary layer.[1]

Recent developments in optical coherence tomography (OCT) have allowed retinal vascular imaging without the need for dye injection. Current spectral domain OCT imaging provides cross-sectional retinal anatomic information with resolution to 4 to 5 microns. Most recently, using split-spectrum amplitude-decorrelation angiography (SSADA) technology, retinal blood flow can be depicted down to the capillary network and in all 3 vascular plexus levels.[2] This imaging technology is termed OCT angiography. Compared with FFA, OCT angiography allows imaging of the retinal vasculature throughout the retinal layers in few seconds, with enhanced resolution and without the need for dye injection. Each vascular layer can be analyzed separately or as a composite. However, current limitations of this technology include the limited field of view (3 or 6 mm) and inability to show vascular leakage, dye pooling, or tissue staining. This technology requires clear ocular media and patient cooperation with artifacts that can be induced by ocular movement and blinking.[3]

In this report, Spaide et al demonstrated the use of OCT angiography to image the retinal vascular layers and compared this technology with the "gold standard" FFA in 12 healthy eyes. They concluded that FFA is not capable of imaging the radial peripapillary capillary network or the deep retinal capillary network, whereas OCT angiography allows imaging of all 3 retinal vascular layers both in a noninvasive manner and with improved resolution. As these vascular networks are affected in a multitude of ocular disorders, OCT angiography could prove useful in the clinical evaluation and management of retinal vascular disorders.

W. A. Samara, MD
C. L. Shields, MD

References

1. Mendis KR, Balaratnasingam C, Yu P, et al. Correlation of histologic and clinical images to determine the diagnostic value of fluorescein angiography for studying retinal capillary detail. *Invest Ophthalmol Vis Sci.* 2010;51:5864-5869.
2. Jia Y, Tan O, Tokayer J, et al. Split-spectrum amplitude-decorrelation angiography with optical coherence tomography. *Opt Express.* 2012;20:4710-4725.
3. Lumbroso B, Rispoli M. Fluorescein Angiography and Optical Coherence Tomography-Angiography: Advantages and Disadvantages. In: Lumbroso B, Huang D, Jia Y, Fujimoto J, Rispoli M, eds. *Clinical Guide to Angio-oct: Non Invasive, Dyeless Oct Angiography.* New Delhi, India: Jaypee; 2015:68-70.

MyD-88 L265P mutations are present in some cases of vitreoretinal lymphoma

Pulido JS, Salomao DR, Frederick LA, et al (Mayo Clinic, Rochester, MN)
Retina 35:624-627, 2015

Purpose.—To determine whether Myd88 L265P mutations occur in diffuse large B-cell vitreoretinal lymphomas.

Methods.—The formalin-fixed paraffin-embedded cells from three patients with classic clinical findings of vitreoretinal lymphoma that also had histologic confirmation were evaluated using a validated amplification-refractory mutation system polymerase chain reaction to determine the presence of the mutation.

Results.—The 74 ± 2 base pair product seen from the mutated Myd-88 protein was noted in 2 of the 3 cases.

Conclusion.—Myd-88 L265P constitutive activating mutations are present in at least some cases of the diffuse large B-cell lymphoma form of vitreoretinal lymphoma. Further studies on the incidence of this mutation in retinal lymphomas are warranted.

▶ Vitreoretinal lymphoma (VRL) is a rare, high-grade, malignant, large B-cell, non-Hodgkin lymphoma.[1] VRL is otherwise known as vitreous large cell lymphoma, vitreous reticulum cell sarcoma, or primary intraocular lymphoma. In addition to the eye, this lymphoma can involve the central nervous system (CNS), which can manifest before, with, or after ocular diagnosis.[2] Historically, VRL has been a clinical diagnostic challenge because it often masquerades as idiopathic uveitis, delaying an established diagnosis for weeks or months. The lack of clinical pathognomonic findings requires reliance on interpretation of malignant cells or tissue.[1] There are no strict treatment guidelines or routinely successful therapies.[1,2] VRL has poor systemic prognosis with a survival rate of only 31 months.[3]

MyD-88 is a protein associated with the innate immune system, specifically in NF-kB signaling. A L265P mutation of this protein has been shown to be present in many cases of Waldenstrom's macroglobinemia and has become a diagnostic criterion for the disease. Recently, this same mutation has been shown to occur in 15% of systemic diffuse large B-cell lymphomas. It has not been previously shown in the vitreoretinal form of diffuse large B-cell lymphoma.

Pulido et al evaluated 3 cases of classic diffuse large B-cell vitreoretinal lymphoma (VRL) for the MyD88 L265P mutation. Clinically and histologically the 3 cases were similar, and all manifested initially with the vitreoretinal component of this lymphoma. The lymphoma tissue demonstrated mutated Myd-88 protein in 2 of the 3 cases. Extraocular involvement occurred in all 3 cases, and, interestingly, there was systemic involvement in the L265P-negative case and CNS involvement in the L265P-positive cases.

Pulido et al concluded that some cases of diffuse large B-cell VRL have the Myd-88 L265P mutation. Further studies are warranted to establish the frequency of this mutation in VRL. This could assist in detection of VRL at an earlier point. Furthermore, specific pharmacologic inhibitors of the Myd-88 L265P mutation are currently undergoing investigation for the treatment of Waldenstrom macroglobulinemia and these could potentially serve as therapeutic alternatives for VRL.[4]

C. L. Shields, MD

Nina Boal, BA contributed to the writing of this review under the direction of Carol L. Shields, MD, Co-Director of the Ocular Oncology Service of Wills Eye Hospital, Philadelphia, PA.

References

1. Levasseur SD, Wittenberg LA, White VA. Vitreoretinal lymphoma: a 20 year review of incidence, clinical and cytologic features, treatment, and outcomes. *JAMA Ophthalmol.* 2013;131:50-55.
2. Rajagopal R, Harbour JW. Diganostic testing and treatment choices in primary vitreoretinal lymphoma. *Retina.* 2011;31:435-440.
3. Grimm SA, McCannel CA, Omuro AM, et al. Primary CNS lymphoma with intraocular involvement: International PCNSL Collaborative Group Report. *Neurology.* 2008;71:1355-1360.
4. Treon SP. How I treat Waldenstrom macroglobulinemia. *Blood.* 2015;126:721-732.

Endoresection technique with/without brachytherapy for management of high posterior choroidal melanoma: Extended Follow-up Results

Garcia-Arumi J, Leila M, Zapata MA, et al (Autónoma Univ of Barcelona, Spain; Research Inst of Ophthalmology, Giza, Egypt; et al)

Retina 35:628-637, 2015

Purpose.—To evaluate the long-term efficacy and safety of endoresection for high posterior choroidal melanoma.

Methods.—Retrospective nonrandomized interventional case series. Forty-one patients had endoresection as primary treatment for posterior choroidal melanoma. Of these, 21 patients had adjuvant brachytherapy. The inclusion criteria were tumor thickness ≥8 mm, base diameter <15 mm, and posterior tumors not extending anterior to the equator. Main outcomes measures were enucleation rate, visual outcome, surgical complications, local recurrence, metastasis, and mortality.

Results.—Mean follow-up time was 102.5 months. Mean preoperative best-corrected visual acuity was 20/100. Mean tumor thickness was 9.8 mm (range, 7.7–13.5 mm standard deviation, 1.7 mm), mean base diameter was 9.9 mm (range, 5–15 mm standard deviation, 2.8 mm). At the latest visit, 36 patients (87.8%) still retained the eye. Mean postoperative best-corrected visual acuity was 20/1, 625. Retinal detachment was the main postoperative complication (28.9%). At completion of follow-up, 12% of patients had phthisis bulbi, and 3 developed chronic hypotony. Five patients (12.2%) had local tumor recurrence none of them had received brachytherapy as initial treatment. At 5 years of follow-up, 3 patients (7.3%) had liver metastasis. On Kaplan–Meier analysis at 10 years, all-cause mortality was 7.3% and specific mortality because of melanoma was 2.4%.

Conclusion.—Endoresection of high posterior melanomas was not associated with a higher risk of metastasis, death, or local recurrence than other reported techniques used to treat similar melanomas.

▶ Endoresection for choroidal melanoma was initially used as a salvage therapy to remove residual melanocytic tumor tissue following ablative photocoagulation therapy. Now, this technique has become a more prominent primary method of melanoma removal. This surgical technique theoretically allows for tumor removal without the potential risks of radiation-induced optic neuropathy or maculopathy that have been commonly seen following plaque radiotherapy. It also avoids the profuse neovascularization and vitreous hemorrhage that have been found after photocoagulation therapy. However, the safety and efficacy of endoresection is still controversial because of the belief that this could disseminate melanoma cells into an extraocular location. This procedure is performed via pars plana vitrectomy and the creation of a retinal flap anterior to the tumor. An incision is made into the healthy choroid around the tumor and the mass is surgically removed. Following tumor excision and reconstitution of the vitreous, a double row of confluent endolaser spots are provided to secure the retina flat and to eliminate residual tumor cells. The eye is then filled with silicone oil for 12 weeks, at which point cryotherapy or plaque radiotherapy may be used if necessary.

The goal of this retrospective, nonrandomized study was to measure the long-term success of endoresection in 41 patients with choroidal melanoma of >8 mm thickness. Endoresection was performed as the primary treatment for each patient.[1] Mean tumor thickness was 9.8 mm, and 21 patients (51%) received additional plaque radiotherapy to prevent local recurrence from tumor seeding. Tumor control was 88% at mean 102 months follow-up, and the recurrences were found only in those who did not receive adjuvant radiotherapy. Enucleation was necessary in 12% of patients. The main complications from this procedure were retinal detachment (29%), scleral bed bleeding (100%), postoperative ocular hypertension (34%), and phthisis bulbi (12%). Despite the magnificent tumor resection, local recurrence and complications remain a problem with mean visual acuity of 20/1625. Prognostically, metastatic disease was similar to those of alternative treatments.

Endoresection for choroidal melanoma is a challenging technique with moderate risk for recurrence, hypotony, visual loss, and enucleation. Despite this, endoresection could be a useful treatment for patients with large choroidal melanoma, particularly if all eyes received a dose of plaque radiotherapy at completion to ensure tumor control.

C. L. Shields, MD

Phillip Gordon, BA contributed to the writing of this review under the direction of Carol L. Shields, MD, Co-Director of the Ocular Oncology Service of Wills Eye Hospital, Philadelphia, PA.

Reference

1. Damato B, Groenewald C, McGalliard J, Wong D. Endoresection of choroidal melanoma. *Br J Ophthalmol.* 1998;82:213-218.

Paraneoplastic sarcoid-like reactions and the eye

Balasubramaniam SC, Salomão DR, Davies JB, et al (Mayo Clinic, Rochester, MN; VitreoRetinal Surgery, Minneapolis, MN; et al)

Retina 35:789-797, 2015

Background.—Sarcoid-like reactions have been reported and confirmed by histopathology in patients with malignant disease. This series demonstrates the complex relationship of malignancy and sarcoidosis as pertaining to the eye, which, to the best of our knowledge, has not been previously reported in the literature.

Methods.—Retrospective case study of five patients with sarcoid-like reactions. Patients 1 to 4 represent patients with ocular sarcoid-like reaction and systemic malignant disease. Patient 5 had ocular malignancy and systemic sarcoid-like reaction; workup revealed renal cell cancer. For each patient, other etiologies of nonnecrotizing granulomatous inflammation were excluded.

Results.—Sarcoid-like reactions have been described in the literature when nonnecrotizing granulomas occur in association with malignancy and in the absence of multiorgan involvement as seen with systemic sarcoid. In our series, sarcoid-like reactions involved the vitreous in three patients, retina in one patient, and the choroid and lung in one patient. Sarcoid-like reaction preceded the diagnosis of malignancy in two patients, was found concomitantly with malignancy in one patient, and followed malignancy in two patients. Two patients had hematologic malignancy, one patient had endometrial carcinoma, one had renal cell carcinoma, and one patient had both renal cell carcinoma and uveal melanoma. Four patients had findings of nonnecrotizing granulomas confirmed by histopathology.

Conclusion.—Sarcoid-like reactions can occur in the eye, and ocular malignancies may incite sarcoid-like reaction. Ocular sarcoid-like reactions have paraneoplastic features in that they can occur at a site distant from malignancy and may precede, occur simultaneously with, or follow malignancy.

▶ Sarcoidosis is a multisystem inflammatory disorder characterized by nonnecrotizing epithelioid granulomas, most often found in the lung and eye. Between 25% to 80% of patients with sarcoidosis will have ocular involvement, with manifestations including uveitis, periphlebitis, papillitis, or conjunctival follicles.[1,2] Malignancy can develop in patients with systemic or localized sarcoidosis, and, in the reverse, patients with cancer can develop sarcoid-like granulomas. Most frequently, these granulomas are observed in lymph nodes draining the malignancy but can also occur in distant organs or in the tumor-affected organ itself. Malignancies with documented sarcoid-like reactions include leukemia, lymphoma, and cancers of the breast, stomach, kidney, colon, lung, bile duct, ovary, and thyroid. Ocular sarcoid-like reaction, however, has not previously been described in relation to malignancies. Sarcoid-like reactions can involute after successful treatment of the primary malignancy or immunosuppression, similar to paraneoplastic syndromes.

In this study, Balasubramaniam et al presented 5 patients with ocular sarcoid-like reactions. Two patients had a known history of systemic malignant disease diagnosed 36 to 40 months before developing the ocular sarcoid-like responses. Diagnoses included B-cell chronic lymphocytic leukemia and endometrial cancer. Ocular sarcoid-like responses included granulomatous vitreitis, phlebitis, and choroidal granuloma, as well as systemic sarcoidosis. Two additional patients had no known history of malignant disease but were found to have malignancy on workup following the ocular sarcoid-like findings. These patients presented with uveitis, periphlebitis, and peripheral retinal neovascularization with vasculitis. The related cancers included renal cell carcinoma and mucosa-associated lymphoma. There was 1 patient with systemic sarcoid-like reaction who had simultaneous uveal melanoma and renal cell carcinoma. Because the patient had 2 separate malignancies, it is difficult to determine whether the ocular malignancy, renal malignancy, or both caused the patient to develop sarcoid-like lymphadenopathy.

This retrospective case series stimulates inquiry into the relationship between malignancy and sarcoid-like reactions, particularly in the eye. There is concern that they might not be related because both conditions are considered relatively common. Further studies evaluating large cohorts of patients with cancer for ocular or systemic sarcoid-like reactions could prove or disprove this relationship.

C. L. Shields, MD

Elizabeth Isaacoff, BS, MBE contributed to the writing of this review under the direction of Carol L. Shields, MD, Co-Director of the Ocular Oncology Service of Wills Eye Hospital, Philadelphia, PA.

References

1. Iannuzzi MC, Rybicki BA, Teirstein AS. Sarcoidosis. *N Engl J Med.* 2007;357: 2153-2165.
2. Rothova A. Ocular involvement in sarcoidosis. *Br J Ophthalmol.* 2000;84: 110-116.

American Joint Committee on Cancer Classification of Uveal Melanoma (Anatomic Stage) Predicts Prognosis in 7731 Patients: The 2013 Zimmerman Lecture

Shields CL, Kaliki S, Furuta M, et al (Thomas Jefferson Univ, Philadelphia, PA)
Ophthalmology 122:1180-1186, 2015

Purpose.—To analyze the clinical features and prognosis of posterior uveal melanoma based on the American Joint Committee on Cancer (AJCC) (7th edition) tumor staging.

Design.—Retrospective interventional case series.

Participants.—A total of 7731 patients.

Methods.—Uveal melanoma management.

Main Outcome Measures.—Melanoma-related metastasis and death.

Results.—Of 7731 patients with posterior uveal (ciliary body and choroidal) melanoma, the AJCC tumor staging was stage I in 2767 (36%), stage II in 3735 (48%), stage III in 1220 (16%), and stage IV in 9 (<1%). Based on tumor staging (I, II, III, and IV), features that showed significant increase with tumor staging included age at presentation (57, 58, 60, 60 years) ($P < 0.001$), tumor base (8, 12, 17, 17 mm) ($P < 0.001$), tumor thickness (2.9, 6.0, 10.1, 10.2 mm) ($P < 0.001$), distance to optic disc (3, 5, 5, 5 mm) ($P < 0.001$), distance to foveola (3, 5, 5, 5 mm) ($P < 0.001$), mushroom configuration (6%, 24%, 34%, 33%) ($P < 0.001$), plateau configuration (3%, 4%, 7%, 11%) ($P < 0.001$), tumor pigmentation (48%, 53%, 69%, 78%) ($P < 0.001$), and extraocular extension (0%, 1%, 11%, 22%) ($P < 0.001$). After therapy, Kaplan–Meier estimates of metastasis at 1, 5, 10, and 20 years were <1%, 5%, 12%, and 20% for stage I, 2%; 17%, 29%, and 44% for stage II; 6%, 44%, 61%, and 73% for stage III, and 100% by 1 year for stage IV. Kaplan–Meier estimates of death at 1, 5, 10, and 20 years were <1%,

3%, 6%, and 8% for stage I; <1%, 9%, 15%, and 24% for stage II; 3%, 27%, 39%, and 53% for stage III, and 100% by 1 year for stage IV. Compared with stage I, the hazard ratio for metastasis/death was 3.1/3.1 for stage II and 9.3/10.1 for stage III.

Conclusions.—Compared with uveal melanoma classified as AJCC stage I, the rate of metastasis/death was 3 times greater for stage II, 9 to 10 times greater for stage III, and further greater for stage IV. Early detection of posterior uveal melanoma, at a point when the tumor is small, can be lifesaving.

▶ The American Joint Committee on Cancer (AJCC) classification system provides a common nomenclature for clinicians to characterize cancer staging, which is noted by tumor (T), node (N), and metastasis (M), the "TNM" convention. Tumor staging is differentiated by 4 stages, designated as I, II, III, and IV. Ocular features related to increased staging include greater tumor size and extent, ciliary body involvement, and the presence of minor or major extrascleral extension. An additional role for the AJCC staging of uveal melanoma is for prediction of tumor-related metastasis and death.

In this report, Shields et al explored the predictive value of the AJCC stage classification for posterior uveal melanoma metastasis and death using a retrospective analysis of 7331 patients with posterior uveal melanoma from 1970 to 2008. The variables evaluated included patient demographic data, tumor characteristics, and tumor treatments. Of the 7731 patients, 36% were identified as stage I, 48% as stage II, 16% as stage III, and less than 1% as stage IV. Increasing stage was statistically associated with older age, larger tumor size, more peripheral location, and extraocular extension. Metastatic disease was found at 10 years in 12% of patients with stage I melanoma, 29% of stage II, 61% of stage III, and 100% of stage IV. All patients with stage IV melanoma developed metastasis by 1 year.

This report confirms the predictive value of the 7th edition of the AJCC scale for posterior uveal melanoma, and underscores its importance as an assessment for melanoma metastasis. On the basis of this predictive classification, patients at high risk for metastasis can be identified so that they can be properly advised for systemic therapy to prevent or reduce the incidence of metastasis.

C. L. Shields, MD

Daniel Taylor, BA contributed to the writing of this review under the direction of Carol L. Shields, MD, Co-Director of the Ocular Oncology Service of Wills Eye Hospital, Philadelphia, PA.

Malignant Lymphoma of the Conjunctiva

Kirkegaard MM, Coupland SE, Prause JU, et al (Univ of Copenhagen, Denmark; Univ of Liverpool, United Kingdom; et al)
Surv Ophthalmol 60:444-458, 2015

Conjunctival lymphomas constitute 25% of all ocular adnexal lymphomas. The majority are B-cell non-Hodgkin lymphomas (NHL) (98%), while T-cell NHLs are rare in the conjunctiva (2%). The most frequent subtype of conjunctival B-cell lymphoma is extranodal marginal zone lymphoma (EMZL) (81%), followed by follicular lymphoma (FL) (8%), diffuse large B-cell lymphoma (DLBCL) (3%) and mantle cell lymphoma (MCL) (3%). EMZL occurs slightly more often in women and, along with FL, presents late in the seventh decade of life, while DLBCL and especially MCL have a predilection for male gender and typically present in the eighth decade. EMZL and FL present most frequently in the forniceal and bulbar conjunctiva. Conjunctival DLBCL, MCL and T-cell NHLs are characterized by a short duration of symptoms before the first ophthalmological consultation. External beam radiotherapy is the treatment of choice for EMZL and FL, while DLBCL, MCL and T-cell NHLs are mainly treated with chemotherapy. Conjunctival T-cell NHLs are associated with a particularly poor prognosis, with 50% of patients having progression or recurrence during a one-year follow-up period.

▶ Conjunctival lymphoma is a malignant neoplasm that constitutes a significant subset of all ocular cancers. Lymphomas are primarily categorized as Hodgkin lymphomas or non-Hodgkin lymphomas (NHL) on the basis of their origin from natural killer cells or B and T cells, respectively.[1] Almost all (98%) lymphomas affecting the bulbar conjunctiva are NHL of B-cell lineage, which are treatable with reasonable prognosis. T-cell lymphomas are much more severe and aggressive than B-cell lymphomas, in general, and have poorer clinical outcomes.

Several different hypotheses regarding the pathogenesis of these diseases have been proposed. In the conjunctiva, it has been suggested that extranodal marginal zone lymphoma (EMZL), a major type (81%) of conjunctival B-cell NHL, can develop as a result of unchecked B-lymphocyte growth and proliferation following chronic antigen stimulation from infectious agents and subsequent inflammatory response. This is supported by the infectious conjunctivitis and chronic inflammation that can sometimes precede EMZL. However, other causal links are also potentially a source, including autoimmune diseases and genetic abnormalities. For example, EMZL is associated with translocations that activate transcription factor kB. Further genetic studies are required to elucidate analogous relationships between genetic abnormalities and other types of conjunctival lymphomas.

The main physical finding of conjunctival lymphoma is a salmon-pink unilateral lesion, which varies in appearance across different subtypes.[2] Patients with low-grade lymphoma rarely complain of other symptoms. In contrast, high-grade types of B-cell NHL (as well as T-cell NHL) present with a greater number of symptoms and more rapid disease progression. These patients consult an ophthalmologist 3 times earlier than those with low-grade lymphoma. Conjunctival lymphoma is infrequently associated with secondary disease, although this differs considerably on the basis of the aggressiveness of the lymphoma subtype.

After ophthalmologic examination, immunohistochemical characterization is the standard for confirming diagnosis of conjunctival lymphoma. Diagnosis is followed by clinical staging. There has been a recent movement away from the conventional Ann Arbor staging system in favor of the new tumor, node, and metastasis (TMN) system proposed by the American Joint Committee on Cancer. Clinical staging, as well as the histopathological subtype, are important indicators of patient prognosis.

A multidisciplinary team should consider individual patient needs, the extent and severity of the tumor, and the histopathological profile of the lymphoma when selecting treatment. External beam radiotherapy (EBRT) is the current therapy of choice for most low-grade conjunctival lymphomas, like EMZL and follicular lymphoma. Patients typically have a remarkably good long-term prognosis following EBRT, with 80% experiencing no recurrence or progression after a 5-year period. The more aggressive types of conjunctival lymphomas, like T-cell NHLs, are managed effectively with chemotherapy, which has been shown to eliminate 65% to 70% of high-grade B-cell and T-cell lymphomas.

In addition to providing a comprehensive and clinically valuable survey of conjunctival lymphoma, these authors highlight areas in which further investigation should be performed. Conclusive data, especially regarding disease etiology and long-term prognosis, are greatly needed.

C. L. Shields, MD

Sara Taylor, BS, BA contributed to the writing of this review under the direction of Carol L. Shields, MD, Co-Director of the Ocular Oncology Service of Wills Eye Hospital, Philadelphia, PA.

References

1. Campo E, Swerdlow SH, Harris NL, et al. The 2008 WHO classification of lymphoid neoplasms and beyond: evolving concepts and practical applications. *Blood.* 2011;117:5019-5032.
2. Shields CL, Shields JA, Carvalho C, et al. Conjunctival lymphoid tumors: clinical analysis of 117 cases and relationship to systemic lymphoma. *Ophthalmology.* 2001;108:979-984.

Development and Validation of a Smartphone-Based Visual Acuity Test (Peek Acuity) for Clinical Practice and Community-Based Fieldwork

Bastawrous A, Rono HK, Livingstone IAT, et al (London School of Hygiene and Tropical Medicine (LSHTM), England; Kitale Hospital and Zonal Ophthalmologist, North Rift, Kenya; NHS Greater Glasgow and Clyde, Scotland; et al)

JAMA Ophthalmol 133:930-937, 2015

Importance.—Visual acuity is the most frequently performed measure of visual function in clinical practice and most people worldwide living with visual impairment are living in low- and middle-income countries.

Objective.—To design and validate a smartphone-based visual acuity test that is not dependent on familiarity with symbols or letters commonly used in the English language.

Design, Setting, and Participants.—Validation study conducted from December 11, 2013, to March 4, 2014, comparing results from smartphone-based Peek Acuity to Snellen acuity (clinical normal) charts and the Early Treatment of Diabetic Retinopathy Study (ETDRS) logMAR chart (reference standard). This study was nested within the 6-year follow-up of the Nakuru Eye Disease Cohort in central Kenya and included 300 adults aged 55 years and older recruited consecutively.

Main Outcomes and Measures.—Outcome measures were monocular logMAR visual acuity scores for each test: ETDRS chart logMAR, Snellen acuity, and Peek Acuity. Peek Acuity was compared, in terms of test-retest variability and measurement time, with the Snellen acuity and ETDRS logMAR charts in participants' homes and temporary clinic settings in rural Kenya in 2013 and 2014.

Results.—The 95% CI limits for test-retest variability of smartphone acuity data were ±0.033 logMAR. The mean differences between the smartphone-based test and the ETDRS chart and the smartphone-based test and Snellen acuity data were 0.07 (95% CI, 0.05-0.09) and 0.08 (95% CI, 0.06-0.10) logMAR, respectively, indicating that smartphone-based test acuities agreed well with those of the ETDRS and Snellen charts. The agreement of Peek Acuity and the ETDRS chart was greater than the Snellen chart with the ETDRS chart (95% CI, 0.05-0.10; $P = .08$). The local Kenyan community health care workers readily accepted the Peek Acuity smartphone test; it required minimal training and took no longer than the Snellen test (77 seconds vs 82 seconds; 95% CI, 71-84 seconds vs 73-91 seconds, respectively; $P = .13$).

Conclusions and Relevance.—The study demonstrated that the Peek Acuity smartphone test is capable of accurate and repeatable acuity measurements consistent with published data on the test-retest variability of acuities measured using 5-letter-per-line retroilluminated logMAR charts.

▶ Visual acuity (VA) is the most common measurement of visual function in clinical practice and helps to screen for patients with eyes that warrant further clinical evaluation. It is estimated that 285 million people worldwide are visually impaired, and 80% have a condition that could be prevented or cured. However, most affected patients live in impoverished areas with minimal access to evaluation or treatment for these conditions.[1] Current visual assessment with Snellen acuity has drawbacks, including nongeometric letter size progression, inconsistent number of letters per line, and crowding phenomenon. LogMAR acuity charts have overcome these obstacles.[2] Using LogMAR framework combined with smartphone technology, visual assessment can efficiently reach globally remote areas.

In this study, Bastawrous et al explore the Peek Acuity smartphone application that was modeled after the Early Treatment of Diabetic Retinopathy Study (ETDRS) VA chart, using LogMAR basis. This chart is widely recognized as the gold standard for VA measurements in clinical trials.[3] As part of the population-based Nakuru Eye Disease Cohort study in central Kenya,[4] they tested 300 consecutive patients aged 55 years or older. On 2 consecutive days, VA measurements were made in the participant's home and in the central clinic. At the participant's home, VA was measured with both Peek Acuity and Snellen acuity in random order. While in the clinic, participants had both Peek Acuity and Snellen acuity tests performed in random order followed by the ETDRS VA test. Results showed that Peek Acuity testing at home was highly correlated to ETDRS testing in the clinic with mean difference of 5 letters (1 line). The clinic measurements of Peek Acuity were even better correlated with ETDRS VA with mean difference of less than 3 letters on a line. Importantly, in both home and clinic measurements of VA, the Peek Acuity test showed a higher degree of correlation with the ETDRS VA than did the Snellen test. Peek Acuity measurements made at home and in the clinic on consecutive days by the same examiner were highly correlated with a small mean difference. The mean testing time for both eyes was 82 seconds for Snellen testing and 77 seconds for Peek Acuity testing, showing no significant difference.

These authors showed that the Peek Acuity test was reliable, fast, and consistent and that this phone-based test performed well against standard clinical and research measures of VA. With the rapid movement toward mobile technologies in health care, a smartphone-based VA application has the potential for vast improvements in health care information delivery, real-time patient monitoring, research data collection, and, most important, early detection of diseases with timely and appropriate treatment.

C. L. Shields, MD

Tony Kang, BS contributed to the writing of this review under the direction of Carol L. Shields, MD, Co-Director of the Ocular Oncology Service of Wills Eye Hospital, Philadelphia, PA.

References

1. Pascolini D, Mariotti SP. Global estimates of visual impairment: 2010. *Br J Ophthalmol.* 2012;96:614-618.
2. Bailey IL, Lovie JE. New design principles for visual acuity letter charts. *Am J Optom Physiol Opt.* 1976;53:740-745.
3. Ferris FL, Bailey I. Standardizing the measurement of visual acuity for clinical research studies. *Ophthalmology.* 1996;103:181-182.

4. Mathenge W, Bastawrous A, Foster A, Kuper H. The Nakuru Posterior Segment Eye Disease Study: methods and prevalence of blindness and visual impairment in Nakuru, Kenya. *Ophthalmology.* 2012;119:2033-2039.

ImmTACs for targeted cancer therapy: Why, what, how, and which

Oates J, Hassan NJ, Jakobsen BK (Immunocore Ltd, Milton Park, Abingdon, Oxon, United Kingdom)

Mol Immunol 67:67-74, 2015

Overcoming immunosuppression and activating a cytotoxic T cell response has the potential to halt the progression of cancer and, in some circumstances, eradicate it. Designing therapeutic interventions that achieve this goal has proven challenging, but now a greater understanding of the complexities of immune responses is beginning to produce some notable breakthroughs. ImmTACs (immune-mobilising monoclonal TCRs against cancer) are a new class of bispecific reagents, based on soluble monoclonal T cell receptors, which have been engineered to possess extremely high affinity for cognate tumour antigen. In this way, ImmTACs overcome the problem of low affinity tumour-specific T cells imposed by thymic selection and provide access to the large number of antigens presented as peptide–HLA complexes. Once bound to tumour cells the anti-CD3 effector end of the ImmTAC drives recruitment of polyclonal T cells to the tumour site, leading to a potent redirected T cell response and tumour cell destruction. Extensive *in vitro* testing coupled with promising early clinical data has provided an enhanced appreciation of ImmTAC function *in vivo* and indicates their potential therapeutic benefit in terms of a durable response and ultimately the breaking of T cell tolerance. This review introduces ImmTACs in the context of immunotherapy, and outlines their design, construction and mechanism of action, as well as examining target selection and aspects of preclinical safety testing.

▶ ImmTACs are soluble biospecific reagents capable of high-affinity tumor antigen binding and subsequent activation of a targeted T-cell immune response. Barriers for antibody-based tumor therapies include the limited number of surface-presenting antigens available and the difficulty of identifying antigens that demonstrate an acceptable degree of localization to the target tissue. ImmTACs, or immune-mobilizing monoclonal T-cell receptors against cancer, represent an attractive alternative or complementary option because of the employment of T-cell receptors (TCR) to target surface or intracellular antigens. Given that the majority of tumor antigens manifest within the cell or on the cell surface, ImmTACs have a large potential and remarkable selection of targets compared with antibody-based therapies.

The ImmTAC basically has 2 receptors, 1 for the cancer cell (HLA receptor) and 1 for the T-cell (CD3 receptor). The mechanism of action of ImmTAC begins with the binding of the ImmTAC to a peptide-HLA complex on a cancer cell surface. The ImmTAC draws a T cell to its CD3 receptor, leading to an immune synapse, activation of the T cell, and destruction of the cancer cell. Dendritic cells uptake the loaded, dead cancer cell, and epitope spreading occurs downstream.

Rapidly evolving technologies have provided previously unavailable options to circumvent barriers to the creation of effective TCRs. By introducing a mutation into 1 of 6 complementary determining regions, affinity of ImmTACs for tumor cell antigens can be increased 1 million fold or greater, compared with wild-type TCRs. Tumor-cell killing using these engineered TCRs has been shown to be particularly effective, even for cells displaying a low number (as few as 10) of antigens.[1] Redirected T cells also secrete cytokines and chemokines related to increased T-cell infiltration into tumor tissue, possibly serving to increase therapeutic benefit. Perhaps the most exciting aspect of ImmTACs is their potential to amplify the body's tumor-specific immune response through antigen cross-presentation and epitope spreading. It is thought that ImmTAC-related tumor cell killing leads to uptake of antigen by dendritic cells. These cells migrate to the lymphatic system where they present antigens to naive T cells. These programmed anti-tumor T cells then undergo clonal expansion and migrate to the site of the tumor, where they can mediate further destruction of the cancer. In this way, ImmTACs present the unique advantage of reprogramming the body to more effectively fight cancer.

The authors conclude that, although ImmTACs are likely to be a powerful cancer therapy, it is unlikely that they or any other therapy will be completely sufficient on its own. This is supported by genomic evidence illustrating the heterogeneity of tumors even within the same patient. Furthermore, similar to antibiotic-resistant bacteria, tumor cells are subject to selection pressures. The implication of this is that treatment may encourage enrichment or emergence of a resistant population. For this reason, therapies will require multifaceted attacks to overcome the variability of resistance profiles of some tumor cells. The challenge moving forward is to define which treatment combinations will be most effective, and this will require a better understanding of the relationship between tumors and the immune system.

C. L. Shields, MD

Jordan Sugarman, BS contributed to the writing of this review under the direction of Carol L. Shields, MD, Co-Director of the Ocular Oncology Service of Wills Eye Hospital, Philadelphia, PA.

Reference

1. Bossi G, Buisson S, Oates J, Jakobsen BK, Hassan NJ. ImmTAC-redirected tumour cell killing induces and potentiates antigen cross-presentation by dendritic cells. *Cancer Immunol.* 2014;63:437-448.

Efficacy of Vismodegib (Erivedge) for Basal Cell Carcinoma Involving the Orbit and Periocular Area

Demirci H, Worden F, Nelson CC, et al (Univ of Michigan, Ann Arbor)

Ophthal Plast Reconstr Surg 31:463-466, 2015

Purpose.—Evaluate the effectiveness of vismodegib in the management of basal cell carcinoma with orbital extension and/or extensive periocular involvement.

Methods.—Retrospective chart review of 6 consecutive patients with biopsy-proven orbital basal cell carcinoma and 2 additional patients with extensive periocular basal cell carcinoma who were treated with oral vismodegib (150 mg/day) was performed.

Results.—Basal cell carcinoma extended in the orbit in 6 of 8 patients (involving orbital bones in 1 patient), and 2 of 8 patients had extensive periocular involvement (1 with basal cell nevus syndrome). Vismodegib therapy was the only treatment in 6 patients, off-label neoadjuvant in 1 patient, and adjuvant treatment in 1 patient. Orbital tumors in all 4 patients who received vismodegib as sole treatment showed partial response with a mean 83% shrinkage in tumor size after a median of 7 months of therapy. In the 2 patients receiving vismodegib as neoadjuvant or adjuvant therapies, there was complete response after a median of 7 months of therapy and no evidence of clinical recurrence after discontinuing therapy for a median of 15 months. The 2 patients with extensive periocular involvement experienced complete clinical response after a median 14 months of treatment. During treatment, the most common side effects were muscle spasm (75%) followed by alopecia (50%), dysgeusia (25%), dysosmia, and episodes of diarrhea and constipation (13%).

Conclusions.—Basal cell carcinoma with orbital extension and extensive periocular involvement responds to vismodegib therapy. The long-term prognosis remains unknown, and additional prospective studies are indicated.

▶ Basal cell carcinoma (BCC) is the most common malignant eyelid tumor in the United States. This cutaneous malignancy generally remains limited to the sun-exposed portions of the ocular region, particularly the lower eyelid. Involvement of both eyelids or invasion into the orbit is uncommon, found in less than 5% of cases. However, the situation is much different in developing countries, where deep orbital involvement can occur in up to 17% of cases, partly due to delay or inadequacy of medical care. Localized eyelid BCC is effectively treated with surgical resection and reconstruction or Mohs micrographic surgery with care to provide tumor-free margin control. Aggressive or neglected cases of orbital or extensive periocular BCC, however, require procedures that can cause facial deformities or visual impairment, and ultimately orbital exenteration might be necessary.

Over the past decade, molecular and genetic studies have shown that the majority of cases of BCC demonstrate mutation in the Hedgehog (Hh) signaling pathway, leading to unrestrained basal-cell proliferation and tumor development.[1] In 2012, the first-in-class Hh signaling pathway inhibitor in the United States was vismodegib (Erivedge), approved by the Food and Drug Administration specifically for adults with metastatic BCC, those with locally advanced BCC recurrent following surgery, or those classified as poor surgical or radiation candidates.[2] Phase II results revealed complete response in 21% and partial response in 22% of 63 patients with locally advanced BCC.[3] A randomized, double-blinded, placebo-controlled study of vismodegib in 41 patients with basal cell nevus syndrome showed favorable results with tumor size reduction.[4]

In this study, the authors evaluated the effectiveness of oral vismodegib in 8 patients with orbital (n = 6) or periocular (n = 2) BCC. Those with extensive periocular BCC showed complete clinical response with median 14 months of medication and showed no recurrence on limited follow-up. Of the 6 patients with orbital involvement, all showed response to vismodegib therapy, and 2 demonstrated complete response combining vismodegib and surgical resection with no evidence of tumor recurrence after 19 and 21 months. Those 4 patients who used vismodegib alone achieved 80% to 95% mass reduction.

Vismodegib appears to be a promising novel therapeutic agent for advanced BCC, demonstrating remarkable tumor response, particularly for those with orbital extension or extensive periocular involvement. Although this medication is relatively well tolerated, adverse effects such as muscle spasms, alopecia, and dysgeusia are commonly reported and in some cases have lead to treatment discontinuation. In addition, a few cases of tumor regrowth, keratoacanthoma, squamous cell carcinoma and resistance to vismodegib therapy have been recognized. Future studies to clarify optimal selection criteria and treatment duration, as well as methods to limit adverse effects will be explored.

C. L. Shields, MD

Marisa Schoen, BA contributed to the writing of this review under the direction of Carol L. Shields, MD, Co-Director of the Ocular Oncology Service of Wills Eye Hospital, Philadelphia, PA.

References

1. Epstein EH. Basal cell carcinomas: attack of the hedgehog. *Nat Rev Cancer.* 2008; 8:743-754.
2. Clozaril [package insert]. San Francisco, CA: Genentech; 2012.
3. Sekulic A, Migden MR, Oro AE, et al. Efficacy and safety of vismodegib in advanced basal-cell carcinoma. *N Engl J Med.* 2012;366:2171-2179.
4. Tang JY, Mackay-Wiggan JM, Aszterbaum M, et al. Inhibiting the hedgehog pathway in patients with the basal-cell nevus syndrome. *N Engl J Med.* 2012;366: 2180-2188.

12 Pathology

Histopathologic Grading of Anaplasia in Retinoblastoma

Mendoza PR, Specht CS, Hubbard GB, et al (Emory Univ, Atlanta, GA; Penn State Milton S. Hershey Medical Ctr, PA)
Am J Ophthalmol 159:764-776, 2015

Purpose.—To determine whether the degree of tumor anaplasia has prognostic value by evaluating its correlation with high-risk histopathologic features and clinical outcomes in a series of retinoblastoma patients.

Design.—Retrospective clinicopathologic study.

Methods.—The clinical and pathologic findings in 266 patients who underwent primary enucleation for retinoblastoma were reviewed. The histologic degree of anaplasia was graded as retinocytoma, mild, moderate, or severe as defined by increasing cellular pleomorphism, number of mitoses, nuclear size, and nuclear hyperchromatism. Nuclear morphometric characteristics were measured. The clinical and pathologic data of 125 patients were compared using Kaplan-Meier estimates of survival. Fisher exact test and multivariate regression were used to analyze the association between anaplasia grade and high-risk histologic features.

Results.—Increasing grade of anaplasia was associated with decreased overall survival ($P = .003$) and increased risk of metastasis ($P = .0007$). Histopathologic features that were associated with anaplasia included optic nerve invasion ($P < .0001$), choroidal invasion ($P < .0001$), and anterior segment invasion ($P = .04$). Multivariate analysis considering high-risk histopathology and anaplasia grading as predictors of distant metastasis and death showed that high-risk histopathology was statistically significant as an independent predictor ($P = .01$ for metastasis, $P = .03$ for death) but anaplasia was not ($P = .63$ for metastasis, $P = .30$ for death). In the absence of high-risk features, however, severe anaplasia identified an additional risk for metastasis ($P = .0004$) and death ($P = .01$).

Conclusion.—Grading of anaplasia may be a useful adjunct to standard histopathologic criteria in identifying retinoblastoma patients who do not have high-risk histologic features but still have an increased risk of metastasis and may need adjuvant therapy (Figs 1, 5 and 6).

► The purpose of this retrospective study was to determine the prognostic value of anaplasia in retinoblastoma. High-risk histologic features, such as massive choroidal or postlaminar optic nerve invasion, have been well shown to be associated with metastasis and death. There are cases, however, in which patients develop metastases or succumb to retinoblastoma despite absence of these

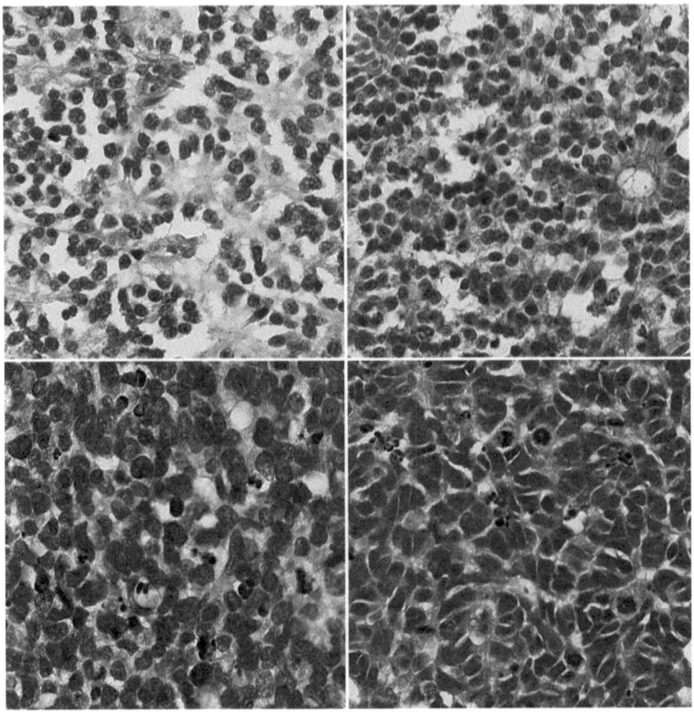

FIGURE 1.—Grading of anaplasia in retinoblastoma. (Top left) Retinocytoma: the nuclei are not enlarged, there is no pleomorphism or mitotic activity, cells have abundant eosinophilic cytoplasm and prominent photoreceptor differentiation (fleurettes). (Top right) Mild anaplasia: the nuclei are not enlarged, but there can be mild pleomorphism, occasional rare mitotic figures, and photoreceptor differentiation (Flexner-Wintersteiner and Homer Wright rosettes). (Bottom left) Moderate anaplasia: there is unambiguous enlargement of nuclei compared to mild anaplasia, definite pleomorphism, frequent mitotic figures, and poor differentiation. (Bottom right) Severe anaplasia: there is enlargement of nuclei similar in size to moderate anaplasia, extreme pleomorphism (angular, rhomboid, or fusiform), cell wrapping, numerous mitotic figures, and poor differentiation. (Hematoxylin-eosin: Top left, 250×; Top right 250×; Bottom left, 250×; Bottom right, 250×.) (Reprinted from Mendoza PR, Specht CS, Hubbard GB, et al. Histopathologic grading of anaplasia in retinoblastoma. *Am J Ophthalmol.* 2015;159:764-776, with permission from Elsevier.)

high-risk features on histology. The authors therefore investigated whether anaplasia is an independent factor in predicting metastasis and/or death, as it is in medulloblastomas, a similar embryonal central nervous system tumor.

Two hundred and sixty-six patients with retinoblastoma who underwent enucleation from 1940 to 2013 were included in the study and evaluated. Histologic sections were reviewed and graded on anaplasia and differentiation as defined in Tables 1 and 2 in the original article. The degree of anaplasia was based on cytologic features that included cell shape, cell wrapping, nuclear size, nuclear contour, nuclear chromaticity, and frequency of mitoses, whereas differentiation was based on 2 schemas based on the types of rosettes/fleurettes (Scheme 1), and the extent of the presence of rosettes/fleurettes in the tumor (Scheme 2). All of the sections were reviewed blindly by 2 ocular pathologists.

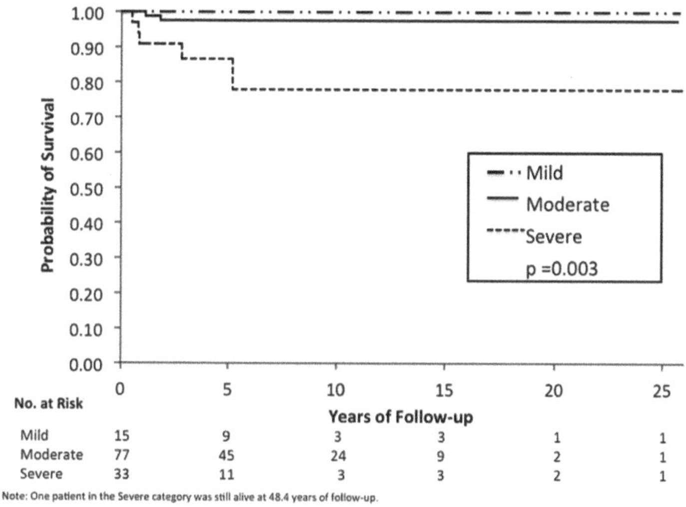

FIGURE 5.—Kaplan-Meier estimate shows that increasing severity of anaplasia grade is associated with decreased survival in retinoblastoma ($P = .003$). (Reprinted from Mendoza PR, Specht CS, Hubbard GB, et al. Histopathologic grading of anaplasia in retinoblastoma. *Am J Ophthalmol.* 2015;159:764-776, with permission from Elsevier.)

Furthermore, 47 cases were chosen for nuclear morphometric analysis to evaluate an objective method for analyzing cytologic features. Statistical analysis was performed between anaplasia grade and high-risk histologic features, as well as anaplasia grade and level of differentiation for all included cases. Out

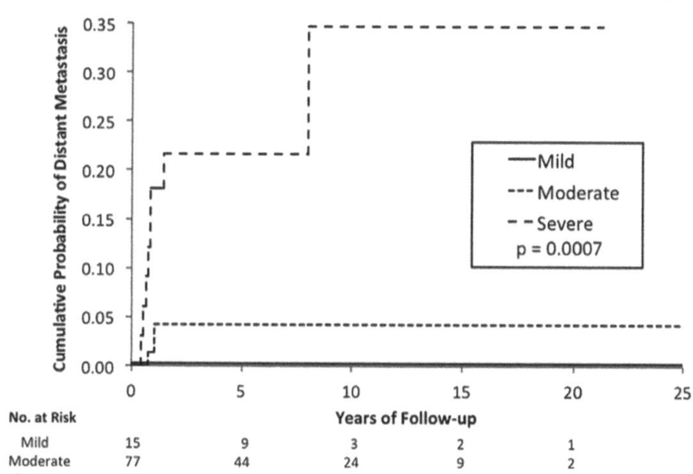

FIGURE 6.—Kaplan-Meier estimate shows that increasing severity of anaplasia grade is associated with increased risk of metastasis in retinoblastoma ($P = .0007$). (Reprinted from Mendoza PR, Specht CS, Hubbard GB, et al. Histopathologic grading of anaplasia in retinoblastoma. *Am J Ophthalmol.* 2015;159:764-776, with permission from Elsevier.)

of the 266 patients, follow-up clinic information was available on 125 patients, and these data were used for Kaplan-Meier estimates of metastasis and survival.

Results show that higher grades of anaplasia were associated with decreased overall survival and increased risk of metastasis (Figs 5 and 6). However, anaplasia alone was not a significant independent prognosticator in the presence of high-risk features. Only when there was an absence of high-risk features was severe anaplasia found to be a significant independent prognostic indicator. Furthermore, level of differentiation did not correlate with level of anaplasia. As for nuclear morphometry, the authors only found the degree of nuclear pleomorphism, such as elongation and angularity, to be correlative with level of anaplasia; size and hyperchromaticity were found to be less correlative.

Ultimately, the authors conclude that microscopic examination of retinoblastoma specimens that includes anaplasia grading may be useful. In particular, patients who lack high-risk histologic features may benefit from anaplasia grading.

V. Lee, MD

Association of Cone-Rod Homeobox Transcription Factor Messenger RNA With Pediatric Metastatic Retinoblastoma

Torbidoni AV, Laurent VE, Sampor C, et al (Pediatric Hosp, Servicios de Atención Médica Integral para la Comunidad, Buenos Aires, Argentina; et al)

JAMA Ophthalmol 133:805-812, 2015

Importance.—Disseminated retinoblastoma is usually fatal. Identification of small amounts (minimal dissemination [MD]) of tumor cells in extraocular sites might be a tool for designing appropriate treatments.

Objective.—To test cone-rod homeobox (CRX) transcription factor as a lineage-specific molecular marker formetastatic retinoblastoma and for evaluation of MD.

Design, Setting, and Participants.—In a prospective cohort design study, we evaluated CRX messenger RNA (mRNA) by retrotranscription followed by real-time polymerase chain reaction as a diagnostic test in samples obtained from bone marrow, peripheral blood, and cerebrospinal fluid (CSF) at diagnosis, after induction chemotherapy, and during follow-up. The study was conducted from June 30, 2008, to June 30, 2014. Seventeen retinoblastoma primary tumors, 2 retinoblastoma cell lines, and 47 samples of bone marrow from other cancers (controls) were studied. Seventeen patients with metastatic retinoblastoma (9 at diagnosis, 8 at relapse; age range: 18-41 months) were included.

Main Outcomes and Measures.—Detection of CRX mRNA as a marker for metastatic retinoblastoma and MD in bone marrow and CSF and its correlation with clinical findings.

Results.—Cone-rod homeobox mRNAwas expressed in all tumors (relative expression levels range, 8.1×10^{-5} to 5.6) and cell lines. In control samples, there was no amplification of CRX; only the housekeeping gene (*GAPDH*) demonstrated amplification. Bone marrow metastatic cells showed expression of CRX mRNA in all 9 children presenting with metastasis at the diagnosis (relative expression levels, 6.0×10^{-5} to 0.67). After induction chemotherapy, no evidence of MD of tumor cells was seen in any of the 8 responding children since only GAPDH showed amplification. In the CSF of children who had a metastatic relapse, CRX mRNA detection was positive in 2 patients in whom no conclusive results were reached by immunocytology for disialoganglioside GD2. Minimal dissemination in the CSF was associated with a clinical relapse in 2 cases. No concomitant MD was evident in the bone marrow in any case.

Conclusions and Relevance.—These data suggest that CRX mRNA is a novel marker for retinoblastoma at extraocular sites. In this study among patients with bone marrow metastasis, there was a quick, complete, and sustained molecular response after induction chemotherapy. In all patients with secondary metastasis, CSF relapse occurred independently from the bone marrow, suggesting a sanctuary site.

► Tumor dissemination has been widely accepted as a major cause of morbidity and mortality in cancer patients, including patients with retinoblastoma. The study of minimal dissemination (MD) by polymerase chain reaction (PCR) or immunocytology has been previously evaluated and now used in other pediatric cancers. The purposes of this study were to (1) determine whether cone-rod homeobox (CRX), a retinal lineage-specific molecular marker, can be detected by reverse transcription PCR (rtPCR) and, if so, (2) could this test be used to identify retinoblastoma patients with MD.

The study was conducted in 2 phases: the first phase involved validating the marker and detection method, and the second phase involved determining the validity of the test in patients. For the first phase of the study, 17 primary retinoblastoma tumors and 2 retinoblastoma cell lines were used to establish the expression of CRX by rtPCR, and 47 bone marrow samples from children with cancer other than retinoblastoma served as controls. High expression of CRX mRNA was detected in all retinoblastoma samples and cells lines, whereas no CRX mRNA could be detected in any of the control samples.

For the second phase, 17 patients with metastatic retinoblastoma were prospectively enrolled. Nine of these patients had metastatic disease upon diagnosis, and the remaining 8 patients were included when they developed evidence of metastatic disease after being originally diagnosed with nonmetastatic retinoblastoma. Bone marrow, peripheral blood, and cerebrospinal fluid (CSF) were obtained from each patient and tested for CRX expression by rtPCR, as well as evaluated by current standard methods that included cytology and disialoganglioside GD2 (GD2) expression by immunostaining or nested PCR. CRX mRNA was detectable in nearly all of the bone marrow samples of patients with metastatic disease to the bone marrow but was only detectable in a third of the same patients in the CSF. After induction chemotherapy, CRX mRNA was undetectable in the bone marrow. For patients with a subsequent diagnosis of metastatic disease, none had metastatic disease to the bone marrow and therefore, as expected, had negative qtPCR results for CRX in the bone marrow. However, CRX detection in CSF samples could only be performed and detected in 2 of 8 patients, whereas GD2 expression could be detected in 5 of 8 patients. Interestingly, the results from the peripheral blood samples were not presented.

The authors conclude that CRX mRNA could be a novel marker for metastatic retinoblastoma. Based on the results of this study, CRX mRNA expression could be useful in detecting metastatic disease in bone marrow samples, which would be advantageous because GD2 can be expressed by normal bone marrow stem cells, leading to false-positive results. However, CRX detection by qtPCR has yet to be optimized for CSF samples. This is an important obstacle given that the patients who were diagnosed with subsequent metastatic disease had evidence of metastatic disease in the CSF but not the bone marrow, possibly suggesting that the CSF may be a sanctuary site. Further optimization of the detection of CRX mRNA needs to be performed with CSF samples, followed by investigation of the predictive value of CRX mRNA expression in identifying patients at risk for developing metastatic disease.

V. Lee, MD

Intraocular Medulloepitheliomas and Embryonal Tumors With Multilayered Rosettes of the Brain: Comparative Roles of LIN28A and C19MC

Jakobiec FA, Kool M, Stagner AM (Harvard Med School, Boston, MA; German Cancer Res Ctr (DKFZ), Heidelberg, Germany; et al)

Am J Ophthalmol 159:1065-1074.e1, 2015

Purpose.—To compare immunohistochemical and genetic overlaps and differences between intraocular medulloepitheliomas and embryonal tumors withmultilayered rosettes of the brain.

Design.—Retrospective histopathologic, immunohistochemical, and genetic analysis of 20 intraocular medulloepitheliomas.

Methods.—(1) Review of clinical data and hematoxylin-eosin-stained sections with (2) immunohistochemical staining of paraffin sections using a polyclonal antibody against the protein LIN28A, and (3) fluorescence in situ hybridization (FISH) testing for the amplification of the genetic locus 19q13.42 involving the *C19MC* cluster of miRNA. Ten retinoblastomas served as controls and to determine the specificity of these biomarkers for intraocular medulloepitheliomas.

Results.—Nineteen of the 20 intraocular medulloepitheliomas were either diffusely or focally LIN28A positive (weak, moderate, or strong). The most intense positivity correlated with aggressive behavior such as intraocular tissue invasion or extraocular extension. None of the cases studied by FISH harbored an amplicon for *C19MC*. The 10 retinoblastomas were LIN28A and *C19MC* negative.

Conclusion.—LIN28A has a putative role in oncogenesis and is found only in embryonic cells and malignancies. Intraocular medulloepitheliomas and embryonal tumors with multilayered rosettes of the brain both display LIN28A positivity. Only the latter, however, display amplification

of the 19q13.42 locus involving *C19MC*, implying that other causative factors are at play in intraocular medulloepitheliomas. More aggressive tumor behavior within the eye can be partially predicted by LIN28A staining intensity.

▶ With growing discoveries in the molecular pathogenesis of diseases, tumors are being reclassified on the basis of immunohistochemical and molecular genetic markers. One example is the reclassification of primitive neuroectodermal brain tumors with multilayered rosettes under the broader category of embryonal tumor with multilayered rosettes, such as brain medulloepithelioma. The reclassification of these tumors is based on the discovery of LIN28A protein expression, as well as C19MC miRNA. The purpose of this study is to investigate whether ocular medulloepitheliomas, a more common variant than its intracranial counterpart, would exhibit similar LIN28A and C19MC expression.

In general, intracranial medulloblastoma share similar histologic characteristics of its intraocular partner, consisting of cords of medullary epithelium and occasional rosettes of neoplastic pseudostratified neuroepithelium. To investigate these commonalities further, the authors performed a retrospective histopathologic, immunohistochemical (IHC), and genetic analysis of 20 cases of intraocular medulloepitheliomas. Ten retinoblastoma tumors were used as controls. After reviewing hematoxylin and eosin–stained slides, unstained slides were further sectioned for IHC staining against LIN28A. Fluorescence in situ hybridization (FISH) was employed to look for amplification of the genetic locus for C19MC. Polyclonal staining against LIN28A was considered positive when cytoplasmic staining was observed and was graded weak, moderate, or strong, as well as unifocal, multifocal, or diffuse. For FISH analysis, signals were tabulated from 200 nonoverlapping intact nuclei, and the tumor was considered positive for C19MC amplification when more than 10% of tumor cells displayed more than 8 signals of the probe or clusters of signals.

The authors confirmed the expression of LIN28A in 19 of 20 intraocular medulloepitheliomas. Moreover, tumors that demonstrated diffuse cytoplasmic staining of moderate to strong intensity correlated with tumors that demonstrated local aggressive behavior (ie, large size, retinal extension, and invasion of local intraocular structures). The 1 tumor that was negative for LIN28A expression appeared more differentiated than the other intraocular medulloepitheliomas, composed of an overabundance of neuropil and neurotubules. However, all of the tumors were negative for C19MC amplification by FISH analysis. Controls were negative for both LIN28A and C19MC expression.

It is believed that LIN28A is expressed early in embryonic development but then disappears with cellular differentiation. Therefore, it is not found in the neuronal cells that comprise the adult central nervous system. However, LIN28A and its homolog LIN28B can be abnormally expressed in tumors, leading possibly to stem cell survival or persistent dedifferentiated state. Similarly, activation of C19MC also encourages stem cell survival and differentiation inhibition, which may work synergistically with LIN28A. This hypothesis is additionally supported by the fact that the authors found no LIN28A staining in the most differentiated tumor sample. Ultimately, the authors conclude that the expression profile of LIN28A in intraocular medulloepithelioma reinforces a strong overlap with other embryonal tumors with multilayered rosettes of the brain. However, the lack of C19MC amplification suggests that the molecular pathways involved in intraocular medulloepithelioma may still differ from other embryonal tumor with multilayered rosettes, which was further supported by a subsequent study by Korshunov et al.[1] Lastly, although the authors noted a correlation between strong LIN28A expression and aggressive tumor behavior, they concluded that LIN28A expression should not replace current anatomic characteristic criteria for predicting aggressive tumor behavior.

V. Lee, MD

Reference

1. Korshunov A, Jakobiec FA, Eberhart CG, et al. Comparative integrated molecular analysis of intraocular medulloepitheliomas and central nervous system embryonal tumors with multilayered rosette confirms that they are distinct nosologic entities. *Neuropathology.* 2015;35:538-544.

Analysis of Varicella-Zoster Virus in Temporal Arteries Biopsy Positive and Negative for Giant Cell Arteritis

Nagel MA, White T, Khmeleva N, et al (Univ of Colorado School of Medicine, Aurora; et al)

JAMA Neurol 72:1281-1287, 2015

Importance.—Giant cell arteritis (GCA) is the most common systemic vasculitis in elderly individuals. Diagnosis is confirmed by temporal artery (TA) biopsy, although biopsy results are often negative. Despite the use of corticosteroids, disease may progress. Identification of causal agents will improve outcomes. Biopsy-positive GCA is associated with TA infection by varicella-zoster virus (VZV).

Objective.—To analyze VZV infection in TAs of patients with clinically suspected GCA whose TAs were histopathologically negative and in normal TAs removed post mortem from age-matched individuals.

Design, Setting, and Participants.—A cross-sectional study for VZV antigen was performed from January 2013 to March 2015 using archived, deidentified, formalin-fixed, paraffin-embedded GCA-negative, GCA-positive, and normal TAs (50 sections/TA) collected during the past 30 years. Regions adjacent to those containing VZV were examined by hematoxylin-eosin staining. Immunohistochemistry identified inflammatory cells and cell types around nerve bundles containing VZV. A combination of 17 tertiary referral centers and private practices worldwide contributed archived TAs from individuals older than 50 years.

Main Outcomes and Measures.—Presence and distribution of VZV antigen in TAs and histopathological changes in sections adjacent to those containing VZV were confirmed by 2 independent readers.

Results.—Varicella-zoster virus antigen was found in 45 of 70 GCA-negative TAs (64%), compared with 11 of 49 normal TAs (22%) (relative risk [RR] = 2.86; 95% CI, 1.75-5.31; $P < .001$). Extension of our earlier study revealed VZV antigen in 68 of 93 GCA-positive TAs (73%), compared with 11 of 49 normal TAs (22%) (RR = 3.26; 95% CI, 2.03-5.98; $P < .001$). Compared with normal TAs, VZV antigen was more likely to be present in the adventitia of both GCA-negative TAs (RR = 2.43; 95% CI, 1.82-3.41; $P < .001$) and GCA-positive TAs (RR = 2.03; 95% CI, 1.52-2.86; $P < .001$). Varicella-zoster virus antigen was frequently found in perineurial cells expressing claudin-1 around nerve bundles. Of 45 GCA-negative participants whose TAs contained VZV antigen, 1 had histopathological features characteristic of GCA, and 16 (36%) showed adventitial inflammation adjacent to viral antigen; no inflammation was seen in normal TAs.

Conclusions and Relevance.—In patients with clinically suspected GCA, prevalence of VZV in their TAs is similar independent of whether biopsy results are negative or positive pathologically. Antiviral treatment may confer additional benefit to patients with biopsy-negative GCA treated with corticosteroids, although the optimal antiviral regimen remains to be determined.

▶ Having investigated the presence of varicella zoster virus (VZV) antigen in giant cell arteritis (GCA) positive temporal artery (TA) biopsies (refer to review of Gliden D et al), the authors analyzed GCA-negative TA biopsies in this study to further examine the association between VZV and GCA. Organized as a cross-sectional study, 70 formalin-fixed paraffin embedded (FFPE) GCA-negative TA biopsies were evaluated for the presence of VZV antigen, and 49 normal, postmortem, FFPE TA biopsies served as a control. The authors also included 93 GCA positive FFPE TA biopsies, 11 more specimens than their original study, as a second experimental arm. Slides were stained for anti-VZV gE immunoglobulin (Ig) G1 antibody, as well anti-CD45, anti-claudin-1 IgG, anti-S100, antimyelin basic protein antibody, and anti-βIII tubulin to characterize cell types identified on hematoxylin and eosin—stained slides. Two independent readers evaluated each slide blindly, specifically evaluating for (1) the presence or absence of VZV staining and (2) the location of the staining.

VZV antigen was 2.86 times more likely to be present in GCA negative TA biopsies, and 3.26 times more likely to be present in GCA positive TA biopsies compared with normal controls (Table 1 in the original article). VZV antigen staining did not differ significantly between GCA-positive and GCA-negative TA biopsies. Positive VZV staining was observed most prevalently in the adventitia of both positive and negative GCA TA specimens (Table 2 in the original article). Further analysis demonstrated the viral antigen around nerve bundles, colocalizing with anti-claudin-1 antibody. Additionally, VZV antigen was detected in skip areas, which recapitulates the known histologic behavior of GCA.

Because of the high frequency of VZV antigen in both positive and negative GCA TA biopsies, the authors suggest the possibility that GCA represents a continuum of VZV vasculopathy in the temporal artery. Therefore, the authors propose treating all patients with clinically suspicious GCA with both corticosteroids and antiviral therapy, even though the authors recognize more definitive studies need to be performed to determine the benefit of antiviral therapy. Although relatively well tolerated, indiscreet use of antiviral medications could result in increased morbidity and mortality in an already elderly, vulnerable population as well as increased health care costs. In addition, although the calculated relative risk was high, the absolute percentages of patients with VZV positive biopsies were only 73% in GCA-positive specimens and 64% in GCA-negative specimens. These relatively low percentages may reflect the fact that many patients are referred for TA biopsy even when clinical suspicion is low. Given the fact that the study did not include clinical information regarding a history of zoster infection, zoster vaccination, or medication, or other valuable clinical information, such vision loss, visual acuity, coexisting medical conditions, it may be at least prudent to conduct a study with clinical histories to identify a subset of patients who may truly benefit from antiviral treatment with corticosteroids.

V. Lee, MD

Varicella Zoster Virus in Ischemic Optic Neuropathy

Golas L, Bennett JL, White TM, et al (Univ of Colorado School of Medicine, Aurora; et al)

Ophthalmology 122:2142-2145, 2015

Background.—Varicella zoster virus (VZV) causes the symptoms and signs of anterior ischemic optic neuropathy (AION), whether it is the arteritic or nonarteritic (NAION) type. VZV is found in the temporal arteries (TAs) of most patients with giant cell arteritis (GCA) and ischemic optic nerve and retinal pathologies. Seven AION patients underwent biopsies of GCA-negative TAs to determine if VZV was present.

Case Reports.—Man, 79, developed acute vision loss in his right eye (OD) and diminished vision in his left eye (OS) after jaw claudication. The TA biopsy was GCA negative after 8 days of oral prednisone. Visual acuity (VA) remained unchanged and the optic nerves developed pallor. TA biopsy was negative for VZV.

Woman, 78, had sudden, painless vision loss in OS after jaw claudication. She was given solumedrol infusions for 3 days with prednisone taper. Bilateral TA biopsies were GCA negative, but VZV antigen was present on immunohistochemical testing. C-reactive protein (CRP) level rose and valacyclovir was added, achieving normal CRP levels 1 week later.

Woman, 53, suffered sudden, painless vision loss in OS. Five months later her VA was 20/25 OD, count fingers (CF) OS, with a left afferent pupillary defect (APD) and diffuse left disc pallor with gliosis. Her TA biopsy was GCA negative but VZV positive.

Woman, 68, reported painless vision loss OD with polymyalgia rheumatic, frontal headaches, jaw tightness, diplopia, and visual field (VF) change OD. After taking prednisone for 2 months, her TA biopsy was negative for GCA. Six months later while on prednisone taper, she had further OD vision loss. Reevaluation of the previous TA biopsy showed VZV antigen and adjacent GCA histopathologic findings.

Woman, 81, developed sudden, painless vision loss OS 3 years earlier but now reported acute vision loss OD. After 1 week on prednisone, her TA biopsy was GCA negative but VZV positive. Oral acyclovir was added to her prednisone taper but vision remained impaired.

Man, 63, reported painless superior VF loss OD and had VA 20/25 OD, 20/25-2 OS, bilateral superior arcuate scotomas, and bilateral inferior disc edema with hemorrhaging. Two months later, his assessment revealed progressive VF loss and additional right superior disc edema with hemorrhaging. After an additional 6 months, he had progressive bilateral superior VF loss, bilateral disc pallor, and left superior peripapillary subretinal hemorrhage. He lost inferior VF OS in 4 months and developed left APD. His TA biopsy was GCA negative but VZV positive.

Man, 49, suffered sudden loss of vision OD. After receiving corticosteroids intravenously, his VA was 20/200 OD. Sudden vision loss OS developed 11 months later, along with left disc edema and hemorrhage. After 4 months he developed bitemporal headache and vesicular lip lesions. Treatment with acyclovir began. A TA biopsy 3 months later was negative for both GCA and VZV.

Analysis.—Five of the patients (71%) with AION had GCA-negative TA biopsies containing VZV antigen. Most of these patients had atypical AION symptoms and signs, suggesting that VZV vasculopathy in AION patients may produce a broader range of ischemia than is seen in classical GCA. Evaluating patients with atypical NAION via TA biopsy for VZV antigen may identify those who may benefit from antiviral treatment.

Conclusions.—TA biopsies in AION patients with or without laboratory and clinical findings for GCA should routinely include virologic evaluation. Extensive serial sections of TA biopsies should be examined for evidence of GCA and VZV antigen to guide treatment decisions regarding the addition of an antiviral agent.

▶ The purpose of this observational study was to explore a possible correlation between varicella zoster virus (VZV) and anterior ischemic optic neuropathy (AION). The basis of the study stems from the observation that VZV vasculopathy produces signs and symptoms that are similar to AION. The study included 7 patients diagnosed with AION with negative temporal artery (TA) biopsies for giant cell arteritis (GCA). Immunostaining with anti-VZV glycoprotein E, a late viral protein indicative of productive infection, was performed on all TA biopsies. Five of the 7 specimens were positive for VZV. However, 1 of the VZV-positive TAs was subsequently found to be positive for GCA. Although the study is far from comprehensive and the sample number is small, the evidence presented is sufficient to warrant further investigation. Much more needs to be elucidated before a causative relationship can be established between VZV and AION, but the authors propose the possibility of AION patients benefitting from antiviral treatment. Consequently, routine testing for VZV could become routine for all TA biopsies. Interestingly, the authors of this study reported this year on the correlation between VZV and clinically suspected GCA as well.[1,2]

V. Lee, MD

References

1. Gilden D, White T, Khmeleva N, et al. Prevalence and distribution of VZV in temporal arteries of patients with giant cell arteritis. *Neurology*. 2015;84:1948-1955.
2. Nagel MA, White T, Khmeleva N, et al. Analysis of varicella-zoster virus in temporal arteries biopsy positive and negative for giant cell arteritis. *JAMA Neurol.* 2015;72:1281-1287.

Correlation of Clinical Profile and Specific Histopathological Features of Temporal Artery Biopsies

Stacy RC, Gilbert AL, Rizzo JF III (Harvard Med School, Boston, MA; et al)
J Neuroophthalmol 35:127-133, 2015

Background.—This study sought to correlate the clinical features of patients with giant cell arteritis (GCA) who present with ophthalmic symptoms and signs, with 2 specific histopathological findings—the presence of giant cells and arterial wall neoangiogenesis. The goal was to assess if these pathological features might be useful in guiding the approach to patient management.

Methods.—Medical charts were retrospectively reviewed from 58 patients who underwent a temporal artery biopsy at a single institution. Detailed information was collected about the clinical presentation and course, with an emphasis on visual function. Histopathological and immunohistochemical techniques were used to examine temporal artery biopsies for evidence of inflammation. Correlations were made between the clinical data and the presence of giant cells and neoangiogenesis.

Results.—Twenty-one (34%) biopsies were positive for inflammation consistent with GCA. Although the percentage of positive biopsies with giant cells was high, neither the presence of giant cells nor neoangiogenesis was predictive of a patient's presenting visual symptoms, severity and bilaterality of vision loss, other ophthalmic manifestations of GCA, presence of headache or jaw claudication, or erythrocyte sedimentation rate. Giant cells were more common in patients with recent weight loss.

Immunohistochemistry confirmed diagnoses but did not alter the clinical course or treatment plan.

Conclusions.—There was no correlation between the clinical, specifically visual, features of GCA and the presence or absence of giant cells or neoangiogenesis in temporal artery biopsy specimens. Although the presence of neoangiogenesis may be important in the pathogenesis of GCA, our study showed no correlation between this finding and the clinical course (Tables 1 and 2).

▶ This study sought to investigate the association of 2 histopathological features, the presence of giant cells and neoangiogenesis, on clinical presentation and management of giant cell arteritis (GCA), as well as determine what ancillary role immunohistochemistry could offer in identifying inflammation in diagnostically challenging cases of GCA. The authors conducted a retrospective chart review of 58 patients suspected of having GCA who underwent temporal artery biopsy at one institution. Data collected included demographic

TABLE 1.—Clinical data of patients with positive and negative temporal artery biopsies

	Positive Biopsy	Negative Biopsy	*P* Value
Number of patients	21	37	
Age, mean, yr	76	73	0.17
Female/male	14/7 (67%/33%)	18/19 (49%/51%)	0.27
Presenting visual symptom			
Permanent vision loss	13 (61%)	26 (70%)	0.57
Bilateral vision loss	3 (14%)	0	**0.04**
Transient vision loss	3 (14%)	6 (16%)	1.00
Diplopia	3 (14%)	3 (8%)	0.66
Constitutional symptoms			
Headache	9 (43%)	17 (46%)	1.00
Jaw claudication	9 (43%)	4 (11%)	**0.01**
Weight loss	11 (52%)	10 (27%)	0.09
History of polymyalgia rheumatica	3 (14%)	2 (5%)	0.34
History of stroke	4 (19%)	3 (8%)	0.24
Examination finding			
Visual acuity ≤20/400	11 (82%)*	9 (35%)*	**0.04**
Optic neuropathy	10 (48%)	3 (17%)†	**0.02**
CRAO	3 (14%)	9 (50%)†	0.07
Laboratory studies			
Erythrocyte sedimentation rate (mean)	77	44	**0.02**
Platelet count, ×1000 (mean)	386	287	**0.002**
Number of days from initiation of steroid treatment to temporal artery biopsy (mean, median)	4, 2	9, 3	0.11
Length of biopsy specimen, postfixation, cm (mean)	1.4	1.5	0.54

Bold values are statistically significant.
CRAO, central retinal artery occlusion.
*Percentages based on the number of patients with permanent vision loss.
†Percentages based on the 18 patients who had known diagnoses other than biopsy-negative GCA.

TABLE 2.—Clinical and histopathological parameters associated with giant cells and neoangiogenesis within the temporal artery specimens

	With Giant Cells	Without Giant Cells	*P* Value	With NA*	Without NA*	*P* Value
Number of patients	17	4		15	6	
Age, mean, yrs	76	75	0.74	76	75	0.82
Female	12 (71%)	3 (75%)	1.00	10 (67%)	4 (67%)	1.00
Presenting symptom						
Permanent vision loss	12 (71%)	1 (25%)	0.25	10 (67%)	3 (50%)	0.63
Bilateral vision loss	3 (18%)	0	1.00	2 (13%)	1 (17%)	1.00
Transient vision loss	1 (6%)	2 (50%)	0.48	2 (13%)	1 (17%)	1.00
Diplopia	1 (6%)	2 (50%)	0.08	2 (13%)	1 (17%)	1.00
Concurrent symptoms						
Headache	8 (47%)	1 (25%)	0.60	7 (47%)	2 (33%)	0.66
Jaw claudication	7 (41%)	2 (50%)	1.00	8 (53%)	1 (17%)	0.18
Weight loss	11 (65%)	0	0.04	9 (60%)	2 (33%)	0.36
History of polymyalgia rheumatica	2 (13%)	1 (25%)	0.48	2 (13%)	1 (17%)	1.00
History of stroke	3 (18%)	1 (25%)	1.0	3 (20%)	1 (17%)	1.00
Examination finding						
Visual acuity ≤20/400†	10 (83%)†	1 (100%)†	1.00	8 (53%)†	3 (50%)†	1.00
Optic neuropathy	7 (41%)	1 (25%)	1.00	7 (47%)	3 (50%)	1.00
CRAO	3 (18%)	0	0	3 (20%)	0	0.52
Laboratory studies						
Erythrocyte sedimentation rate (mean)	77	60	0.43	81	64	0.11
Platelet count, ×1000 (mean)	‡	‡	‡	403	333	0.09
Days from initiation of steroid treatment to temporal artery biopsy (mean, median)	4, 2	4, 2	0.98	4, 2	2, 1	0.31
Transmural inflammation	17 (100%)	3 (75%)	0.19	15 (100%)	4 (50%)	0.07
Accessory vessel involvement	8 (47%)	1 (25%)	0.60	5 (33%)	4 (67%)	0.33
Giant cells	—	—	—	14 (93%)	3 (50%)	0.05
NA	14 (82%)	1 (25%)	0.052	—	—	—

Bold value is statistically significant.
CRAO, central retinal artery occlusion.
*NA, neoangiogenesis.
†Percentages based on the number of patients with permanent vision loss.
‡Not analyzed due to insufficient data (see text).

information, clinical presentation, and progression. Histopathological and immunohistochemistry studies were also performed to detect evidence of inflammation, which included stains against CD3 and CD68/CD163 and neo-angiogenesis, specifically anti-CD31. Two examiners reviewed all 58 biopsies in a blind fashion.

All re-reviews of the specimens confirmed the initial histologic diagnosis. Twenty-one of 58 biopsies were positive for GCA, and 37 of 58 biopsies were negative. Typical microscopic findings of positive biopsies included the presence of T lymphocytes, epithelioid histiocytes, and giant cells, the latter which are not necessary for diagnosis. Although immunohistochemistry staining did not change the final diagnosis, it did confirm and localize more subtle inflammation, and highlighted neoangiogenesis not visible on hematoxylin and eosin staining. Patients with positive biopsies were more likely to have permanent vision loss with visual acuity ≤20/400, bilateral vision loss, jaw claudication, optic neuropathy, elevated mean erythrocyte sedimentation rate (ESR), and elevated platelet count (Table 1). Although 80% of positive biopsies had giant cells and 71% had neoangiogenesis, these histopathological findings were not predictive of initial visual complaints, severity of symptoms, bilateral visual loss, or other associated signs and symptoms of GCA including headache, jaw claudication, or ESR (Table 2). However, there was an association between the presence of giant cells and recent weight loss, a clinical symptom found to be negatively associated with irreversible vision loss in a prior study.

There was no correlation between the presence of neoangiogenesis and patient clinical course. This is in contrast to previous findings in the literature that there may be a protective characteristic to the presence of neovascularization. The study found no statistical difference between permanent vision loss and the presence or absence of neoangiogenesis, 67% vision loss with neoangiogenesis versus 50% without ($P = .63$). However, there was a statistically significant association between the presence of giant cells and neoangiogenesis, as well as a trend between transmural inflammation with neoangiogenesis. These findings may be of significance in corroborating the proposition of vasogenic messengers released by macrophages.

In summary, the study demonstrated no correlation between clinical presentation with the presence or absence of giant cells or neoangiogenesis. However, the secondary findings, which include a correlation between vision loss and neoangiogenesis and a correlation between the presence of giant cells and neoangiogenesis, contribute to the existing literature about the clinical significance of neoangiogenesis and its pathophysiologic mechanism.

A. A. Nti, MD
V. Lee, MD

Fine-needle aspiration biopsy of uveal melanoma: outcomes and complications

Singh AD, Medina CA, Singh N, et al (Cleveland Clinic, OH)

Br J Ophthalmol 1-7, 2015

Purpose.—To report outcomes and complications of fine-needle aspiration biopsy (FNAB) of uveal melanoma performed for diagnostic and prognostic purposes.

Methods.—Prospective interventional case series of 150 consecutive patients with a clinical diagnosis of uveal melanoma. The FNAB approach (transcorneal (TCO), transscleral (TSC) and transvitreal (TVT) was primarily determined by the location of the tumour. The FNAB was performed using a 25-gauge needle using a previously published technique. Prognostication was done using fluorescent in situ hybridisation detection of monosomy of chromosome 3.

Results.—FNAB was obtained via TCO (8), TSC (71) and TVT (64) approach and impression smear in seven cases. Diagnostic yield was 92%. False-negative results were observed in 8%. Diagnostic yield was significantly correlated to biopsy approach (TCO 100%, TSC 96%, TSV 86%; $p = 0.029$) and tumour size (basal diameter >5.0 mm; height >2.5 mm). Persistent haemorrhage (subretinal haemorrhage or vitreous) requiring surgical intervention (1%) and rhegmatogenous retinal detachment (1%) were rare. Endophthalmitis, hypotony, tumour recurrence, episcleral seeding were not observed over the average follow-up of 37 months. Prognostication could be performed in 85% of cases. Overall, only 47% of eligible patients enrolled into the adjuvant therapy trial.

Conclusions.—FNAB for uveal melanoma with 25-gauge needle is a safe procedure that can yield diagnostic and prognostic information in vast majority of cases (92% and 85%, respectively). Even so, only about half of the eligible cases eventually enrolled into the adjuvant therapy trial. Possibility of negative FNAB yield should be considered when counselling patients with small tumours. Alternative means of diagnostic biopsy and methods of prognostication need to be assessed for small tumours (Figs 5 and 6, Table 3).

▶ To identify patients for enrollment in a concurrent uveal melanoma adjuvant therapy trial, the authors conducted a prospective study to assess the diagnostic and prognostic utility of fine needle aspiration biopsies (FNAB) of clinically suspected uveal melanomas, as well as to determine related procedural complications. One of 3 routes was implemented as indicated by the location of the tumor: transcorneal (TCO) (5%), transscleral (TSC) (50%), and transvitreal (TVT) (45%). All FNABs were performed using a 25-gauge needle. One to 2 passes were made for anteriorly located tumors, whereas only 1 pass was made for choroidal tumors. Biopsies were analyzed by a single investigator for features of uveal melanoma and were categorized in 1 of the following classifications: (1) unsatisfactory for interpretation, (2) negative for melanoma, (3) atypical cells not diagnostic or consistent with melanoma, and (4) positive for

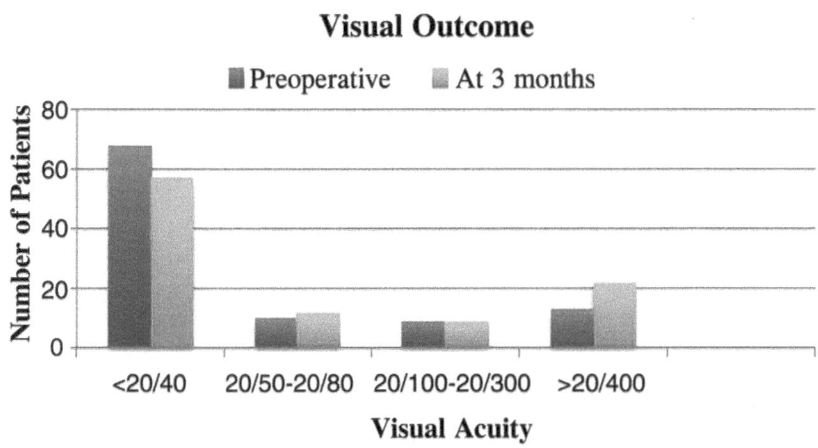

FIGURE 5.—Visual outcome following fine-needle aspiration biopsy (FNAB). Note worsening of visual acuity at preoperative visit and at 3 months following plaque radiation therapy and FNAB. (Reprinted from Singh AD, Medina CA, Singh N, et al. Fine-needle aspiration biopsy of uveal melanoma: outcomes and complications. *Br J Ophthalmol.* 2015;1-7, with permission from BMJ Publishing Group Ltd.)

melanoma. Samples that were positive for melanoma with adequate cellularity (at least 200 cells) underwent subsequent fluorescent in situ hybridization (FISH) analysis for chromosome 3 monosomy using direct labeling for CEP3 and 3p25 loci. A tumor was considered monosomy for chromosome 3 if 20% or more cells demonstrated loss of chromosome 3. Patients underwent ophthalmic examinations at each visit and were followed every 3 months in the first year and every 6 months thereafter.

One hundred and fifty patients underwent FNABs and were followed on average for 2 years. Tumors were treated by plaque radiation therapy, tumor resection, or enucleation. Overall, 92% of the samples were found to have enough cellular material to undergo cytologic diagnosis. Of those samples, 86% were positive for melanoma, whereas 5% had atypical cells consistent with melanoma. False-negative results were calculated to be 8% of the cases. Forty-one eyes out of the 150 were enucleated, and FNABs were performed after enucleation using a TSC approach. There was 100% correlation between cytological and histological diagnoses on all enucleated specimens. Greater tumor height (average 6.2 mm) and, to a lesser degree, larger basal diameter (average 13.4 mm) were found to positively correlate with diagnostically adequate biopsies (Table 3). In addition, 100% of the TCO approach provided adequate yield, followed by 97% for TSC and 84% for TVT. Prognostication with FISH analysis was achievable on 121 samples, resulting in a yield of 84.6%. Enucleation, tumor size (> 5 mm in basal diameter and > 2.5 mm in height), and location (> 3 mm from fovea) were associated with higher prognostic yield.

Complications from FNAB were only assessed in 102 eyes, which exclude the eyes that underwent FNAB after enucleation. Mild vitreous or subretinal hemorrhage occurred in all cases, which resolved spontaneously (Fig 6).

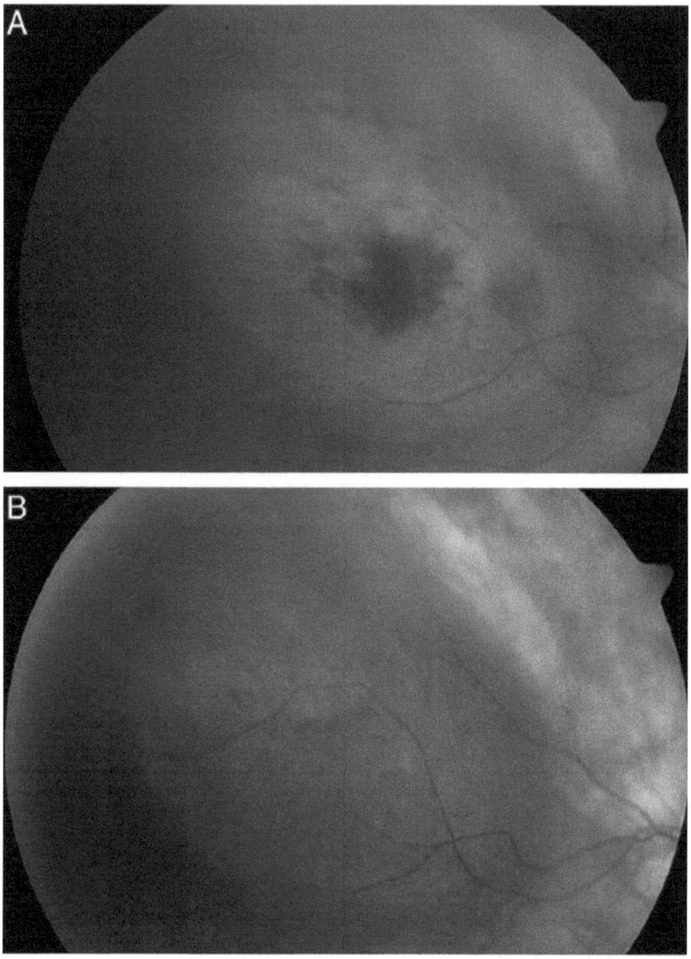

FIGURE 6.—Typical localised preretinal haemorrhage at the fine-needle aspiration biopsy (FNAB) site present at the first postoperative visit (1 week) (A). Such haemorrhage is not visually significant and underwent total spontaneous resolution within 6 weeks (B). (Reprinted from Singh AD, Medina CA, Singh N, et al. Fine-needle aspiration biopsy of uveal melanoma: outcomes and complications. *Br J Ophthalmol.* 2015;1-7, with permission from BMJ Publishing Group Ltd.)

Persistent hemorrhage requiring surgery and rhegmatogenous retinal detachment occurred rarely (1% respectively), and there were no cases of endophthalmitis, hypotony, episcleral seeding, or tumor recurrence. Visual acuity at 3 months was measured to be ≤20/40 in 57% of eyes and ≥20/400 in 22% of eyes, which worsened in 13% (Fig 5). The authors deduce the decline in vision was unlikely from tumor or radiation-related complications because of the short time interval.

Ultimately, the authors conclude that FNAB with a 25-gauge needle is a safe and useful modality to obtain diagnostic and prognostic information for a

TABLE 3.—Fine-needle aspiration biopsy of uveal melanoma: comparison of positive and negative diagnostic samples (n = 143)

Feature	Positive (n = 131)	Negative (n = 12)
Tumour height (mean)	6.2 mm	3.3 mm
Largest basal diameter (mean)	13.4 mm	11.6 mm
Treatment		
Plaque	91	11
Enucleation	40	1
Location		
Iris	5	0
Iridociliary	4	0
Ciliary	3	1
Ciliochoroidal	26	0
Choroidal	93	11
Approach*		
Transcorneal	8	0
Transscleral	68	3
Transvitreal	55	9

p value = 0.029 by Fisher's exact test.
*Positivity of sample for diagnostic cytology: relationship to biopsy approach.
Reprinted from Singh AD, Medina CA, Singh N, et al. Fine-needle aspiration biopsy of uveal melanoma: outcomes and complications. *Br J Ophthalmol.* 2015;1-7, with permission from BMJ Publishing Group Ltd.

majority of patients clinically diagnosed with uveal melanoma. However, smaller tumors (height < 2.5 mm) are likely to produce inadequate specimens. Therefore, alternative methods should be explored for small tumors. This information may become increasingly more important as customized systemic surveillance and treatments are developed for specific chromosomal and genetic mutations associated with uveal melanomas.

M. Lau, MD
V. Lee, MD

Diagnostic Cytologic Features of Uveal Melanoma

Medina CA, Biscotti CV, Singh N, et al (Cleveland Clinic Cole Eye Inst, OH)
Ophthalmology 122:1580-1584, 2015

Purpose.—To report the cytologic characteristics of uveal melanoma.

Design.—This is a prospective, single-center study of consecutive patients.

Subjects.—All patients with a clinical diagnosis of uveal melanoma from May 2009 to July 2013 who underwent prognostication fine-needle aspiration biopsy (FNAB) were included.

Methods.—The cytologic characteristics of uveal melanoma were analyzed for 150 consecutive patients with a clinical diagnosis of uveal melanoma who were treated at the Cleveland Clinic Cole Eye Institute between May 2009 and August 2012.

Main Outcome Measures.—Cellular features of all cases were analyzed for cell type, presence of melanin, nuclear grade, tumor-infiltrating lymphocytes, and necrosis. Cytology was then correlated with histopathology in enucleated eyes.

Results.—A total of 150 patients were included. Seven samples of tumor resections were excluded from the study because they were studied by impression smears. A total of 143 FNAB samples of 143 patients formed the basis for analysis. Fifty-three percent of the patients were male, and the average age for all patients was 60 years. Transcorneal (n = 8), transscleral (n = 71), and transvitreal (n = 64) approaches were used. Of 143 samples, 131 were adequate. Among these, spindle cells were observed in 98% (63% mixed and 35% spindle only), whereas only epithelioid cells were observed in 2 samples. Melanin granules were observed in 80% of samples. Tumor nuclear grade (atypia) increased with tumor height and by tumor location (least atypia with iris tumors).

Conclusions.—Cytologic features such as spindle cells and melanin granules, present in 98% and 80% of samples, respectively, are important cytologic diagnostic features. Tumor nuclear grade (atypia) increased with tumor height. Iris melanoma has bland features compared with ciliary and choroidal melanoma (Figs 3-5, Table 2).

▶ This prospective, single-center study describes diagnostic cytologic characteristics of uveal melanoma from prognosticated fine-needle aspiration biopsies (FNAB). FNAB samples from 143 patients with a diagnosis of uveal melanoma were analyzed for cytologic characteristics, which included cell type, presence of melanin, nuclear grade, presence of tumor-infiltrating lymphocytes, and necrosis. Tumor location included iris (3%), iridociliary (3%), ciliary, ciliochoroidal (18%), and choroidal (74%). Samples were obtained via transcorneal, transscleral, and transvitreal approaches. Cytology was then correlated with histopathology in 41 enucleated eyes.

Of the 143 patients, 131 FNAB samples were found to be adequate, defined as those with sufficient cellularity to ascertain a diagnosis. Cell type was classified as spindle cell type if cells demonstrated spindle-shaped cytoplasm (Figs 3 and 5); otherwise, cells were classified as epithelioid type (Fig 4). Grade 3 nuclear atypia had conspicuous nucleoli when viewed through the 10× objective, 4-fold nuclear pleomorphism, hyperchromasia, and coarse chromatin (Fig 4). Grade 1 tumors had none of these features, and all other tumors were categorized as grade 2 (Fig 3). For statistical purposes, grade 3 was defined as high grade, and grades 1 and 2 were defined as low grade. Tumor-infiltrating lymphocytes were considered positive when there was either lymphocyte-infiltrating aggregates of melanoma cells or lymphocytes intimately associated with melanoma cell cytoplasm. Melanin (Fig 4) and necrosis were also documented.

There were 63% mixed and 35% pure spindle cell tumors, and only 2% pure epithelioid cell tumors. Melanin granules were observed in 80% of samples but were absent in the 2 purely epithelioid cell tumors. Tumor height and largest basal diameter correlated with nuclear grade. However, there was no significant correlation between tumor height or basal diameter and cytologic type. Tumor

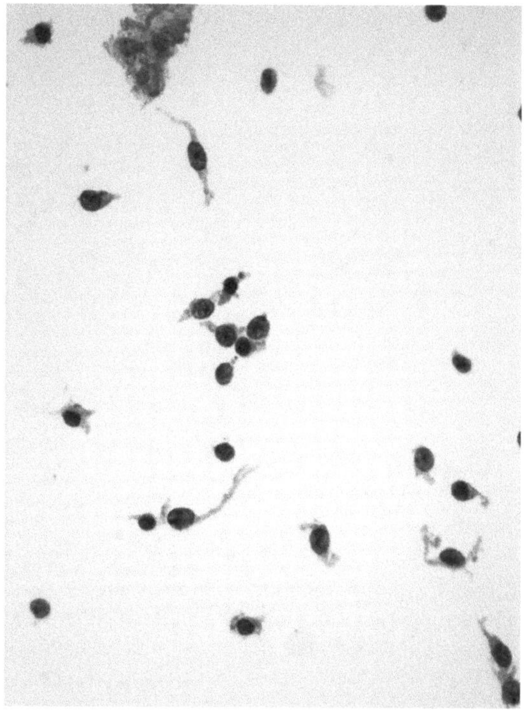

FIGURE 3.—This uveal melanoma illustrates the characteristic cellular features. Note the spindle cell shape characterized by elongated, often caudate cytoplasm. Note also the relatively bland nuclear features, grade 2 by our criteria (Papanicolaou stain). (Reprinted from Medina CA, Biscotti CV, Singh N, et al. Diagnostic cytologic features of uveal melanoma. *Ophthalmology.* 2015;122:1580-1584, with permission from American Academy of Ophthalmology.)

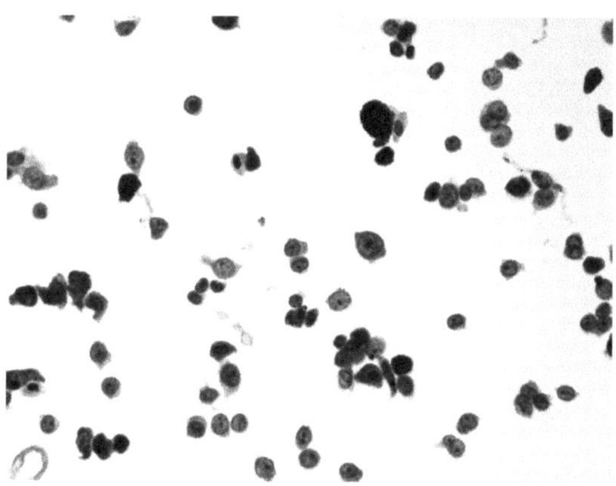

FIGURE 4.—Most of the cells in this uveal melanoma have an epithelioid appearance. Note the higher-grade nuclear atypia compared with the example in Figure 3. (Reprinted from Medina CA, Biscotti CV, Singh N, et al. Diagnostic cytologic features of uveal melanoma. *Ophthalmology.* 2015;122:1580-1584, with permission from American Academy of Ophthalmology.)

FIGURE 5.—The spindle-shaped melanoma cell to the *upper right* has prominent melanin pigmentation. (Reprinted from Medina CA, Biscotti CV, Singh N, et al. Diagnostic cytologic features of uveal melanoma. *Ophthalmology.* 2015;122:1580-1584, with permission from American Academy of Ophthalmology.)

nuclear grade varied by tumor location; the least atypia was seen with iris lesions. Tumor infiltrating lymphocytes were present in only 31% of samples. There was 100% correlation between cytologic and histologic diagnosis in all 41 enucleated eyes.

The authors conclude that certain cytologic features, such as spindle cells and melanin granules, are important and may be helpful for establishing diagnostic criteria. They point out that FNAB has an adequacy of 88% to 95%. Therefore, negative FNABs should not be taken as unequivocal proof that

TABLE 2.—Diagnostic Cytologic Features of Uveal Melanoma: Adequate Samples (n = 131)

Features	Adequate Samples (n = 131), %
Cell type/pattern Mixed	
Mixed	63
Spindle	35
Epithelial	1.75
Nuclear grade	
Low	79
High	21
TILS	
Yes	31
No	69
Necrosis	
Yes	4
No	96
Distribution of melanin	
Yes	79.8
No	20.2

Reprinted from Medina CA, Biscotti CV, Singh N, et al. Diagnostic cytologic features of uveal melanoma. *Ophthalmology.* 2015;122:1580-1584, with permission from American Academy of Ophthalmology.

intraocular malignancy does not exist. As techniques for FNAB improve and become used more frequently, it will be important to have defined descriptive cytologic diagnostic features for intraocular malignancy.

N. Fuerst, MD
V. Lee, MD

American Joint Committee on Cancer Staging and Clinicopathological High-Risk Predictors of Ocular Surface Squamous Neoplasia: A Study From a Tertiary Eye Center in India

Chauhan S, Sen S, Sharma A, et al (All India Inst of Med Sciences, New Delhi)
Arch Pathol Lab Med 138:1488-1494, 2014

Context.—Ocular surface squamous neoplasia (OSSN) is the most common tumor of conjunctival epithelium associated with risk of permanent visual impairment. It includes conjunctival intraepithelial neoplasia and squamous cell carcinoma. Although American Joint Committee on Cancer–TNM (AJCC-TNM) staging is commonly used in various tumors, it has only recently been described for OSSN.

Objectives.—To evaluate the prognostic relevance of AJCC-TNM staging and the clinicopathological features in OSSN.

Design.—Sixty-four histopathologically proven cases of OSSN (20 conjunctival intraepithelial neoplasia and 44 squamous cell carcinoma) were included in the study. The AJCC-TNM staging and clinicopathological features of OSSN cases were recorded. Patients were followed up for 17 to 40 months (median, 32 months). Univariate and multivariate analyses were performed to determine the prognostic value of various clinicopathological features.

Results.—Longer sunlight exposure ($P = .01$), diffuse growth pattern ($P = .02$), larger tumor size (≥2 cm) ($P = .03$), histopathological diagnosis of squamous cell carcinoma ($P = .02$), and orbital invasion or invasion of adjacent structures (T3 or T4) ($P < .001$) emerged as significant predictors of reduced recurrence-free survival. Using multivariate analysis, a higher T category (T3 or T4) was the most important prognostic indicator of a poor outcome.

Conclusions.—A higher T category (T3 or T4) is an important predictor of clinical outcome, and the use of the AJCC-TNM staging system is recommended in the management of all patients with OSSN. Longer sunlight exposure, larger tumor size (≥2 cm), orbital invasion or invasion of adjacent structures (T3 or T4), and a histopathological diagnosis of squamous cell carcinoma are other clinicopathological features of prognostic relevance in patients with OSSN (Tables 1 and 2).

▶ The seventh edition of the American Joint Committee on Cancer (AJCC) included the tumor, node, and metastases (TMN) staging classification for conjunctival squamous carcinomas, also known as ocular surface squamous

TABLE 1.—AJCC-TNM Classification of 64 Patients With Ocular Surface Squamous Neoplasia

AJCC-TNM Classification	No. (%)
T1N0M0	4 (6)
T2N0M0[a]	**38 (59)**
T2N1M0	1 (2)
T3N0M0	4 (6)
T4N0M0[a]	**12 (19)**
T4N0M1	1 (2)
T4N1M0	3 (5)
T4N1M1	1 (2)

Abbreviation: AJCC, American Joint Committee on Cancer.
[a]Most of the patients belonged to T2N0M0 or T4N0M0 category.
Reprinted from Chauhan S, Sen S, Sharma A, et al. American joint committee on cancer staging and clinicopathological high-risk predictors of ocular surface squamous neoplasia. *Arch Pathol Lab Med.* 2014;138:1488-1494.

neoplasia (OSSN; Table 1).[1,2] The purpose of this study is to correlate AJCC–TNM staging and clinicopathologic features of OSSN to clinical outcome. Sixty-four histologically confirmed cases of OSSN (20 conjunctival intraepithelial neoplasia (CIN) and 44 squamous cell carcinoma (SCC)) were enrolled in the study. Clinical features, including history of ocular trauma and duration of sunlight exposure as reported by the patient or implied by occupation, were recorded (Table 2). Histopathological features, such as largest tumor diameter, severity of dysplasia, and invasion, were also recorded (Table 2). Tumors were all staged according to AJCC–TNM classification. Forty-eight of 64 patients had follow-up data, ranging from 17 to 40 months, which were correlated to the preceding factors.

The majority of the tumors fell into 2 AJCC–TNM classifications: (1) T2N0M0, 59%; (2) T4N0M0, 19%. Of the patients where follow-up information was available, 8 patients had recurrence, and 4 other patients succumbed to their disease. Risk for recurrent disease was greatest when (1) lesions exhibited a diffuse growth pattern, measured larger than 2 cm, or diagnosed as SCC; or (2) patients had a history of longer sunlight exposure; or (3) lesions with intraocular or orbital invasion, which correlated to T3 or T4 of the AJCC–TNM classification.

The authors concluded that a higher AJCC–TNM T category was a significant prognostic indicator of a poor outcome, in addition to other previously recognized clinicopathologic features associated with poor outcome (ie, large tumor size, SCC, intraocular/orbital invasion). Of interest, there was a subset of patients that were younger (< 50 years old) with lesions involving the palpebral conjunctiva who exhibited higher rates of metastasis and death. These patients were not immunosuppressed (ie, HIV positive or status post transplant), which is a risk factor for the development of OSSN. However, 3 of the patients enrolled in the study had xeroderma pigmentosum and 6 patients reported a history of ocular trauma to the affected eye, which have been associated with higher risk of developing OSSN. Although it is unclear whether the high-risk patients were also the patients with these known risk factors, it does underscore the practice of prudence when caring for younger patients with any atypical

TABLE 2.—Correlation of Clinicopathological Features With a Histopathological Diagnosis of CIN or SCC in 64 Patients With Ocular Surface Squamous Neoplasia

Variable	Total Patients, No. (%)	Patients With CIN, No. (%)	Patients With SCC, No. (%)	*P* Value[a]
Age, y				
≤50	18 (28)	7 (39)	11 (61)	.55 (NS)
>50	46 (72)	13 (28)	33 (72)	
Sex				
Male	50 (78)	20 (40)	30 (60)	.003
Female	14 (22)	0	14 (100)	
Laterality				
Left eye	41 (64)	15 (37)	26 (63)	.26 (NS)
Right eye	23 (36)	5 (22)	18 (78)	
Duration of sunlight exposure				
Less	30 (47)	6 (20)	24 (80)	.10 (NS)
More	34 (53)	14 (41)	20 (59)	
Socioeconomic status				
Poor	54 (84)	13 (24)	41 (76)	.007
Other	10 (16)	7 (70)	3 (30)	
History of ocular trauma				
Yes	6 (9)	1 (17)	5 (83)	.65 (NS)
No	58 (91)	19 (33)	39 (67)	
Associated ocular pathology				
Yes	13 (20)	1 (8)	12 (92)	.04
No	51 (80)	19 (36)	32 (64)	
Clinical appearance				
Gelatinous	19 (30)	14 (73.6)	5 (26)	<.001
Leucoplakic	9 (14)	4 (44)	5 (56)	
Papillomatous	4 (6)	2 (50)	2 (50)	
Ulcerative	20 (31)	0	20 (100)	
Fungating mass	12 (19)	0	12 (100)	
Tumor location				
Limbus	35 (55)	18 (51)	17 (49)	<.001
Bulbar conjunctiva	6 (9)	0	6 (100)	
Palpebral conjunctiva	23 (36)	2 (9)	21 (91)	
Growth pattern				
Nodular	42 (66)	20 (48)	22 (52)	<.001
Diffuse	22 (34)	0	22 (100)	
Orbital invasion or invasion of adjacent structures				
Present	24 (38)	0	24 (100)	<.001
Absent	40 (63)	20 (50)	20 (50)	
Management				
Wide surgical excision	46 (72)	20 (44)	26 (57)	
Exenteration	18 (28)	0	18 (100)	<.001
T category				
T1 or T2	44 (68)	20 (46)	24 (55)	
T3 or T4	20 (20)	0	20 (100)	<.001
Largest tumor diameter, cm				
<2	27 (42)	13 (48)	14 (52)	
≤2	37 (58)	7 (19)	30 (81)	<.001

Abbreviations: CIN, conjunctival intraepithelial neoplasia; NS, not significant; SCC, squamous cell carcinoma.
[a]χ^2 Test.
Reprinted from Chauhan S, Sen S, Sharma A, et al. American joint committee on cancer staging and clinicopathological high-risk predictors of ocular surface squamous neoplasia. *Arch Pathol Lab Med.* 2014;138:1488-1494.

lesion. Nevertheless, AJCC–TNM staging should be performed when evaluating OSSN, as it should for all other available tumors.

V. Lee, MD

References

1. Edge SB, Byrd DR, Compton CC, Fritz AG, Greene FL, Trotti A. *AJCC Cancer Staging Manual*. 7th ed. New York, NY: Springer; 2010.
2. Miller CV, Wolf A, Klingenstein A, et al. Clinical outcome of advanced squamous cell carcinoma of the conjunctiva. *Eye (Lond)*. 2014;28(8):962-967.

High-Resolution Optical Coherence Tomography as an Adjunctive Tool in the Diagnosis of Corneal and Conjunctival Pathology

Nanji AA, Sayyad FE, Galor A, et al (Univ of Miami, FL; et al)
Ocul Surf 13:226-235, 2015

Purpose.—To evaluate the use of a commercially available, high-resolution, spectral-domain optical coherence tomography (HR-OCT) device in the diagnosis of corneal and conjunctival pathologies, with a focus on malignant lesions.

Methods.—Eighty-two eyes of 71 patients were enrolled in this prospective case series, including 10 normal eyes, 21 with ocular surface squamous neoplasia (OSSN), 24 with a pterygium or pingueculum, 3 with lymphoma, 18 with pigmented conjunctival lesions (nevus, flat melanosis, or melanoma), and 6 with Salzmann nodular degeneration. Subjects were imaged using photography and HR-OCT (RTVue, Optovue, Fremont, CA). When clinically indicated, surgery was performed and histopathologic specimens were correlated with OCT images.

Results.—HROCT was useful in differentiating among various lesions based on optical signs. Specifically, in OSSN, HR-OCT findings included epithelial thickening and hyper-reflectivity, whereas pterygia and pinguecula showed a subepithelial mass under thinner epithelium. In lymphoma, a hyporeflective, homogenous subepithelial mass was observed. Differentiating between pigmented lesions with HR-OCT was more difficult, but certain characteristics could be identified. Eyes with nevi and melanoma both displayed intensely hyper-reflective basal epithelial layers and discrete subepithelial lesions, but could be differentiated by the presence of cysts in nevi and intense shadowing of sublesional tissue in most melanomas.

Conclusion.—We found that a commercially available HR-OCT was a useful noninvasive adjunctive tool in the diagnosis of ocular surface lesions (Fig 1, Table 2).

▶ The authors of this study conducted a prospective, pilot study examining the clinical application of a commercially available, Food and Drug Administration (FDA)-approved, high-resolution optical coherence tomography (HR-OCT) in the diagnosis of corneal and conjunctival lesions. Although similar preliminary

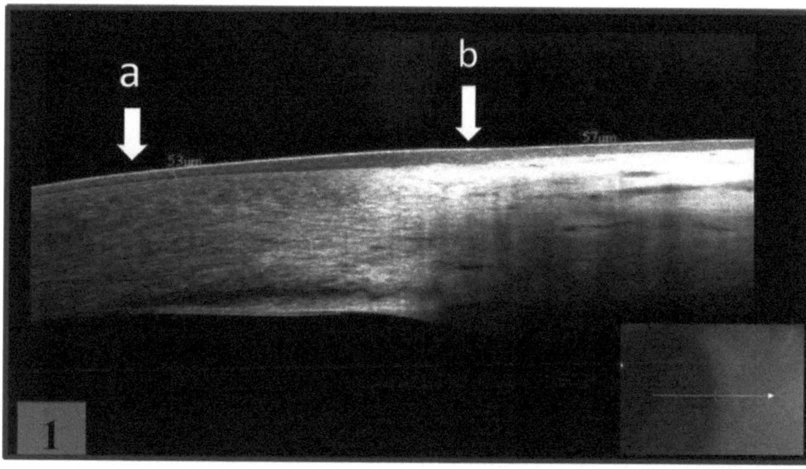

FIGURE 1.—HR-OCT of a normal eye. The top, hyper-reflective layer represents the tear film. The normal cornea, by HR-OCT, has a thin and dark epithelium (a) overlying a regularly-structured stroma. The epithelium becomes brighter (slightly hyper-reflective) over the limbus and conjunctiva but remains thin (b). (Reprinted from Nanji AA, Sayyad FE, Galor A, et al. High-resolution optical coherence tomography as an adjunctive tool in the diagnosis of corneal and conjunctival pathology. *Ocul Surf.* 2015;13:226-235, with permission from Elsevier Inc.)

studies have been previously reported, this is the first such study using equipment that is readily available commercially and FDA approved. Eighty-two eyes were included in the study, consisting of 8 types of lesions: pterygium, pinguecula, ocular surface squamous neoplasia (OSSN), lymphoma, Salzmann nodular degeneration, flat melanosis, nevus, and melanoma. Subjects were enrolled as a prospective case series, and lesions were imaged using Optovue RTVue HR-OCT. The images were correlated to standard clinical findings and, when available, histologic findings.

Optical coherence tomography (OCT) scans were evaluated for thickness and reflectivity. The general OCT characteristics of each type of lesion are listed in Table 2. Among the lesions studied, OSSN appeared to benefit the most from HR-OCT. OSSN lesions exhibited a thick epithelium on OCT, as well as abrupt transition from unremarkable epithelium and neoplastic epithelium. Pigmented lesions, however, profited the least from OCT imaging. Although variability in epithelial thickness was observed, in addition to hyperreflectivity of the basal epithelium, significant shadowing prevented analysis of deeper levels. Nonetheless, OCT images helped in 3 diagnostically challenging cases and in monitoring treatment response. In addition, the histologic findings whenever available, albeit in a smaller subset of the lesions included in the study, correlated to the OCT findings, leading to confirmation of the clinical diagnosis.

The clinical presentation of many such anterior segment lesions often involves a differential diagnosis with nontrivial management implications. Strategies to economize clinical evaluation and conserve time, resources, and risk to patients would be beneficial.

Although, as recognized by the authors, there are several limitations of the study, the utility of OCT in the evaluation and management of anterior segment

TABLE 2.—Optical Signs of Ocular Surface Lesions

Lesion	Epithelial Layer: Thickness	Epithelial Layer: Reflectivity	Subepithelial Layer
Normal	Thin epithelium (about 45-70 μm)	Dark corneal epithelium; mild hyper-reflectivity over limbus and conjunctiva	No masses, no shadowing, anterior portion of conjunctival epithelium hyper-reflective
OSSN	Severely thickened; inferior border of lesion may be partially obscured by shadowing in very thick lesions	Strongly hyper-reflective, usually with abrupt transition from normal to abnormal	Not involved in CCIN; unable to comment for SCC (none in current study)
Pingueculum	Normal to slightly thickened epithelium	Mildly hyper-reflective	Dark subepithelial tissue mass near limbus
Pterygium	Normal to slightly thickened epithelium	Mildly hyper-reflective	Highly hyper-reflective subepithelial lesion; hyper-reflective layer seen between Bowman's and corneal epithelium in corneal scans
Lymphoma	Normal thickness	Normal	Hypo-reflective and homogenous subepithelial mass; surrounding hyper-reflective layer of uninvolved tissue and shadowing of underlying tissue
Salzmann's nodular degeneration	Thin epithelium, usually thinner than normal	Normal	Dense, subepithelial, hyper-reflective material just anterior to Bowman's layer
Flat melanosis	Normal thickness	Hyper-reflectivity of the basal epithelium ± patchy hyper-reflectivity within epithelium	No involvement
Nevi	Normal thickness	Mildly hyper-reflective but often with strong reflectivity of basal epithelium	Subepithelial mass with mild shadowing of the underlying tissue; cysts often seen
Melanoma	Normal thickness to somewhat thickened epithelium	Mildly hyper-reflective but often with strong reflectivity of basal epithelium	Hyper-reflective subepithelial mass with obscuration of the underlying tissue (and in some, the posterior portion of the lesion) due to shadowing; rarely cysts.

OSSN, ocular surface squamous neoplasia; CCIN, corneal and conjunctival intraepithelial neoplasia; SCC, squamous cell carcinoma.

Reprinted from Nanji AA, Sayyad FE, Galor A, et al. High-resolution optical coherence tomography as an adjunctive tool in the diagnosis of corneal and conjunctival pathology. *Ocul Surf.* 2015;13:226-235, with permission from Elsevier Inc.

pathologies seems irrefutable. The results presented in the study reveal the potential to obtain collateral information noninvasively, which can be clinically relevant but far from substituting sound clinical evaluation and judgment. As these technologies continue to be enhanced and refined, it will be critical to continue to rigorously assess the value of HR-OCT and its applications to patient care.

K. Willett, MD
V. Lee, MD

Impression cytology diagnosis of ulcerative eyelid malignancy

Sen S, Lyngdoh AD, Pushker N, et al (All India Inst of Med Sciences, New Delhi, India)

Cytopathology 26:26-30, 2015

Objective.—The utility of impression cytology in ocular diseases has predominantly been restricted to the diagnosis of dry eye, limbal stem cell deficiency and conjunctival neoplasias. Its role in malignant eyelid lesions remains largely unexplored. Although scrape cytology is more popular for cutaneous lesions, impression cytology, being non-traumatic, has an advantage in small and delicate areas such as the eyelid. The present study has been designed to evaluate its role in the diagnosis and management of malignant eyelid lesions.

Methods.—Thirty-two histopathologically proven malignant eyelid lesions diagnosed over a 2-year period, including 13 basal cell carcinomas, 11 sebaceous carcinomas, four squamous cell carcinomas, two malignant melanomas and two poorly differentiated carcinomas, formed the study group.

Results.—The results of impression cytology were compared with those of histopathology in the study group and with an age- and sex-matched group of benign cases as controls. The sensitivity of impression cytology was 84% (27/32) for the diagnosis of malignancy and 28% (9/32) for categorization of the type of malignancy.

Conclusions.—Impression cytology is a simple, useful, non-invasive technique for the detection of malignant ulcerative eyelid lesions. It is especially useful as a follow-up technique for the detection of recurrences.

▶ The purpose of this prospective study is to investigate the utility of impression cytology in ulcerative eyelid malignancies. Often used for conjunctival lesions and corneal infections, impression cytology is a valuable and cost-effective technique for sampling lesions without inducing tremendous tissue injury. Essentially, it entails just touching the surface of the lesion of interest with filter paper, followed by fixation, filter paper dissolution, then staining. Current methods, such as scrape or incisional biopsies, often induce tissue injury or loss, which could be a disadvantage with regard to the delicate tissue surrounding the eyelids. For that reason, the authors wanted to explore whether impression cytology could be extended for diagnosing ulcerative eyelid lesions.

Over 2 years, 32 patients with presumed eyelid malignancy with ulceration of skin, conjunctiva, or lid margin were evaluated with impression cytology. Twenty age- and sex-matched patients with benign eyelid and conjunctival lesions were also evaluated and served as controls. Two to 5 impression cytology samples were taken from the area of ulceration, depending on the size of the lesion. Patients were excluded if they did not have subsequent diagnosis by routine histopathologic examination.

Twenty-seven of 32 patients in the study group were found to have a malignant eyelid tumor, whereas all of the control cases were not. However, only 9 of the 27 cases could be definitively diagnosed; diagnoses included basal cell carcinoma, sebaceous carcinoma, squamous cell carcinoma, malignant melanoma, and poorly differentiated carcinoma. Cytologic diagnosis could not be made in the remaining 5 of the 32 cases, which were subsequently found to be basal cell carcinoma, squamous cell carcinoma, and malignant melanoma.

Although the authors acknowledged even before conducting the study the likely poor sensitivity of impression cytology, they thought this method could still serve a purpose in ulcerative eyelid lesions. The authors concluded that because of its low specificity, impression cytology should not be used for primary diagnosis of eyelid malignancies. However, the authors believe it may still have a role as a screening technique. As a relatively atraumatic, cost-effective, and portable technique, the scope of impression cytology should be considered. However, more definitive studies need to be conducted comparing impression cytology to other methods, such as scrape and fine-needle aspiration biopsies, as well as clinical suspicion alone, before impression cytology can be confidently employed.

V. Lee, MD

Epithelial downgrowth in the vitreous cavity and on the retina in enucleated specimens and in eyes with visual potential

Rachitskaya AV, Dubovy SR, Hussain RM, et al (Univ of Miami, Miller School of Medicine, FL; et al)

Retina 35:1688-1695, 2015

Purpose.—To report clinical course and visual and anatomical outcomes of six eyes with histopathologically confirmed vitreous cavity and retina epithelial downgrowth.

Methods.—This is a retrospective 15-year review of archived pathologic slides and corresponding medical records of patients with vitreous cavity and retina epithelial downgrowth. Posterior segment epithelial downgrowth was defined as epithelial or goblet cells in the vitreous cavity or on the surface of the retina.

Results.—Histopathologic diagnosis of epithelial downgrowth was made in 122 patients. Of those, 6 patients (5%) had vitreous cavity and retina epithelial downgrowth. Three patients developed blind painful eye, and epithelial downgrowth was identified in enucleated specimens. The other three eyes with visual potential presented with tractional retinal detachments. Epithelial downgrowth was identified in epiretinal membranes obtained during pars plana vitrectomy. The latter group had more previous surgeries ($P = 0.03$), and all had keratoprosthesis implantation as their last surgery. All three had pathologic specimens obtained at the time of the keratoprosthesis implantation; no anterior segment epithelial downgrowth was noted in two patients, and one patient had involvement of corneal button, iris, and posterior capsule. Final visual acuity ranged from hand motion to light perception.

Conclusion.—In the current study, vitreous cavity and retina epithelial downgrowth occurred after multiple intraocular surgeries, including repair of the open globe injuries both in enucleated specimens and in eyes with visual potential. In eyes with visual potential, keratoprosthesis implantation seems to predispose the development of posterior segment epithelial downgrowth.

▶ The authors report a retrospective review of histopathologically confirmed vitreous cavity and retina epithelial downgrowth. A review of all archived pathology slides within the Florida Lions Ocular Pathology Laboratory database spanning a 15-year period was performed, and 122 cases of epithelial downgrowth were identified; 6 of these cases were found to have vitreous cavity and retina epithelial downgrowth. Epithelial downgrowth typically involves sheets of 1 to 3 layers of nonkeratinized, stratified squamous epithelium of conjunctival or corneal origin.[1] Current theory dictates that epithelium finds entry anteriorly, and reaches posterior structures by crawling along the ocular surfaces, as well as the vitreous body.

Three of the 6 cases involved enucleated globes with a clinical history of a blind and painful eye; the other 3 cases involved eyes with visual potential, and the diagnosis of epithelial downgrowth was made from retinal membranes submitted for histopathology. All specimens were stained with immunohistochemical stain for cytokeratin (AE1/3) for confirmation of epithelial origin.

Although both groups had a history of multiple ophthalmic surgeries, interestingly, the eyes with visual potential had more surgeries than the enucleated group (3 vs 9, respectively). The former group all had a history of corneal decompensation, and all of them underwent placement of a Boston Type I KPro (KPro) implant. Each patient presented with decreased visual acuity and were found to have peripheral retinal membranes causing tractional retinal detachments. Patients subsequently underwent a pars plana vitrectomy and membrane peel, which were described as dense and difficult to peel because of tight adhesions to the retina. The membranes were referred to as "trampoline-like" because of their tendency to recoil. In addition, the authors point out that all 6 cases discussed involved eyes with aphakia or an anterior chamber intraocular lens and disruption of the anterior hyaloid.

In conclusion, the authors reaffirm the rarity of posterior epithelial downgrowth. They also propose that epithelial cells grow along vascularized surfaces and vitreous strands, entering the posterior segment of the eye. Although a history of multiple ophthalmic surgeries is a proposed risk factor, the authors highlight KPro as a specific predisposing risk factor for epithelial downgrowth. They specifically recommend that when evaluating retinal detachments in eyes with a history of multiple surgeries and a KPro, retina surgeons consider the possibility of peripheral membranes secondary to epithelial downgrowth.

B. J. Kim, MD

V. Lee, MD

Reference

1. Weiner MJ, Trentacoste J, Pon DM, Albert DM. Epithelial downgrowth: a 30-year clinicopathological review. *Br J Ophthalmol.* 1989;73:6-11.

Yellow-Orange Palpebral Spots

Belliveau MJ, Odashiro AN, Harvey JT (Univ of Toronto, Canada; McMaster Univ, Hamilton, Ontario, Canada)

Ophthalmology 122:2139-2140.e1, 2015

Background.—An entity termed "orange palpebral spots" has recently been described, consisting of discoloration of the eyelid, increased adipose tissue and pigment-laden macrophages in the superficial dermis, and largely normal findings otherwise. Three patients with a similar finding but yellowish discoloration were reported, prompting the suggestion to change the entity's name to "yellow-orange palpebral spots."

Case Reports.—Case 1

Man, 57, was referred for a 3-year history of xanthelasma of both upper eyelids. The only medication he took was finasteride. The yellowish skin did not have the elevated look of xanthelasma, and a diagnostic biopsy revealed increased adipose tissue in the superficial dermis, lymphocytic infiltrate near the adnexal structures, and pigment-laden macrophages, especially in the superficial dermis, with positive staining for melanin pigment.

Case 2

Man, 61, had a history of 6 months with yellowish discoloration of both eyelids. He was taking acetaminophen with codeine and caffeine. The appearance of the lesions did not resemble xanthelasma plaque, and a diagnostic biopsy demonstrated various amounts of increased adipose tissue and pigment-laden macrophages in the superficial dermis. Staining for melanin was positive; staining for iron, mucin, and amyloid was negative, as was polarization.

Case 3

Woman, 79, was incidentally noted to have bilateral yellowish discoloration of the upper eyelids while being evaluated for tearing.

She had cataracts and macular degeneration and was taking levothyroxine, alendronate, and acetylsalicylic acid. No other areas of yellowed skin were identified.

Analysis.—In addition to these three patients, two series of patients with orange discoloration demonstrated similar findings. Although the underlying cause for the disorder has not been identified, the histopathologic findings are similar whether the spots are yellow or orange, suggesting that it may be appropriate to term the disorder "yellow-orange palpebral spots." Theories of causation include local trauma. It is possible that the lesions are often overlooked.

Conclusions.—With an awareness of the entity, clinicians should be able to recognize it in patients. Although no unifying cause has been identified and no links to underlying systemic illness have been uncovered, further cases should help to narrow down the possible cause.

▶ This succinct case report highlights an interesting entity that can be confused with xanthelasma, a common ophthalmic diagnosis. Xanthelasma clinically present as yellow plaques located in the periorbital area. Histologically, these lesions are composed as lipid-laden histiocytes in the dermis. However, as the authors astutely point out, not all yellow lesions around the periorbital area are presumed xanthelasma. Other similar lesions have been presented in the literature, including "orange palpebral spots"[1] and "fatty nodules of the dermis",[2] that should be included in the differential. The authors here suggest a new variant, "yellow-orange palpebral spots," to the previously described dermatologic entity of "orange palpebral spots." All 3 patients described in this case report presented with prominent yellowish discoloration of the upper eyelid. Histologic examination revealed increased adipose tissue and pigment-laden histiocytes in the superficial dermis. The authors regard this entity distinct from the previously described "fatty nodules of the dermis" by Jakobiec et al[2] because of the lack of giant cells. Time will tell whether or not these entities are distinct from each other or related, but nonetheless, this case report stresses the importance of pathology to confirm the clinical diagnosis.

V. Lee, MD

References

1. Assouly P, Cavelier-Balloy B, Dupré T. Orange palpebral spots. *Dermatology.* 2008;216:166-170.
2. Jakobiec FA, Mendoza PR, Hatton MP. Fatty nodules of the dermis of the upper eyelids: a new entity. *Graefes Arch Clin Exp Ophthalmol.* 2013;251:2823-2825.

Article Index

Chapter 1: Cataract Surgery

Chapter 2: Refractive Surgery

Chapter 3: Glaucoma

Chapter 4: Cornea

Chapter 5: Retina

Chapter 6: Uveitis

Chapter 7: Oculoplastic Surgery

Chapter 8: Pediatric Ophthalmology

Chapter 9: Neuro-ophthalmology

Chapter 10: Imaging

Chapter 11: Ocular Oncology

Chapter 12: Pathology

Author Index

I

J

K

L

M

Kolibri 360 GmbH
Ferdinand-Jühlke-Straße 7
99095 Erfurt, Deutschland
produktsicherheit@kolibri360.de